modified

modified

GMOs AND THE THREAT TO
OUR FOOD, OUR LAND,
OUR FUTURE

CAITLIN SHETTERLY

G. P. Putnam's Sons
New York

G. P. PUTNAM'S SONS
Publishers Since 1838
An imprint of Penguin Random House LLC
375 Hudson Street
New York, New York 10014

Library of Congress Cataloging-in-Publication Data

Names: Shetterly, Caitlin, author.
Title: Modified : GMOs and the threat to our food, our land, our future / Caitlin Shetterly.
Other titles: GMOs and the threat to our food, our land, our future | Genetically modified
organisms and the threat to our food, our land, our future
Description: New York : G. P. Putnam's Sons, [2016]
Identifiers: LCCN 2016011424 | ISBN 9780399170676 (print)
Subjects: LCSH: Genetically modified foods.
Classification: LCC TP248.65.F66 S384 2016 | DDC 664—dc23
LC record available at http://lccn.loc.gov/2016011424
p.   cm.

Printed in the United States of America
1 3 5 7 9 10 8 6 4 2

BOOK DESIGN BY TANYA MAIBORODA

Penguin is committed to publishing works of quality and integrity.
In that spirit, we are proud to offer this book to our readers;
however, the story, the experiences, and the words
are the author's alone.

For my sweet Rabbit and my tender Lion,
for you two shall inherit this earth

contents

"There is, in fact, no distinction between
the fate of the land and the fate of the people."

—WENDELL BERRY, 2012 JEFFERSON LECTURE

PART 1

Flyover Country

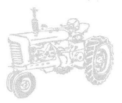

"Man is a part of nature, and his war against
nature is inevitably a war against himself."

—RACHEL CARSON, 1963 INTERVIEW ON THE
CBS PROGRAM *The Silent Spring of Rachel Carson*

"In the Great Plains the vistas look like music,
like Kyries of grass . . ."

—GRETEL EHRLICH, *The Solace of Open Spaces*

chapter 1

The blue Nebraska sky stretched above my car like a tight rubber band; the wind held its *My Ántonia* constancy and the sun beat down. All around, as far as the eye could see, were dusty brown fields of dried soybeans and golden fields of dried corn. There were no trees. Just that huge, open expanse of soy and corn crop after soy and corn crop, alternating gold and brown and open to the big blue sky. Tractors glinted in the sunlight like ships at a distance sailing up and down, methodically cutting ribbons out of a sepia ocean while dust billowed like a thick and impenetrable storm behind them. Harvesttime.

THE DAY BEFORE, I had landed in Denver, Colorado, in the late afternoon. When I deplaned and exited the airport, standing for a moment on the hot, dry concrete sidewalk outside the baggage claim, my rolly suitcase gripped in my right hand and my black L.L. Bean backpack on my shoulder, I was suddenly and immensely thirsty. I looked up and saw the Rocky Mountains rising, snowcapped and gleaming, before me; they seemed so close. I wondered if I could just reach my arm through that horizontal and relentless sun, if I'd be able to dip my hand into that snow, bring a handful to my mouth, and cool off. As I turned away from the mountains toward the rental-car lots, the land before me stretched as flat as paper across the Great Plains of eastern Colorado and into Nebraska, where I was headed.

I had come to Denver to start somewhere—to start telling a story, a story that I'd stumbled upon in that life-becomes-art-and-art-becomes-life kind of way. Two months earlier, I'd published an article in *Elle* magazine about a long and tedious illness that had plagued me for nearly four years, until I met Dr. Paris Mansmann, an allergist and immunologist. Mansmann is based in the suburban town of Yarmouth, Maine—a short distance outside Portland, our state's biggest city and cultural center, where I lived. Mansmann had asserted that, in his opinion, I had developed a sensitivity to the proteins that are created from the DNA inserted into GMO corn to make it herbicide-resistant and, also, to carry its own pesticide; these genetic aberrances, he posited, had caused my immune system to go haywire.

Although his theory seemed unorthodox, perhaps crazy—and, it turned out, also majorly controversial—I decided to trust in it. I was too desperate not to. I'd been sick for so long—during the first year of my marriage and for the entire first two years of my son Marsden's life. And by "sick," I don't mean that I was just "not feeling great" or that I was a little queasy. I mean that I was so sick that I was often unable to get out of bed because arthritic pain radiated throughout my body, making my thighs and ankles weak and causing me to hobble around like a ninety-year-old. (My ankles, I'd joke to Dan, my husband, felt like they'd been "Kathy Batesed," a reference to the movie *Misery*.) I was exhausted—yet my body was in such a state that I felt like I'd been plugged into an electrical outlet and couldn't relax enough to sleep. I had horrible headaches; a constant head cold; tingling and numbness in my feet, legs, and arms; and rashes splattered like pizza sauce across my face. During this time, I had tried every diagnosis—or theory—that came my way, including hormone treatments, vitamin injections, iodine pills, elimination diets, and a long and debilitating course of powerful antibiotics aimed at curing me of chronic Lyme disease. Everything seemed to make me sicker, not better. I felt like Christina in the famous Andrew Wyeth painting; the world was just out of reach. My life was passing me by while we spent thousands and thousands of dollars we really did not have to consult with anyone who would see me—from Harvard-educated MDs to shamans. All the while, we were just hoping someone would find a key to unlock this puzzle and make me well.

But desperation wasn't the only reason I was game to trust Mansmann's theory. In 2010, long before I was even thinking about genetically modified organisms, known in common parlance as GMOs, and before I had any inkling about what might be wrong with me, Marsden, then one year old, started to have episodes at bedtime when he would cry so hard that he would stop breathing and turn blue. The first time it happened, Dan and I raced to the car and then to the ER where they hooked our baby up to an EKG. The diagnosis: "He has a behavioral problem called 'breath-holding syndrome.'" We looked blankly at the doctor. "It's like a tantrum," she continued. "Kids do it to get their way sometimes. You need to be more sure in your parental decisions—if it's bedtime, it's really bedtime." A nurse piped up then: "I knew a kid who had these until she was five! The family would say, 'Oh here she goes again. . . . '" The ER doctor suggested distractions, which might help him "forget" to hold his breath. In a bizarre twist of this-must-be-dark-theater-not-my-life, I found myself following the ER doctor's advice and for the next three nights I was singing "If you're happy and you know it, clap your hands!" as Marsy screamed inconsolably and turned blue and then white in my arms.

Call it a mother's instinct, but after three nights of this stopbreathing routine—the surest way to turn a new mother into a grayhaired one-hundred-and-fifty-year-old is to scare her shitless—I was convinced that something else was at play, bigger than my son having "behavioral problems." Here's what I know: When he was born, he radiated goodwill; he took one look around and gave Dan and me an expression that seemed to say, "What's all the fuss, guys?" He rarely cried; he was fascinated by our big, complicated world. At two months old, when the recession flattened us, we drove him across the country from our apartment in Los Angeles to move in with my mother in Maine. That whole trip he'd been cool as a cucumber. Up until now, he had been a good sleeper and a happy, mild-mannered baby.

Thankfully, our pediatrician also wasn't convinced that these symptoms were a behavioral problem or some defect in Marsy's character that we needed to eradicate. Sometimes, she told us, breath-holding syndrome, or "spells," can be the result of iron deficiency, fear, trauma, or pain a toddler can't express.[1] She said she wanted to revisit his perennial eczema, which he'd had since he was a tiny baby. The eczema had progressed like California wildfire since the introduction of solid foods, going from little sore patches behind his knees and elbows to covering his trunk and legs and climbing up his cheeks. At night, I slathered him in organic oils and rubbed zinc oxide on the worst bits, to little avail. She suggested an elimination diet because food allergies, she said, can also affect behavior.

Over the next few months of winter and into the spring, we put our son on an austere diet that avoided—all at once—wheat, eggs, dairy, corn, soy, nightshades, fish, shellfish, peanuts, and nuts. We ate a lot of turkey, brown rice, and broccoli, as I remember it. Interestingly, corn, at that time, like nightshades, was not on most elimination diet programs (though the baby guru Dr. William Sears recommends including it). But our pediatrician said it was possible—however, like nightshades, unlikely—so we added it to the list just to be thorough. In a matter of days, the death-imitating tantrums stopped and the eczema began to abate.

Eventually, when we thought that Marsy seemed much better, we

---

[1] These days, there's a lot more information about breath-holding spells than there was even as recently 2010. The idea that they are, themselves, "tantrums" without some physiological underpinning is being phased out of the medical literature.

started to reintroduce foods. First up: corn, our most American and wholesome of foods, the one food I assumed would be the safest, because who in the world could have a problem with corn? I loved corn. I loved the way it looked growing green and leafy and innocent and all-American in fields across our landscape. I loved to eat it: corn chips, sprouted tortillas, popcorn, nachos, soft polenta with Parmigiano and butter thrown in at the very last second of cooking and topped with baked crispy kale (this was the first meal I'd ever made for Dan), creamed corn. . . . And I'd put pureed frozen sweet corn into most of my homemade veggie baby food mixtures, thinking I was adding extra fiber and goodness. Being a person who loved to cook and eat—a self-professed foodie—I didn't like to think that anything was off-limits. Instead, I liked to think in terms of textures and flavors, colors and bounty. And corn—and corn products—were included in my food landscape.[2]

My dad, who is a Fritos nut, even has a family story that he liked to share, when I was growing up, in late August when local corn on the cob was ready. He'd tell us about the gadget we had in our kitchen that my great-grandfather Orton Galloway invented in order to scrape a corncob free of fresh, juicy kernels to make creamed corn. The gadget looked like a little wooden bench with some nails sticking up in the center, and there was a little narrow opening just after the nails for the kernels to fall through. When my great-granddad Orton got to the U.S. patent office to register his invention, the story goes that he found a room full of people all waiting to register variations on the exact same corn-scraping device. Apparently, Orton took in his competition and decided it was pointless to wait to patent his invention. He left the office deflated and trudged home to Wyoming, Ohio. Nonetheless, in our family, my dad used his grandpop's invention faithfully every summer, cooking the fresh, juicy kernels in a double boiler so the corn

---

[2] I'm almost embarrassed to write this, but I do believe I made it through the Honors English program in college thanks to coffee, Doritos (an entire bag per all-nighter), and Oreos (again, whole package).

didn't burn and adding butter, salt, and pepper. Sometimes we'd have this as a kind of porridge for breakfast and sometimes we'd eat it alongside fish or hamburgers.

In recent years, these creamed-corn devices seem to have gone the way of the dinosaurs. One summer, my dad was on a business trip down in Kentucky and was out walking on a Sunday morning when he walked by the window of an old junk shop. In the window was a corn scraper just like the one his grandfather had made, and underneath it was a small, cardboard sign with the words "What is this?" written in black Sharpie. When Dad got back to Maine the next day, he called up the shop and told the proprietor what it was. Then he bought the scraper and had it sent to my brother as a gift.

Coming off the elimination diet, our pediatrician had told us that we should deluge our fasting patient—every meal should contain the food specimen we were scrutinizing for three full days, as this was the best way to really get it into his system. Lo and behold, over the test period for corn, eczema splotched and then raged, red and painful, over Marsy's limbs and cheeks. His nose ran like a faucet and the mucus made him gag and choke. He was crankier, slept fitfully and had runny bowel movements, and his breathing sounded raspy at night. Again, he cried inconsolably at bedtime. At that point Mars was only fifteen months old, so he couldn't tell us much—if his belly or head hurt or if he itched all over. However, Dan and I could see with our own eyes that *something* was happening and that he was miserable.

With our pediatrician's guidance, we took corn back out of Marsden's diet—or at least we thought we did. The FDA, it turns out, doesn't require that corn be labeled as an allergen on any packaging. And 80 percent of packaged food contains ingredients made from GMO corn or soy. In fact, there are more than 250 nonorganic substances—often chemicals—that are legally allowed as additives in "organic foods," many of which are made from industrial, or GMO, corn. GMOs, as of this writing, still require no labeling in the United States (and there is a huge Washington push from the chemical companies to make it impossible for the states to regulate labeling on their own[3]). But, oddly, even so, in the face of the increasing cacophony around GMOs and our industrial food system, more and more manufacturers are starting to label corn or omit GMOs altogether. (Just yesterday I looked at a label for Whole Foods brand "Organic Black Pepper & Sea Salt Potato Chips" and I almost fell over. There, in huge print, under the ingredient list, which included the words "organic dextrose" and "organic maltodextrin," it said "DERIVED FROM CORN" in reference to the maltodextrin [although dextrose is often made from corn, this one is, apparently, not]. This is new.[4])

As time marched on, Dan and I discovered with dizzying helplessness that corn is in everything—it was our Waldo, popping up everywhere we least expected it: in baking powder, cheese, vitamins, medications, tea bags, juice, dish soap, preservatives, the lining of paper coffee cups, the waxy coating on the outside of store-bought fruit. You name it, almost everything my family used, no matter how piously natural and organic it was, could be traced back to some corn-field in Iowa. It came disguised as dozens of names, such as "xanthan

---

[3] In late 2015, the Safe and Accurate Food Labeling Act, known by its opponents as the Deny Americans the Right to Know, or DARK, Act, was passed in the House, denying states the right to label and regulate GMO foods. It was largely understood that the bill was sponsored by "Monsanto and its agribusiness cronies," said Andrew Kimbrell, the executive director of the Center for Food Safety. He said that the bill would effectively "crush the democratic decision-making of tens of millions of Americans." Furthermore, he said, "Corporate influence has won and the voice of the people has been ignored." When the DARK Act was initiated—and because of popular pressure in the wake of the FDA's late-2015 approval of a genetically modified salmon (bred by a Massachusetts company called AquaBounty to grow twice as fast as "natural" salmon)—Congress asked the FDA to come up with a better labeling rubric for GMOs before the salmon could be sold in supermarkets. The FDA proposed that manufacturers no longer put "GMO-free" or some such on their labels; they wanted slightly longer wording, such as "Not genetically modified through the use of modern biotechnology." That's gonna take a mom an extra second to register! Update: In early 2016, the DARK Act was narrowly rejected by the Senate. As a Campbell's Soup exec reportedly told a political staffer I spoke with, whether or not the government makes a labeling law, that "train has left the station." People want labels.

[4] A quick organic chemistry lesson, just to hit home this point: most of the chemicals out there (which are not organic in the same way that food can be certified as organic) are started with petroleum; they are "carbon based." Since the advent of the wonder product GMO corn, more and more chemicals and products are begun with a corn base.

gum,"[5] "vegetable starch," "modified food starch," "citric acid," "natural flavors," and "vitamin C." Almost daily, we'd turn a corner and realize, "This toothpaste is full of corn!" And then, the next day, "Wait, our dish soap is made from corn!" A week later, "Oh my God, iodized salt has dextrose in it!" And, "This kiddie ibuprofen is full of corn!" Even baby food labeled as "100% organic" and "non-GMO" often has citric and ascorbic acids added as preservatives, both of which are made from GMO corn.

One night, overwhelmed, I said to Dan, "This is impossible." We somehow agreed—though viewed through the lens of time this seems crazy, if not irresponsible—to accept defeat. We were exhausted, we were confused, we couldn't stand it anymore. If providing our son with food, clothing, and shelter were our three most important jobs, it felt like we were failing at the first one. We decided finally that we'd make our son "well enough." Corn was too formidable an opponent to truly eradicate.

But to add to the overwhelming stress of that confusing period when we were trying to stick our fingers into a leaky silo from which corn seemed to flow unendingly into our lives, the illness I was suffering from—the one that no one could quite pinpoint—started to get worse. Some of my symptoms were not unlike my son's: the facial rashes, constant head cold, and irritable bowel syndrome (IBS). But it was the bodily pain and achiness that was the hardest for me to handle, and it was getting worse. It had traveled, most depressingly, to my hands, which were so stiff and painful that they became completely useless for tasks such as buttoning Marsy's little sweaters, applying Band-Aids to his delicate skin, opening jars of baby food, or finely chopping parsley, which I like to add to just about everything I cook. My hands hurt when I tried to walk Hopper, our big, sleek, Rotty-shepherd

---

[5] Xanthan gum is technically made from a bacteria grown on corn, and in harvesting, some people say, some corn is retained. Some manufacturers of it, however, promise they have removed the corn from it and sell a "corn-free" xanthan gum. When I eventually stopped eating gluten and needed to use xanthan gum for baking, I found that I had no reaction to the "corn-free" xanthan gum.

mix, and frozen hands did not prove ideal for my career as a writer, either. For months, I had been trying to push these symptoms to the side—take a few Advil, take my vitamins (fistfuls of them, all promising to make me strong as an ox), eat as healthily as I could manage, and drink some coffee to get my energy up—and focus on my child. Whatever was going on with me physically, I didn't feel like facing it.

I told almost no one—even friends and extended family—how sick I was, because I didn't have any way to explain what was wrong: I had no diagnosis, just a collection of symptoms. "It's stress," Dan said to me at night.

"It's stress," I told my mother.

Looking back, I realize now that Dan and I spent an extraordinary amount of time pretending to the rest of the world that "we're fine over here," even though at home in private moments we drained hours worrying, researching, and then just plain praying that my illness would go away.

Finally, one hot summer night in August 2010, after a particularly hard day when I could barely get out of bed, Dan and I looked at each other and said, "This is something. It's real. Nothing is working. We can't keep on like this." I remember that moment so clearly, because it was the turning point: we started fearing the worst. The illness had gotten hold of us and taken up residence in our lives. Whatever it was, even if it wasn't life threatening, then it was surely life ruining. And just in admitting our fear, it seemed we were already done in by whatever it was. I remember that night feeling my knees buckle beneath me—I was standing in our small pantry and Dan was standing in the kitchen as we talked—and as I crumpled down to the floor, I was overwhelmed with unhappiness, tears springing from my eyes, kind of like in those old black-and-white movies when the heroine faints and has to be revived with smelling salts. (Just call me Scarlett.)

A few weeks later, I started going back and forth to Boston's Mass General Hospital. I had batteries of new tests checking for every conceivable allergy, condition, or disease out there. With each test, Dan and I girded ourselves for something terrible. But my symptoms were perplexing—even vexing—to every specialist who saw me. I got the same stumped looks, all of which led to more referrals. In the next few months, one hunch after another was posited and then debunked: I had brain scans and neurological workups, and I tried a bevy of drugs aimed at all sorts of things, including conditions like fibromyalgia, even though my GP told me that fibromyalgia was a "bucket illness" and that no one knew what the hell it was or what would fix it. Nothing made me better. I kept getting worse.

Then in February 2011, I made my way to Dr. Mansmann's office. It sits on the banks of the Royal River, a wide waterway that originates north in the town of New Gloucester and winds south, through Yarmouth, until it splashes into Casco Bay. The river was frozen and white and the bare trees stood silver sentry on its shores. Dr. Mansmann has a helmet of graying, thick hair and an intensely serious air. He speaks softly and at a measured, almost monotonous pace. On that February day, after his wife, Leslie, checked me in, he led me through the waiting room lined with filing cabinets and piles of medical journals and thick books with titles like *Immunology*, *Rhinitis*, and *Stedman's Medical Dictionary*. We walked through his small lab, where he has a microscope, beakers, and bottles of solutions. He led me into a little exam room equipped with a metal table and a wooden desk.

Mansmann is a third-generation allergist who began working in his father's allergy clinic at Jefferson Medical College in Philadelphia when he was in high school. He told me modestly that he had helped his father develop "a couple" of asthma drugs when he was in college at St. Joseph's University in Philadelphia. (The drugs, Slo-Bid and Aerolate, were used to treat asthma for years.) After undergrad, Mansmann went on to pass three medical boards—general medicine, pediatrics, and, finally, allergy and immunology—which he completed at Duke University on a fellowship from the National Institutes of Health. From Duke he went to West Virginia University, in Morgantown, where he headed an allergy and immunology clinic and worked with the National Institute for Occupational Safety and Health, studying respiratory disease caused by workplace exposure. In 2000, he and his family moved to Yarmouth, Maine, to be closer to his parents, who had moved to the Rangeley Lakes area and needed a family member close by.

Mansmann and I sat down together and he promptly pushed my thick tome of medical files to the side and pulled out a blank piece of paper. He told me he'd already read through everything but that he wanted to start at the beginning and hear it from me. "You've had every test I could ever think of running," he told me. "So now I just have questions." And then he began asking me questions, questions I'd never been asked in quite the same perfunctory, logical way: When did my rashes seem to flare? Was the pain an ache in my muscles or did it feel deeper? Did my hands feel tight and stiff, or was it my joints that hurt? Was I worse after I slept or at the end of the day? Were there good periods and bad? Did I always have that cold? Did I ever have trouble breathing? He seemed, as we spoke, to have all the time in the world. I began to relax a bit because I felt like someone was really hearing me for the first time in four years; someone was able, at least on the face of it, to put my symptoms into a list that made sense.

I told him how frustrated I was—that I was missing time with my kid, that this had gone on for too long. And then, in a moment of vulnerability, I told him I was afraid. He nodded and informed me, with little emotion, that autoimmune diseases could sometimes take at least eight years to diagnose. "That being said, however"—he spoke casually and with no pyrotechnics—"I think it's possible you've developed a reaction to genetically modified corn."

I looked at him dubiously. "What?"

Couldn't I just be tired? I asked. I mean, I had just finished writing a book . . . almost a year ago. But still. Wasn't it George Orwell who wrote, "Writing a book is a horrible, exhausting struggle, like a long bout of some painful illness"? Or could it be stress? Whatever he was talking about seemed too strange to even consider.

He shook his head. He said he'd come to believe, in the years since GMOs were first introduced, that some people might be developing a kind of chronic allergic response that was caused not by the corn itself, but instead by the proteins created by both the enterotoxins, bred into the corn to make it pest-resistant, and the proteins created from making it "Roundup Ready" (or impervious to the herbicide glyphosate, marketed by Monsanto as Roundup). He said he thought these small genetic modifications that are made in the DNA of GMO corn can cause the immune system to overreact—and a faucet gets turned on. This specific reaction, he believes, causes the body to release an avalanche of eosinophils—a kind of white blood cell—from the bloodstream into the mucus membranes, muscles, fascial system, and bowels. As this reaction progresses, he said, it tends to look much more like an autoimmune disease or something that used to be called chronic "serum sickness."[6] Chronic serum sickness is described as a kind of hypersensitivity, or the immune system on overdrive, often in reaction to medications or drugs, and includes the following symptoms in its diagnosis: "rash, arthritis, arthralgia, and other systemic symptoms." Specifically, Mansmann said he believes that the DNA changes bred into GMO corn could actually cause serum sickness—much like a drug or medication could. In his opinion, my body had become "primed," or in a state of constant reaction, and therefore it seemed to be allergic—or sensitive— to pretty much everything I ate or came into contact with.

To test his theory, he took a swab of some mucus from inside my nose. If the eyes are the windows to the soul for most of us, then the nose is the window to the immune system for Dr. Mansmann.[7] He smeared the mucus on a small glass slide and then took it with him to his sink. There he doused it in Hansel stain, a blue medical dye used to

---

[6] A 2009 study published in the *Journal of Crop and Weed* found that the herbicide glyphosate, or Roundup, caused "severe mucus secretion" in the stomachs of fish and also damaged their epithelial cells, esophagi, and intestines.

[7] He was even, at a later point, able to diagnose me with a pernicious case of acid reflux by looking at my nasal mucus, which was full of "fat cells" from food that was literally backwashing into my nose. (So gross!)

identify eosinophils, then rinsed it off, leaving a pinkish smear on the slide. He placed the slide under the microscope, then stood back and said, "Take a look." On the slide were hundreds of pink circles, which, he told me, were eosinophils. My nose was chock-full of them. When the immune system is working properly, he told me, eosinophils swarm certain invading substances, be they parasites or viruses, and work to eliminate them. Sometimes, however, an allergenic protein can prompt the immune system to release eosinophils. Then, if the allergen can't be detected and eliminated by the patient, the eosinophils just keep coming, creating a chronic condition. He felt if we could calm my body down with the elimination of corn, my whole being would come back into balance.

Mansmann told me to take all corn out of my diet—no matter if it was organic (organic, just in its nature, according to USDA labeling laws, cannot be GMO) or not. His reasoning was that it's difficult to find a clean source of non-GMO corn in the United States (or anywhere) because, since the late eighties and early nineties when genetically modified corn was first planted in field trials across the United States and then deregulated by the USDA to become a legitimate crop (now comprising over 90 percent of all corn planted in this country—more than 90 million acres), all corn has become contaminated due to wind pollination, birds, bees, and simple human error. "Not everyone is allergic," he said, "but it's an exposure issue. You expose somebody to an allergen and then they can develop an allergy to it." The problem with America, he said, "is that we've got a very corn-driven food system—it's in everything, and so the exposure levels are very high, day in, day out." What about soy? I asked. I knew just in a cursory way that GMO soy, too, was ubiquitous. He told me that was a good question and that although soy has not proliferated to the same degree into every corner of American lives, trying to stay away from GMO soy would be a good idea. Cornstarches carried more allergenic proteins and were less refined, he told me, than corn sugars, which are so refined they carry almost no proteins from the original plant. He recommended that Dan and I start making pretty much everything we ate from scratch and that we get very familiar with our farmers market and seasonal vegetables. And he told me how to keep an eye out for hidden corn in vitamins. He extolled the virtues of eating seasonally and was practically rhapsodic about "spring vegetables," making my mouth water. Mansmann said it would take my body a year to fully heal. But there was good news, too: in two to three years of living corn-free, he said, my body might be able to tolerate small amounts.

Dan and I threw ourselves into the corn-free diet with gusto, following Mansmann's advice. We began baking all our bread, we learned how to make our own flour tortillas, baking powder, pasta, and sweet treats such as muffins and cakes. We made our own mayonnaise, bean dips, and ice cream.[8] And we started hitting the Portland Farmers Market with a new attitude: this was our food for the week, not just a lovely Saturday night supper. We made friends with the vegetable rock stars at the market: Daniel of Freedom Farm, Chris and Galit of Fishbowl, Simon of Thirty Acre Farm, Jan of Goranson's, and the guys at Uncle's farm stand. We started buying larger quantities of everything at the end of the summer—Maine-grown dried beans (black, Jacob's cattle, Marfax, yellow eye, and navy), tomatoes, broccoli, cucumbers, stone fruits, berries, cabbages, celery, squashes, ginger, and pumpkins—and we canned, jammed, pickled, and froze them at night and on weekends through September and into October. We joined a local buying group that sourced fresh, local whole foods from around Maine. We started gardens to grow our own tomatoes, herbs, lettuces and spinaches, zucchinis and peppers. In the fall, we picked a huge amount of apples at Ricker Hill, an old orchard in the hills near Lewiston, and canned them as applesauce. One year I was even

---

[8] Dan and Marsy bought me a Cuisinart ice cream maker. And we all found that it was so incredibly easy to make ice cream that we now do it regularly. (I make a mixture in a bowl of cream, a little of the cream top of yogurt, sugar, scraped vanilla bean, and whatever my flavor is, like stewed rhubarb and strawberries, for instance, and throw it into the maker while we eat dinner. It's done in twenty minutes for dessert.)

forward-thinking enough to make six fresh apple pies and freeze them for the coming winter. We bought Maine-grown grains.

By luck, we met an intrepid farmer trying to raise corn-free chickens (harder than you might guess, because chickens have literally been bred to get fat fast on corn) and began buying his meat chickens. We started gathering grass-fed beef from a young Cornell graduate who had taken up farming outside of Portland. His meat came as hamburger, pot roasts, steaks, stew beef (which I use to make a Texas chili during the cold winter months, usually serving it atop toothsome rice—brown or white—with a generous spoonful of guacamole on top), and brisket for New England boiled suppers or for slow roasting with tomatoes, wine, mushrooms, celery, and spices. We bought wild fish (never buying farm raised, which is often fed GMO soy and corn), and we found a local farmer who produced grass-fed dairy. Marsy and I stopped taking every medicine or supplement with corn in it, which was most of them (and we had a local apothecary mix up corn-free acetaminophen and Benadryl).[9] Wherever we went, we took our own stainless-steel water bottles and coffee cups (to avoid the paper cups that are lined with a wax made from corn).

In a matter of months, we estimated that at least 85 percent, if not more, of our food became locally sourced and everything we ate was organic. Now, it's important to remember that it's not like we were doing this on some trust-fund budget, where the sky was the limit on what we could spend, and that we had some capacious and bucolic land around us in which to garden and cavort. We were living in an apartment for part of this time, and then, as years passed, renting a house with a little sandy yard for another chunk of time. At the house, we put in raised beds to grow what we could and plugged in a big freezer. In the meantime, we were allocating a good portion of the money we made to our food, at the expense of skiing weekends, gadgets, and cool Patagonia vests. Furthermore, we had to completely

---

[9] In 2011, this was much harder to do than it is in 2016. Many vitamins now come labeled as "corn-free" or "GMO-free."

upend the dictum that many of us in America live by: time is money. For us, time spent = food to eat. We jettisoned the desire for expeditious meals and slowed down to slow research every little thing we bought to eat, then slow cooked, and slow ate it. This pace could sometimes feel really arduous at eleven on a school night when we still had to can 40 pounds of tomatoes before they went bad. But if Hippocrates's statement "Let food be thy medicine" were words to live by, we were holding on to them like a lifeline.

As we cleaned out for real this time, undaunted by the Sisyphean task of it now that we had a doctor's order behind us, Marsden's eczema completely disappeared. His nose stopped constantly running and his whole body seemed to calm down noticeably. For myself, the first thing I noticed was that my own seemingly untreatable and just unbearable skin rashes began to dissipate. Slowly, my body stopped aching, and I could walk distances or even jog easily without limping for the first time in years. I started to have more energy, and I slept better at night. The head cold went away—*poof*—and I wasn't going through a box of tissues a day. Almost four months later, in late May, I felt pretty much like my old self.

During this trial our control group was Dan. He had no problems— that he knew of—with corn. And he, like us, had never tested positive on an allergy test for corn. But he has struggled his whole life with an autoimmune blood disorder known as ITP, or idiopathic thrombocytopenic purpura, that causes his white blood cells to attack his platelets, making him have fewer platelets than what is considered normal. Most of us walk around with anything from 150,000 to 450,000 platelets in a given sample. Dan's, however, have been as low as 7,000, which, for some people, can be life threatening. (We later learned that although this dip had made Dan very sick when it happened, Dan was still kicking due to the fact that he has unusually large platelets that compensate, to some degree, for the dearth in numbers.) As he remembers it, that lowest number of his—7,000—was during a period when we were eating a ton of corn—polenta, tortillas, popcorn, fake butter made with corn oil—and eschewing dairy and gluten because we thought those things, just from popular wisdom, were bad for us. A year into living corn-free, Dan's platelet count rose dramatically, going above 45,000, which was higher than he'd ever had in his life. Was this coincidence? Perhaps. We don't know. Our health is such a mystery, isn't it?

In the meantime, I was so startled by my physical well-being that I didn't know how to enjoy it. Each night I'd go to bed preparing myself for the possibility that I might wake up the next morning and be sick again. And I found myself asking Dan over and over like a broken record, Could GMO corn really be my problem? What if it isn't and this comes back? Will this blessed state really last? I couldn't let go; I had to know more.

The first question to tackle: What *is* genetically modified corn? Like many people, I had read Michael Pollan's *The Omnivore's Dilemma* and seen Aaron Woolf's documentary *King Corn* and had learned from both about the proliferation of corn into our food and everyday products. But I'd be lying if I didn't admit that the GMO thing was, at best, a little fuzzy for me still. I'd honestly never stopped to think about the fact that the corn I was eating wasn't the same old corn my parents and grandparents grew up eating (or the corn my great-grandfather invented that doohickey for). And even though I'd known, I suppose, in some recessed crunchy granola part of my brain that "GMO" was a term to regard suspiciously, I realized, suddenly, like a child first figuring out the "F" word, that I'd never stopped to think about what it meant.

A little bit (and then a lot, as time went on) of research led me to the following information: To genetically engineer a food, a scientist takes two different species—for instance, a flounder and a strawberry (this is not just pulled out of a hat—it's a real example!)—and splices, or "meshes," as some scientists have described it, their DNA together. This meshing is done, most often, with gold bullets—yes, real bullets—which have been dipped in strands of the DNA that carry the desired traits and, sometimes, tungsten powder. The bullets are then actually shot out of a gene gun, which is, for all intents and purposes, a real gun.[10] The Crosman air pistol was used to make some of the first GMOs. It looked kind of like this:

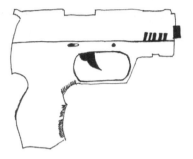

These days, the gene guns effectuate the power of .22 caliber guns and look either like clunky, white, space-age guns, more appropriate for *Star Wars* than real life, or the barrels are built into sophisticated-looking machines that resemble those ice machines you see in bars—big, top-opening, stainless-steel vaults of hard, glassy ice. They still shoot their bullets into Petri dishes containing sample cells, and helium is now used as an accelerator. Once they hit the Petri dish, the bullets break the nuclei of the host DNA and affix themselves into the host's now broken double helix. Okay, so somehow, whenever I hear this explanation of genetic modification, I imagine the song from *Annie Get Your Gun*: "Anything you can do, I can do better; I can do anything better than you." Anyway, it's a pretty imprecise science in that it's unclear *exactly* where the genes land in the host plant and *exactly* how they will get expressed. But what is clear is that the host plant—strawberry, corn, cotton, soy, what have you—will then, by some scientific miracle, begin to manufacture the inserted DNA. Some scientists posit that it's more accurate to call GMOs "transgenics,"

---

[10] Monsanto now uses an agrobacterium method of gene transfer for some of their products. In these cases, a bacterium actually transfers the genetic material by invading the host plant's DNA and delivering the desired DNA into its nucleus. This method works "especially well for plants like potatoes, tomatoes, and tobacco," according to GMO Compass, an online resource, and less well for grains like corn and wheat.

because they, in fact, carry genes that have been transferred across two phyla. For obvious reasons (too similar to transgender, anyone?) this word has not stuck with the pro-GMO camp, who prefer, these days, to just call GMOs, simply, GM (genetically modified) in an effort to get away from the negative connotations associated with the now fairly well-known acronym GMO. To wrinkle this further: many people opposed to GMOs have also adopted this nomenclature because they say that the pro-GMO camp accuses the anti-GMO camp—you still following me?—of being "anti-science" when they use the acronym GMO, because GMOs increasingly are being used in medicine to find cures for diseases (or, for instance, to engineer super-mosquitoes, which might help eradicate the Zika-carrying mosquitoes). GM, both camps agree, now just refers to the crops. And, to make things more complicated, the FDA now calls GMOs just simply GE, for "genetically engineered." For our purposes we'll just go with GMO, since it's what everyone understands, more or less.

An important point to remember that is rarely discussed in this argument of what's inserted into what and how, is that not only is the DNA of, say, the flounder being inserted into the strawberry, but there's also the following: (1) the "promoter," a section of DNA from a plant virus that acts as an "on switch" and enables the inserted gene to function in a foreign environment; and (2) the "marker gene," which will indicate whether the inserted DNA survived the transfer— these genes are usually antibiotic resistant, which has led some scientists to posit that they might increase antibiotic resistance in people; and then there's (3) a "terminator sequence," or the "off switch," which tells the DNA when to stop transcribing and prevents extraneous DNA from being transcribed.

In terms of corn, one of the insertions—or "the flounder" in this case—is a gene from a bacterium (not a plant) called *Bacillus thuringiensis*, or Bt. Just so we're clear on this: a bacterium is not the same species as a plant. You would never—in nature—be able to make a bacterium and a corn plant mate, just like you couldn't make a strawberry and a flounder mate, no matter how randy that flounder was and how juicy the strawberry looked. This is not the same as hybridizing an apricot and a plum—or getting a peach to mate with a plum and then for whatever that is to mate with an apricot to make a Pluot. I find that people like to say that farmers have been "genetically modifying" our food for ten thousand years. This is just not accurate. It is only true in a really fuzzy way: for instance, you can take the branches from a McIntosh apple tree and splice them onto a Cortland to get another McIntosh tree (above the graft only), but you are never making a *transgenic*. To emphasize, a GMO, most often, carries the genes from two different species—and only technology (except in rare occurrences) can make this happen. No farmer or plant breeder or botanist can do this outside of a lab. Again, GMOs can only be made in the laboratory. Nature will never make a GMO on her own and you can't make one out in the field, no matter how brilliant a farmer you are. Furthermore, a GMO will never be "organic" in the literal sense or the USDA-labeling sense, despite the fact that Biotech reps repeat the mantra that the two are essentially the same thing.[11] Michael Pollan writes in *The Botany of Desire*, "The deliberate introduction into a plant of genes transported not only across species but across whole phyla means that the wall of the plant's essential identity—its irreducible wildness, you might say—has been breached, not by a virus, as sometimes happens in nature, but by humans wielding powerful new tools."

Now, back to corn: Bt is an interesting bacterium. It was first discovered by a Japanese biologist, Ishiwata Shigetane, in 1901. It's primarily a soil-dwelling bacterium that can also occur on leaf surfaces, in animal feces, and in insect-rich environments—in short, it's all around us. Some Bt produces crystal proteins called endotoxins, or Cryproteins, which have been found to have an insecticidal action

---

[11] There are now smartphone apps that help the discerning shopper identify bar codes in the supermarket for foods that contain GMOs and those that are organic.

against a variety of moths, beetles, wasps, wild bees, ants, flies and mosquitoes, and roundworms. Bt is closely related to *B. anthracis*, which causes anthrax—however, it differs in its plasmid (which is a "short, circular piece of DNA that occurs in bacteria and acts like a tiny bacterial chromosome," according to the reference book *Botany: An Introduction to Plant Biology*). In the case of Bt, the protein the plasmid creates targets only the caterpillar; in anthrax, it targets humans and livestock.

In 1911, a German scientist was able to isolate the bacterium as the cause of a disease called *Schlafsucht*, or septicemia, in flour moth larvae, and in the following decades the first research was accomplished that indicated that if the bacterium were introduced into the environment of some insects, it would work like an insecticide. In 1962, Rachel Carson wrote optimistically about Bt in her pioneering book *Silent Spring*, which elucidated the dangerous risks of the pesticide DDT: "High hopes now attend tests of . . . *Bacillus thuringiensis*. . . . Within its vegetative rods there are formed, along with spores, peculiar crystals composed of a protein substance highly toxic to certain insects, especially to larvae of the mothlike lepidopteras. Shortly after eating foliage coated with this toxin the larva suffers paralysis, stops feeding, and soon dies."

In the years after *Silent Spring*, Bt began to be manufactured by various companies across the United States as an agricultural alternative to some pesticides because insects were becoming resistant. Early studies seemed to show that when used as a sprayed insecticide on crops, Bt would be effective for a little while and then would eventually dissipate with time, rain, sun, and air. It was decided that because of this, it had little effect on pollinators, the environment, or humans and wildlife. So, eventually, some strains of Bt were also approved for use on organic crops. Then, in 1995, the first genetically engineered Bt corn, which carried the DNA of Bt, was registered with the EPA by Monsanto, the largest and most famous chemical and biotech company, based in St.

Louis, Missouri, and known for being the co-creators with Dow Chemical of Agent Orange, and the makers of saccharin, RgBH (bovine growth hormone), PCBs, Roundup, and some of the first GMO products.[12] Monsanto's goal was to incorporate the Bt into the plant so that a corn borer caterpillar would take one bite of the corn (or anywhere on the corn plant) and die. A corn borer, by the way, looks like this:

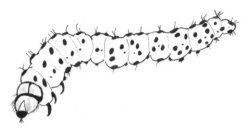

So this is the little critter that encouraged the first GMO and started the big war. Kind of an ugly dude, right?

Monsanto's Bt corn worked so great at killing the corn borers that the company knew they had a hit on their hands. Without further ado, in 1996, Monsanto's Bt corn was approved for sale in the United States, even though no independent tests had been done by the EPA, USDA, or FDA to determine the safety of this product for human consumption. (Monsanto claimed they had done lots of in-house testing of the product and that they had sent their reports to the government regulatory agencies. In a 2013 email to me, they wrote, "USDA reviews GM plants to ensure they are safe for agriculture and the environment. Applicants typically submit a 400-page document that contains

---

[12] I tried to get in touch with Monsanto a few times and was rebuffed and told my questions didn't merit an actual interview. I later learned that a cadre of 4,600 emails released from the U.S. Right to Know campaign to the *New York Times* (through the Freedom of Information Act) exposed that some scientists received unrestricted grants and perhaps other monetary or non-monetary perks directly from Monsanto or indirectly from grants that Monsanto made to their universities or university foundations in order to support their messaging. Apparently my work on the subject of GMOs in *Elle* magazine had been discussed by the company in these emails. More specifically, according to Eric Lipton, the *Times* reporter, Monsanto asked Kevin Folta, a scientist whose pro-GMO proselytizing was subsidized indirectly by Monsanto, to, in the words of Lipton, "intervene on Monsanto's behalf and criticize" my piece. Which Folta dutifully did. Ka-ching!

data from both laboratory and field experiments. For products that contain traits to protect the plants from insect pests and disease, there is an EPA review. Applicants typically submit about twenty study volumes containing thousands of pages of data to address the safety of the introduced protein.") Later, in 1999, the Bernsteins, an allergist team made up of two brothers and their father, at the University of Cincinnati, did a study that suggested that Mexican farmworkers who were exposed to Bt as a spray suffered some allergic response. That is the only independent test I'm aware of that even came close to addressing the possibility that Bt could be an allergen when people are exposed to it at high levels—either as farmworkers or within food.

Today many strains of Bt are incorporated into genetically modified crops—soy, cotton, corn, potatoes, etc.—with different Cryproteins, which have been developed and targeted for different kinds of insects. Suffice it to say that at this point, Bt-modified crops are ubiquitous across the American landscape and within the average American diet. So ubiquitous that, according to a Canadian study published in the journal *Reproductive Toxicology* in 2011, Bt toxin has even been found in the cord blood of pregnant mothers.

Now most GMO corn plants are engineered to carry many different strains of Bt, in the form of the Cryproteins (I like to call them the "cry babies"), to target a variety of insects. And they will *also* carry a "Roundup Ready" gene, which makes the corn plant resistant to Monsanto's herbicide Roundup, so the two can be used together. (In that same Canadian study, glyphosate was found in blood samples from nonpregnant women.) Corn may carry even more transgenic insertions—the options with corn are, frankly, dizzying. Right now Big Pharma is (according to activists) researching the ways that corn might be engineered to carry birth control hormones, antibiotics, and any number of pharmaceuticals. Though we have not seen sound evidence of this yet, it is intriguing to think about, for sure. (Not to mention the brave new frontier of using plant RNA to combat cancer.) Note: Soy, too, carries both Bt and Roundup Ready DNA, as do potatoes, beets, and cotton. The fact is, once you figure out how to modify these plants, you can start tinkering on a lot of different levels.

As I was getting rapidly well on my corn-free diet, and all the while trying to learn as much as I could about GMOs in order to convince my inner skeptic, I found myself lowering into a very nuanced and complicated cauldron (or cesspool) of scientific theories, anecdotal evidence, public opinion, and everything in between. With the goal being to someday write about what had happened to me and how I'd gotten well, I started talking to people. And each interview I did seemed to leave me with more questions. Like a chameleon, I'd find myself alternately convinced of the benefits or dangers of GMOs, depending on whom I was talking to, and then in the next conversation I'd find myself changing tack again. Late at night, when I was lying in bed and trying to fall asleep, my mind would finally stumble into a gray area in the middle of the two camps. There, in the soothing peace of nighttime, I'd find myself running through the things I still wondered about, despite interviewee X's assertions in one direction or the other. I was realizing that the more I got into this topic, the more I found an awful lot of people—even experts—who still did not know exactly how GMOs might eventually affect humans, plants, animals, and the environment at large.

Eventually, my illness and some of the complicated issues surrounding GMOs that came to light through my subsequent research led to the article I wrote that was published by *Elle* in August 2013. While the support for the piece was overwhelming, the backlash on some Internet news sites like *Slate* and *Forbes* was also fast and furious—it became a lightning rod in the larger and extremely incendiary debate on GMOs. Overnight I was both lauded by the anti-GMOers as the poster child for what was wrong with genetic modification and summarily attacked by the pro-Biotech forces for being an idiot with no journalistic credibility. Both adulation and scorn came to me in not only the disembodied venues of Twitter (where a group debated and then determined that my problem was just that I was allergic to corn, despite the fact that I had been allergy-tested for corn protein) and Facebook but also through a deluge of emails and a few nasty attack articles online. And although a part of me wanted to run away and hide—because every direction on this issue seemed to portend more contentious interviews—I pushed my discomfort to the side and decided that what was needed was more information. Why had my article hit such a nerve?

In early October 2013, I got on an airplane and flew west from my hometown of Portland, Maine, to Denver, Colorado, so that I could drive across America's breadbasket. On my trip I planned to meet up with a young farmer named Zach Hunnicutt, who grows popcorn and GMO corn and soy in the middle of Nebraska. And from Zach's I had loosely thrown together an itinerary: I would drive farther east to Iowa, where I planned to meet up with Lisa Stokke and Dave Murphy, the founders of Food Democracy Now!,[13] one of the leading activist groups vociferously decrying GMOs. I hoped, also, that I might be able to make a detour on the way to Iowa to meet a former Monsanto seed scientist and researcher named Richard Goodman, who currently works at the University of Nebraska–Lincoln. That last one depended on how much time and gumption I had. We'll get to that.

But more than anything, before I wrote another word on this GMO subject, I felt I needed to see the plains and the heartland—or, as some call it, the Corn Belt—for myself. I had to witness those GMO corn and soybean fields that are at the center of the incendiary debate I had stumbled into, first as a patient and mother and then as a writer. I needed to know what it would feel like to see, as far as my eye could focus, nothing but waves of amber, undulating in the prairie winds, until they seemed to dissolve into the baby blue edges of a large, flat sky.

---

[13] Yes, that exclamation point really is part of their name.

chapter 2

In Denver, I rented a silver Volkswagen Bug with Colorado plates, which ended up being just about the silliest midget of a car to drive across the plains, as the roads there are populated almost exclusively by tractor trailers, monster trucks, and SUVs roaring down the straight-as-a-pin highways. Then I found a supermarket where I stocked up on coffee for the first leg of my drive and hummus, crackers, a box of salad mix, some potato chips, a box of organic buckwheat hemp cereal, a box of organic soymilk (because real milk would need a cooler), a jar of salad dressing, and a bag of grass-fed beef jerky. I was anticipating something of a food desert (at least for me) for a few days and I needed to be prepared. As the sun began to slant behind me, I set off driving east.

As I drove beyond the city limits of Denver, construction gave way to huge sand and gravel pits off the sides of the road, which soon became long stretches of arid scrubland covered with sagebrush and horses. On the radio, I played Ryan Adams through my iPhone, his music filtering a rush of emotions through me—love, nostalgia, deep sadness, and joy—making me feel alive. And then I turned to Lucinda Williams, her voice as gravelly and dry as the landscape outside my window. I've always said about myself, quoting Tennessee Williams's play *The Glass Menagerie,* that I do best in motion; I am always "attempting to find in motion what was lost in space."

Seeing America this way—on a road trip alone across our land—felt like I was tapping into some untethered part of my soul I hadn't seen for years—since getting married and becoming a mother and tying my life down to the routine of other people's lives and needs. The last time I'd been wild like this, driving across America, Dan and I had been moving to Los Angeles in the midst of the recession.

As THE SUN began to slide toward the horizon, I noticed a harshness to the land, as if somehow this western edge of the Great Plains had never quite recovered from the Dust Bowl. Eastern Colorado remains arid and rough ground to farm. Here, ranches with grazing black Angus cattle stretch over the land and marauding northern harriers sit on fence posts, surveying the scrub for prey. The smell of sagebrush in the wind unleashes wildness and Home on the Range notions of Americana.

Soon, the cowboy country of Colorado gave way to Nebraska and Route 76 turned into 80, and the land became tamed and heavily irrigated: I saw crop circles and silos, sugar beet farms (all, most likely, the GMO beets used these days for anything from common table sugar and molasses to animal feed[1]), and factories where the beets are processed. I saw a greasy-spoon restaurant with a huge sign above it that towered over the highway, reading F-O-O-D. At the border where Colorado and Nebraska meet, the air changed so dramatically, it was as if a storm front had come in, and a thick, pungent smell of hay and the dry smell of harvest dust penetrated the car, making my nose stuff up immediately and my eyes weep. As it got dark, I followed big trucks laden with grapefruit-sized white GMO sugar beets along the interstate, until I got too tired to go any farther and pulled over at a Hampton Inn in North Platte, Nebraska.

---

[1] Indeed, 60 percent of American sugar—or 8.8 million pounds—is now made from GMO sugar beets.

North Platte sits in the southwestern part of the state where the north and south Platte rivers join up to form the Platte River—which, in fact, gives the state its name: the Native American tribes the Otoe, Pawnee, and Omaha all called the river "flat water," and the Otoe word for "flat water" was "nebrathka." The French explorers renamed the Platte "Riviere plate" (pronounced "platte," which means "flat" in French) and it stuck. It is here, in the Platte, that more than 500,000 sandhill cranes take refuge during their springtime migration from southern Texas and Mexico northward as far as Alaska or Siberia, where they will breed. Here the cranes eat small invertebrates in the marshes around the river and kernels of GMO corn from the fields that surround the river.[2] After two or three weeks of rest and food, the cranes continue pushing north.

Historically a railroad town, North Platte has the feeling of being a gateway, straddling the divide between the wilder, less tamed west and the large-scale industrial agriculture that has come to define Nebraska and, indeed, the farming "breadbasket" in the middle of this country. Farming and businesses tied to agriculture have conventions all year long in North Platte, especially during the winter after harvest is completed. The conventions tend to take over the hotels and motels in town, filling them with plainspoken farmers and their wives. The night I got to the Hampton Inn, some wives of farmers sat in the lobby, knitting together and drinking decaf coffee while their husbands talked farming. As cozily homey and welcoming as this scene was, North Platte feels like a town where you visit, not where you stay.

In my room, I unpacked my bags and pulled out the two books I'd brought along: Ian Frazier's hypnotic road story, *Great Plains*, and *The*

---

[2] In 2013, the American Bird Conservancy published a report that begins to document the toll on birds from just one class of pesticides, neonicotinoids, used on GMO corn. The scientists describe eggshell thinning and breaking, and, even more alarmingly, that "a single corn kernel coated with a neonicotinoid can kill a songbird. . . . As little as 1/10th of a corn seed per day during egg-laying season is all that is needed to affect reproduction with any of the neonicotinoids registered to date." And, even more damningly, the report states, "EPA risk assessments have greatly underestimated this risk, using scientifically unsound, outdated methodology that has more to do with a game of chance than with a rigorous scientific process."

Sibley Field Guide to Birds of Western North America. Then I took out my bathing suit. No matter where I travel, I always bring both my running shoes and a bathing suit. My preference is to run in new places, getting to know them a bit from the ground. But with long travel days and unpredictable roads, my next hope is that wherever I stay might have a pool. I swim to unwind, the water washing over me in little chlorinated rivulets, a kind of evening ablution. After a swim back and forth across the quiet blue pool of the Hampton Inn, I showered and got into bed. I was tired. My journey had begun. As my eyelids began to drop closed, I opened my *Sibley's*, turning the pages slowly and methodically, as I tried to identify some of the hawks I'd seen flying overhead while I crossed the western edge of the plains.

The next morning, I awoke with my nose stuffed and swollen and looked out my window to see recently harvested fields of corn, now brown and stubbly, planted right up to the edges of the parking lot of the hotel. After eating a breakfast of cereal and soymilk, I packed my bags and went to my car. I pulled out my road snacks and arranged them on the passenger seat for easy access, filled up with gas, and then continued driving east.

The land in Nebraska is flat and wide, and that open space conjures a feeling of freedom, and even joy. Ian Frazier wrote, "Joy [on the Great Plains] seems to be a product of the geography, just as deserts can produce mystical ecstasy and English moors produce gloom." It turns out, however, I wasn't looking at the same plains Frazier had zigzagged across in the late 1980s on his wild driving trip, visiting towns and hollows in order to record for the rest of us the landscape of that part of the country. And, it goes without saying, that the plains the pioneers—and Laura and Mary and Ma and Pa—traversed and settled are so far gone, they are not even a whisper of a memory on the wind.

Since the intensive cultivation of mostly GMO corn and soy (and some non-GMO wheat and milo, or sorghum) began a short twenty years ago, the landscape has become one enormous breadbasket.

(Though "breadbasket" is probably the wrong word, as it conjures satisfied feelings of food security. In fact, almost all this corn and soy is used for a myriad of other things, like plastics, chemicals, pharmaceuticals, animal feed, and biofuel or ethanol.[3]) Little else, human or otherwise, remains. And this increase in industrial-scale agriculture needs the constant IV of the extremely compromised and shallow Ogallala Aquifer. The Ogallala, named for the town of Ogallala, Nebraska, and in turn named after the Oglala Sioux tribe (while gaining a mysterious "al"), stretches 174,000 square miles underneath the Great Plains, from South Dakota to Texas, and is one of the world's the largest aquifers. It supplies all the states it touches with water for both agriculture and domestic use. Because of the irrigation, there's an unexpected aspect of lushness to the landscape of Nebraska—as Frazier writes of the aquifer, "Its water has turned a number of Dust Bowl counties greener than they ever were before."

The Ogallala, however, is likely to be empty, or close to empty, within the next twenty to fifty years, scientists posit.[4] The aquifer, only 100 feet deep to begin with, has already lost more than 50 feet due to irrigation, which was begun in the 1950s. Without the Ogallala, drought will be imminent. For example, Zach Hunnicutt told me that in 2012, any crops that he knew of in Nebraska that were not planted on irrigated land (or that missed the path of the irrigation pivot) were dead by July fourth.

In addition to the unexpected and antithetical lushness here, alongside the roads you find sloughs—depressions or hollows in the landscape, like ponds, but usually shallower—that are filled with water and aquatic vertebrate and invertebrate animals, which interrupt the crops.

---

[3] These days you can buy sneakers, toys, dishes, and cutlery made from GMO corn. Or, if you want a two-fer, you can pick up a Coca-Cola made with high-fructose corn syrup from GMO corn contained inside a "biodegradable" bottle made from GMO corn. The options with corn are frankly endless. It's the wonder seed.

[4] NASA has been studying the world's aquifers from a satellite in space—and the news is not good. We are draining our underground water supply at an alarming rate, making the idea that there's an infinite supply of water not much more than a mirage.

The sloughs teem with migrating ducks rising up and down in waves as musical as the fluctuations in a Beethoven sonata. On the fields, cattle lazily glean the harvested corn and soy (making me wonder if the "grass-fed" beef from Nebraska I've seen sold at Whole Foods is actually turned out and finished in the fall on the harvested—GMO—fields). Closer to the center of the state, any green lushness I perceived earlier gave way to miles and miles of monocultured corn, a different kind of man-willed abundance, punctuated by gleaming, spider-legged irrigation pivots and small cities of enormous grain silos and their accompanying elevators. I found myself thinking of the photographer Frank Gohlke's silver-gelatin prints in his book *Measure of Emptiness*, in which he photographed grain elevators across the Midwest. There is a loneliness to the empty spaces and the shadows that surround the monolithic structures of the elevators in his images, as if in their physical being they elucidate the loss of some important connection to the earth as our farming becomes bigger and more industrial.

In the wide-open terrain of the plains, the edges of farms butt up against big-box stores, express stops, and, sometimes, little copses of trees. An image from my trip that has stayed with me: a town surrounded by fields and fields of nutritious soybeans and corn as high as elephants' eyes is a town full of, presumably, food. But in that town there is no grocery store or farm stand, just a Walmart to do one's shopping. There is a deep disconnect, I say to myself out loud in the car, when the food that is being grown in one's own town cannot feed the town, and the people of the town must buy their food shipped in from somewhere else—maybe China or Mexico?—at Walmart.

The wind, knowing nothing of the changes that have come to the plains in the last hundred or so years, comes across the land with a constancy that is slightly unnerving. If the wind could be described as "whispering" in the pine trees back home in Maine, the wind across the prairie is more like a long and protracted Indian whoop; it is a call to action, rolling over the land like a biblical reminder that Nature is more powerful than man. But then, when you supplant in your mind the acres and acres of golden corn and brown soy with the rich and diverse mixture of prairie grasses that once blanketed this earth and had wonderful names like big bluestem, purple love grass, stinkgrass, bearded sprangletop, hairy crabgrass, squirrel tail, porcupine grass, threadleaf sedge, soapweed, and American bulrush, the wind, all of a sudden, becomes friendly, even playful. Writing this today, I try to close my eyes and imagine crossing this prairie 150 years ago, skimming my eyes across the softness of multicolored grasses rippling in the wind; I imagine that the differences in greens—from dark to light and hues that vibrated with Nature's accents of purples and browns and reds and blues—must have been something!

But that was before the tractor, the Dust Bowl, before the Ogallala, before the advent of biotechnology, and before cultivation was ramped up, heedless of both history and the future, occupying every square inch of prairie. Sandra Steingraber describes the loss of prairie in her home state of Illinois this way in *Living Downstream*: "Of the original 281,900 acres of tall grass prairie in my home county, an official 4.7 fragmented acres remain (.0017 percent). I have never found them. . . . I have no real relationship to the native plants of my native state." And Aldo Leopold wrote in his elegiac meditation on nature, *The Sand County Almanac*, published in 1949 and yet already at that time tragically prescient of things to come, "No living man will see again the long-grass prairie, where a sea of prairie flowers lapped at the stirrups of the pioneer." In a recent depressing moment with Marsden, I showed him a photo of myself in Kansas. In the photo, I am holding him—he's a tiny baby then, barely three months old—and Hopper is at our feet, his ears cocked while he gazes up at Madonna and child, the perfect attendant. I said, "See, that's us. We're on the Kansas prairie." He looked at me like I was insane and said, "That's not the prairie. There's a store right there and a gas station and an eighteen-wheeler." This picture was not jiving with the Laura Ingalls Wilder books that he and I had devoured first on the page at bedtime and then, again, on audio, read by Cherry Jones. "Ah, yes," I said, seeing his problem.

"That's what remains of much of the prairie, unfortunately." Indeed, even though Franklin Delano Roosevelt made an important gesture during the Dust Bowl to save some of the prairie, conserving 4 million acres, a recent report found that nearly 24 million acres of prairie land have been plowed under just between 2008 and 2011; roughly 19 million of those acres—in landmass, the size of my home state of Maine—have gone to corn, soy, and wheat.

Let's hover for a second on the Dust Bowl, that severe period in our country's history when the droughts of the 1930s, coinciding with the Great Depression, caused the overplowed land to lift in the wind, creating huge billows of dust called black rollers and black blizzards, forcing many people who lived and farmed the middle of this country to go broke and then go west to California. The Dust Bowl—also known as the Dirty Thirties—becomes an important guide to understanding not only this landscape but also the emotional and physical climate that was ripe for the introduction of GMOs and the chemicals that are part and parcel with them. For many farming the Great Plains today, the Dust Bowl and the Depression are not such a distant memory; they still cast a pall over the land, haunting the citizens.

In the opening montage of the Ken Burns documentary *The Dust Bowl*, the narrator informs us that the Dust Bowl "was the worst man-made ecological disaster in American history. When the irresistible pressure of easy money and the heedless actions of thousands of farmers, encouraged by their government, resulted in a collective tragedy that nearly swept away the breadbasket of the nation." Or, to put it another way, from the author Timothy Egan, on whose book *The Worst Hard Time* Burns based his documentary: "It was a classic tale of human beings pushing too hard against Nature and Nature pushing back."

Some refer to the disaster as "The Great Plow-Up" because farmers, encouraged by the government to grow as much wheat as they possibly could, decided to make a go of it, forging forward with an exuberant heedlessness, plowing up almost the entire prairie. Frazier writes in his book, "Prairie is much easier to plow under than it is to restore." And at first the farmers were rewarded: crops were bountiful, and farming became so lucrative that so-called suitcase farmers, or businessmen from other parts of the country, came in, bought an acre or two of land, and planted it with wheat, then left until harvesttime. In this manner, the irretrievable process of rending the land for agricultural production was begun.

Before the Great Plow-Up, the prairie grasses that had evolved over centuries held down the soil and protected it from the wind like a thick and dense carpet, locking moisture into the beautiful, rich, and loamy soil as deep as 12 feet down. It was great "grass country"— perfect food for ruminants, horses, goats, and buffalo, who got the benefit of a diverse mix of grass species that gave full nutritional benefit. Once all the dirt was exposed for crop production, however, there was nothing there to protect the land from the wind, sun, and drought; it was all laid bare. As L. Frank Baum writes in *The Wizard of Oz*, the sun, like the wind, was also a formidable opponent, one you had to be mindful of as you set up a homestead and farm on the prairie: "When Dorothy stood in the doorway and looked around, she could see nothing but great gray prairie on every side. Neither a tree nor a house broke the broad sweep of flat country that reached the edge of the sky in all directions. The sun had baked the plowed land into a gray mass, with little cracks running through it. Even the grass was not green for the sun has burned the tops of the long blades until they were the same gray color to be seen everywhere."

A few foresighted pioneers to the plains understood the challenges, calling it one of the "riskiest" places in the world to attempt large-scale agriculture. But the heedless American thirst for "progress" was too great to listen to this kind of reason. When the decade of dust and drought began to set in, "experts" advised the farmers to keep plowing. They told them that rain would surely come and, in fact, that the more prairie grasses they removed, the more they increased their chances for rain! In American farming it's said that the answer to every problem is *always* more production. And so, even though the writing was on the wall, farmers kept plowing, and the blowing continued and the drought worsened and more and more topsoil blew off the land and it became almost impossible to survive, let alone farm. To make matters worse, what little the farmers could grow was plagued by sieges of grasshoppers, then rabbits, which had multiplied because the bigger predator animals had been shot by settlers. These pests came in waves, eating everything green—kitchen gardens, hopeful crops, grass.

And then, well, we all know the stories—they are iconic in our American history: Many Dust Bowl farmers lost their farms (and some, their lives) after Jobian battles against all kinds of adversaries. Many tried desperate westward migrations to California, the whole family packed into the car with every belonging tied to the roof, hoping to hold on by picking grapes or oranges in the sunny groves of the Golden State. For many across America—and especially for those who suffered across the middle of our country, trying to grow the nation's food—the Depression was like a sharp slap across their faces, forcing them to realize that the American Dream was forever irretrievable.

As I was driving across the plains and thinking about the Dust Bowl, I found myself remembering that incredible scene in John Steinbeck's *The Grapes of Wrath* when a neighbor's son, decked out in goggles, a dust mask, and gloves, drives up in a tractor to a tenant farmer's small piece of arid land, ready to plow it under. Steinbeck writes of the driver: "He could not see the land as it was, he could not smell the land as it smelled, his feet did not stomp the clods or feel the warmth and power of the earth. He sat in an iron seat and stepped on iron pedals." When the tenant confronts the goggled man, "Goggles" tells him that he needs to feed his family, too, needs the three dollars a day that he'll get from the bank—tells him he'll get two more bucks if he levels the house, too. The tenant farmer is desperate, then enraged, then impotent: "There's some way to stop this," he says. "It's not like lightning or earthquakes. We've got a bad thing made by men, and by God that's something we can change."

What we might not have considered—and didn't occur to me until I was driving across the arid, depressing scrubland of Eastern Colorado and cascading into the irrigated lushness of Nebraska—is how deeply that experience of painful desperation has stuck in the psyches of the farmers on the plains today. As Frazier writes, "The Great Plains have plenty of room for the past." Even though times have gotten better, it is a nightmare that, for some, seems only a hairsbreadth away.

By 1940, when the rains had surely come to stay, soaking the hard pans of earth and returning them to viable soil, farmers became cautiously optimistic again: the worst was behind them. By then the federal government had entered agriculture—never to leave, it turned out—but that extra insurance made people feel safer, like they had someone behind them. And they did have someone behind them: Franklin Delano Roosevelt, who came to the drought-ravaged plains twice, showing people just in his physical personhood that even if God had given up on them, he had not. On his first trip, in 1936, he took a 4,000-mile whistle-stop tour, a journey that allowed him to talk with farmers and families and to see and hear about for himself the incredible hardship folks were enduring. Then he went back to Washington and told Americans what was happening to their fellow countrymen. In 1938, FDR came again. He was in Texas giving a speech meant to boost people's sprits, letting them know they hadn't been abandoned, when suddenly, in the middle of his speech, some dark rainclouds came out of nowhere and it began to pour. As it rained, Roosevelt kept speaking, the rain hitting him and drenching his clothes. To many there that day, it felt like Divine Intervention. And the story goes that FDR took credit for that rain.

As if in punishment for optimism and relief, drought hit the plains again in the 1950s. When it was over, farmers didn't want to gamble anymore with the weather; they didn't want to be dependent on Nature ever again. They turned to the Ogallala Aquifer. They figured out how to tap it so that they would no longer have to wait for rains that may or may not come, depending on the capricious heavens above. Over the next fifty or so years, people on the plains reveled in the providence of this incredible godsend of water, using it with nary a thought for the future. Lessons that might have been learned were jettisoned—there was no going backward. Trees, which had been planted in one of FDR's Dust Bowl relief programs, the Shelterbelt Project—under the Emergency Relief Appropriation Act of 1935—and were meant to create shelterbelts from the wind, were cut down to make room for more crop production. With water everywhere, this kind of protection from the wind was now seen as unnecessary. Because of the aquifer, the Plains states became greener, lusher than they had ever looked.

It was in this climate of a rueful assurance that the worst had come and gone that genetically engineered crops came onto the horizon in the late eighties and early nineties. It was then that the huge multinational chemical companies like Monsanto and Dow approached the farmers of the plains and the heartland and promised genetically engineered seeds that would be drought- and pest-resistant, as well as give higher yields, making the vulnerable memories of the past something no one had to lose sleep over anymore. Tillage—a practice farmers have used for years to pop out weeds by digging in between rows of crops—would no longer be needed. In fact, it was now a bad thing to do to your land; you might get another Dust Bowl if you did! Roundup, the weed killer made from glyphosate and manufactured by Monsanto, would take care of the weeds, and the topsoil would need never be disturbed. Crop rotation—from corn to oats to alfalfa—would no longer be necessary, either. Monocropping (growing only one thing and never allowing the soil to rebound with rotation) would make more money and the pesticides and chemical fertilizers would take care of any problems. Money and power, it was understood, could finally concentrate here on the plains for good. In Steinbeck's still relevant story of America, *The Grapes of Wrath*, he writes, "She's a nice country, but she was stole a long time ago." Although he was writing about the Depression and the Dust Bowl, he could just as easily have penned those words half a century later when the big multinational companies decided to set up camp in the middle of America, taking food production out of the hands of farmers for good.

In response to these promises from the experts at Monsanto, the land was put into even more production—stretching into wetlands, surrounding and then suffocating the small family farms, encroaching on both sides of every road, taking up millions of acres of land (worldwide, GMOs are cultivated on at least 448 million acres). But by now, people felt that they had the extra insurance of a powerful company behind them—much like when the government came to the plains to help during the Dust Bowl and people felt that they weren't going at this farming thing alone. This company promised seeds that could endure any calamity at all, and the corresponding chemicals to go with them.[5] Dr. Eric Chivian, a physician and former professor at Harvard Medical School, where he founded and directed the Center for Health and the Global Environment,[6] says that the mentality in the plains is complicated, if not quixotic: "There's a sense of infinite space, that Nature is so vast there is no way we can damage it. At the same time, there is often a 'frontier mind-set,' that Nature can be an enemy, dangerous and brutal, wiping out one's livelihood, if not one's family, and that it therefore must be conquered and controlled."

As I drove east toward Zach Hunnicutt's farm, seeing GMO field after GMO field, I wondered, *Can GMOs really save the plains from the perhaps unavoidable destiny of another severe drought? What about the other problems wreaked from monoculturing, intense pesticide use, and overuse of the land? Can GMOs be made to somehow protect us from those, too?* Probably not, the cynic in me answered. But the belief and the hope are

---

[5] As Abbie Hoffman is remembered to have said: "An expert is a guy from out of town in a cheap suit."

[6] He is also a farmer, running a small heirloom fruit orchard and keeping bees, as well as having shared the 1985 Nobel Peace Prize for cofounding International Physicians for the Prevention of Nuclear War.

there, and they whisper over the Great Plains like a wish coming in with the wind.

Soon, it was time for me to turn off the highway in the town of Phillips, Nebraska, as Zach had instructed. He had told me that he would be working at harvesting soybeans all afternoon, and could easily make time for me to hang out with him on his tractor while he worked. Suddenly I found myself lost on unnamed dusty dirt roads that checkerboarded across the landscape, cutting the fields of soy and corn into big, neat squares.

chapter 3

As I drove down the dusty roads in what I hoped was the right direction, there was a moment when I started to wonder if this guy, Zach, had put me on; he'd simply told me to meet him somewhere on a road called "F-Road." ("It's only in the last twenty years that we've had road names," he explained.) GPS, however, was not equipped to find an "F" road lost in a sea of corn and soy fields, right smack in the middle of Nebraska. Looking for anything that might approximate an "F" road, it quickly became the "F'ed" road, because that's just about how I felt. As dust billowed behind me, I was completely walled in by fields of corn plants on either side of the road, many marked with "trial" signs from the various chemical companies—Syngenta, Pioneer, Aventis—that signified that the seed companies were working with a farmer to try out a new GMO variety or a new pesticide. Before I flew out there, I had heard about these fields of experimental crops from a scientist in Cincinnati, but I wasn't prepared for the fields upon fields that I'd witness in trials.

· · ·

I FIRST CAME ACROSS Zach Hunnicutt on Twitter, where he posts images and thoughts from his life as a young farmer with a family growing GMO corn, GMO soy, and popcorn (which is technically non-GMO because no one has considered it a big enough cash cow to modify it)[1] on 2,500 acres in the flat-as-a-pancake town of Giltner, Nebraska. What had made me stop on his handle and then inspect his bio ("We turn sun, rain, soil & seed into corn, popcorn, & soybeans") was his open-faced embracement of social media. In retrospect this seems a little silly, but I was surprised that tweeting about farming—which involves comments on weather, the soil, crops, tractors, and harvesting—could generate traffic. Yet I found not only that he had close to four thousand followers (which isn't a ton, but is noticeable for a regular guy who's living a pretty regular all-American farming life) but also that he's followed by heavy hitters in the GMO debate, like Monsanto's director of millennial engagement and the Big Ag lobbying organization CropLife America. In Zach's tweets I noticed a folksy-yet-young tone, whether he was mentioning storm clouds rolling in, sunsets over "drying down" corn (corn that's drying at the end of the growing period before it's harvested, as you don't harvest fresh or "wet" corn), agricultural policy, or sports. And I couldn't help but like him, even from afar. I decided to call him up and see if I liked him as much on the phone as online. When he answered, he said he was on his tractor harvesting corn that day but that he had time to talk. The machine, he told me, does most of the work; "It's another employee that just needs management," he said with a chuckle.

I told him that I was writing a book about GMOs and that I was

---

[1] I later learned that under stress (such as drought, depleted soil, and insect infestations) even popcorn plants, technically a type of flint corn, will breed at odd times, trading pollen and genetic material with the nearby GMO flint (or industrial) corn varieties, making it possible that some popcorn kernels—both organic and inorganic—could contain GMO DNA. (Notable: Inorganic popcorn is often coated with the pesticides called neonicotinoids, and is almost always sprayed with atrazine, so though it may not be GMO, it's not "clean.")

interested in his Twitter presence because he seemed to be such a regular guy, yet he was tweeting from the epicenter of one of the largest debates in America about who gets to grow our food and how. He laughed and told me that he had turned to social media because, until recently, most of America hadn't been inspecting the work of farmers like him. He said, "We know that here in flyover country, for the most part, we don't get paid attention to. Life happens on the coasts where the news gets made and the movers and shakers are. We've kind of been left alone out here—good, bad, or indifferent, that's just how it's been." Similarly, Ian Frazier wrote, "The Great Plains are like a sheet Americans screened their dreams on for a while and then largely forgot about."

Until now. The recent interest in agricultural practices and policies has ignited national—and international—debates about CAFOs (concentrated animal feeding operations, or feedlots), water use, GMOs, and pesticides,[2] bringing a level of scrutiny to the job that many farmers were just not prepared for. Zach was personally concerned that the disparity between the "image people had in their heads of what farming is [i.e., the storybook white farmhouse, red barn, cows and chickens running across a green yard] and what it's becoming" (i.e., Big Ag and industrial farming) was a problem, one that those movers and shakers on the coasts couldn't reconcile very easily on their own. He said, "It's similar to seeing someone for the first time since high school and you're shocked at how they've changed. . . . The thing is, we're proud of what we've done, how we use the technology and the resources." So intrepid, charming, coach-dad Zach decided to jump into the fray on Twitter, his goal being to change—for the better—how America sees farmers like him.

---

[2] As a term, "pesticides" covers herbicides, fungicides, and insecticides. Though we will get more specific in this book and make points that separate the three, in general it suffices to say that the entire class of chemicals that target undesirables in one's field or household garden is called a "pesticide."

And who are farmers like him? I wanted to know. Well, his family, he told me, were originally called the Huncotes. They came to Amer ica from England in 1634 and settled in Virginia until they eventually moved down to the Carolinas and Georgia, where they changed their name to Hunnicutt. When the Civil War broke out, however, his great-great-grandpa, a blacksmith and farmworker, migrated to the Nebraska Territories, which included parts of the current states of Colorado, North Dakota, South Dakota, Wyoming, Montana, and, obviously, Nebraska. Zach told me he wasn't sure why, exactly, his family had fled the Southeast, and though he has found some Hunnicutts listed on both sides of the war, he assumes his great-great-grandfather simply saw more opportunity on the frontier than in the war. In Nebraska, Great-Great-Grandpa Hunnicutt claimed a quarter section, or 160 acres, put down roots, and took up homesteading. His son, Otto, was born there in 1898. Otto, Zach's great-grandpa, eventually married a woman named Bessie Detamore, whose family was homesteading their own claim near Giltner. Otto moved there with her, and the Hunnicutts have been farming that land ever since. Otto and Bessie survived the Dust Bowl and managed to hold on to most of the family's land for the duration. When it came his turn, Otto's son, Zach's grandfather, began to expand the farm, little by little, from the original 160 acres.[3] By the time Zach's dad got into farming, he had taken up 3,500 acres, which he now shared with his own father and two brothers, each overseeing a little under 1,000 acres. This one farm supported four family units, Zach said.

Eventually Zach's grandfather quit farming and his three children broke up the acreage equally, each going out on their own. When Zach's brother, Brandon, came back home after college fifteen years ago, he and his dad started gradually expanding again—buying some land and renting more from retired neighboring farmers. Brandon

---

[3] Ian Frazier writes in *Great Plains* that to expect a person to be able to survive on 160 acres—"a little square of this vast region where animals and Indians used to travel for hundreds of miles looking for food . . . was like expecting a fisherman to survive on just a little square of ocean."

then took over the old family homestead, working from there. A few years later, after graduating in 2004 with a degree in agriculture from the University of Nebraska–Lincoln, Zach decided to come back home and farm, too. He bought a house in Giltner, where he now lives with his family—his wife, Anna, and their three kids, Everett, Adeline, and Houston. Zach now runs the farm business with Brandon and their father.

After hearing his family's story, I wanted to know more about his farm and his beliefs about GMOs. Good-naturedly, Zach invited me to come out to Nebraska to meet him and see what farming was to him and his family. Which was how I ended up somewhere in the middle of a sea of corn, feeling totally lost.

Just as I was becoming desperate, an SUV driven by a woman with long, flaxen hair went bombing past and turned right up a dirt road. Wondering if that was Zach's wife, I turned my small car around and followed her. She pulled off the road into a field and parked. I got out and yelled, "Hey, I'm looking for Zach Hunnicutt?" She yelled back, "You got the right place . . . he's out in the tractor!" Indeed, on a big green tractor following a big green combine, I could see the blurry image of a man.

ZACH HUNNICUTT DROVE toward me across an endless swath of brown soybeans, turned his huge green John Deere tractor around in a plume of Nebraska dust, and pulled up next to my small rental car, now covered with a thick layer of prairie dirt. He opened his cab door and called out to me, "Come on up," while tipping up his University of Nebraska–Lincoln baseball cap with a smooth, brown forearm to show me his face: startlingly handsome, one blue eye and one almond brown, a tuft of short, dark brown hair. Zach's Deere was the size of an army tank, and built just like one, too. It made my VW look like an actual bug, a small and irritating pest that had appeared in his fields without invitation. But his genuine smile belied the metallic ruthlessness of the machine, so I clambered up its side, got in, and took a look. Here was the face of America's young, industrial-scale farmer growing GMOs for our nation. An apple-pie-you-could-be-my-kid's-football-coach kind of guy, totally down-to-earth and familiar, as if you've known him your whole life but only now finally woke up enough to notice his incredible sparkle. Along with his baseball cap, he wore a zipped-up maroon fleece (even though the temperature outside his acclimatized tractor was in the high seventies), a pair of shorts, and hiking sneakers. Safely secured and sealed in the cab of Zach's tractor, he turned us around and we took off across his field to catch up with his brother, Brandon, driving the combine.

Michael Pollan, in *The Omnivore's Dilemma*, quotes a farmer in Iowa named George Naylor who tells him that industrial agriculture is growing food for "the military-industrial complex." And it wasn't until I was on Zach's tractor that I understood what Naylor meant: the manner in which we fight wars and how we farm our food are inextricably linked. Farming is one of the most oil-guzzling activities that exists, and we fight our wars to protect that very same oil. And, like our machines of war, the tractors and combines of today are so high-tech that they barely need any human help; they are automated to do their jobs—harvesting, separating, combining—from within the steely distance of a machine.[4]

Huge machine rolling over the land aside, Zach looked every bit like he'd just come from a quick, invigorating hike up Cadillac Mountain. An insulated thermos on his dashboard was full of tea, which filled the tractor cabin with a homey aroma as he sipped it. He's soft-spoken and thinks as he's speaking—he doesn't rush to anything and he has a

---

[4] For those of us who might not know this—I didn't—a combine is simply, as Zach explained to me, a machine that "combines several actions that used to have to be done way back when by hand. . . . It's cutting the plants off, it's gathering [them] into the machine, it's threshing [them], and taking . . . basically, the chaff off the seed, and taking all that stuff that's not seed back and spraying it out on the field, essentially compost." So, in this case, Brandon's combine was cutting and gleaning the soybeans, while Zach and I followed along to catch and carry the harvest in our wagon.

Midwesterner's polite habit of stopping when a pushy Easterner interrupts, and then he tries to thoughtfully and gamely answer the next question. Sitting there on that tractor, he made me feel like we had all the time in the world to talk as we followed Brandon, who was driving the combine up and down the rows of beans. Every so often we pulled up next to Brandon so he could fill the wagon on the back of the tractor with soybeans. Once we were full up, we made our way to the other end of the field, where an eighteen-wheeler hovered with its motor running, also waiting to be filled up. Once the truck was full, it would take the load to some grain bins Zach's family owns a few miles to the south and from there it goes—perhaps now, or perhaps later, when he can get a better price—to the co-op, an entity that buys farmers's grain at harvesttime. Other than that, there was little else to do. Since the automated tractor technology would take care of most of the work, Zach just needed to sit there and make sure the internal computer did what it was supposed to do—which is how he is able to spend a good deal of his time in the tractor cab on his iPad, counting and recording yields, posting on Twitter and Facebook, and, sometimes, reading.

It goes without saying, perhaps, that Zach has embraced the available technology—whether it's the farm equipment or the GMO seeds. According to him, the adoption of technology has been really widespread from twenty- to eighty-year-old farmers alike. And it was the technology, in fact, that convinced him to come back home to farm. When he was in college, the idea of farming was, at first, not at all appealing. What ended up piquing his interest, though, was the technology of everything from genetically engineered crops to tractor advancements. "The number one specific problem I had with making the decision to come back and farm was if it was the kind of thing where I'd have to come back and do it the same way for the next forty years. I wouldn't want to do that. The ability to constantly adapt and improve and change was a big part of it." He did allow that in tacking in favor of technology "you lose some of the romance, you know, the backbreaking work of the farm and stuff," but that "if I were to bring my great-grandpa out here and show him what we're able to do and the tasks that have been either automated or made it so that we're basically not spending as long working and breaking down our bodies physically, I think he would think every single thing is a great idea." Although to a bystander it might seem awfully cushy to be riding around inside a big machine with the temperature set to 72 degrees, drinking tea and listening to the radio, Zach says it's still a lot of work: "It's still gonna be a sixteen-hour day. There's still gonna be breakdowns and things we have to deal with. There's still the mental side to hard work."

I asked Zach then if, even so, because of the technology, he felt some kind of substantial disenfranchisement from the actual dirt of farming? "So before," he answered, "before we had Roundup Ready soybeans, we'd have to go walk the fields with a machete and go chop out some sunflowers and cockleburs and nightshades and anything else that was out there. You know, my social security statement goes back to 1987—and I was born in 1982." He looked at me for emphasis; he was five years old when he started working his daddy's farm. "You know, that was hard work and seemed like it went on forever—it was probably only about two weeks—but it was the first start of getting out there in the fields." I tried to think of my own five-year-old, Marsy, out in the fields cutting down sunflowers and cockleburs, and though I imagined it might be tiring at times, I figured he'd actually like to be involved that way. Already at a young age he is such a hard worker, loving tasks that can be completed with his bare hands, especially those that involve being outside in the natural world and getting dirty. So, I asked Zach, "Don't you think that job taught you to work hard?"

"It did," he said, nodding and taking a sip of fragrant tea.

The parent in me perked up with a question that was as much about my own parenting as his—and also about my fears that the world we're living in is so full of gadgets and so much less connected to anything that's real than I remember as a child. "Are our kids going to understand work the same way that you did when you were five?" As

I asked this, I was watching a red-tailed hawk hunt in the field; as the combine went through, critters that could escape moved to the uncut fields, and, as they did, the hawk followed them. The hawk still knew that life was work, that the knife's edge of survival was sharp.

"You know," Zach said, "I had a similar conversation with my wife the other day. I've got my Bible app on here"—he slapped his iPad on his knee—"and it's got every version of the Bible in the English language and in forty languages; it's a free app. I can take notes on it, I can do whatever. But, you know, I did a Bible study group with a group of guys and a lot of these guys are sixty and above and they have these Bibles they've been using forever. They've got notes they've taken in it and things they've highlighted, lessons they've learned. And there's something to having the actual physical thing. So, actually, I just got a new Bible the other day, it's got lines in the margins to make it easier to write notes and stuff."

Ultimately, despite the lesson of the Bible, Zach told me that because his job has become much less of a physical-labor job, he likes that he can have all three kids in the tractor "pretty easily" so that they can be on the farm with him. He said that when he was a child, it wasn't unusual to go several days without seeing his dad during planting and harvest: "My dad was gone before I got up and until after I went to bed." These days, because of the technology, the tasks on farms just simply don't take as long as they used to. This freedom has allowed Zach to coach his son's T-ball team during planting season, for instance, something his own father had to delay until late summer, when the plants could be left alone. All that being said, after a quiet pause in our conversation, Zach hinted at a primal discomfort with the possibility that his own children would have no relationship with the land he himself farms because not only have they never witnessed their father out toiling and working the land the way he did, but they, unlike Zach, had never been called upon to engage with the land: "What you're saying, about keeping ourselves connected, and keeping the kids connected. I've wondered about that—you know, if we need to make a more intentional effort to do those things, like to bring my kids out with me whenever I can and explain to them what's going on, you know, and get out [of the tractor] and run through the soybeans and have that time of being out there figuring out what those jobs are going to be that they're going to do, that will teach them the same things, as, you know, going out and cutting sunflowers."

But it was those sunflowers, actually, and nightshades and cockle-burs that made Zach interested in the first GMOs. He told me that when GMOs were introduced to his farming family and their friends, "everyone was excited about it" because "weeds mean you have to do more to the soil and to the environment to get rid of them. . . . To have a relatively safe option to control the weeds so you can spend less time getting rid of weeds and more time building up your soil . . . was a no-brainer for us." Although I'd later learn that there were many farmers across the Great Plains and the Midwest who scoffed at the promises Big Biotech extolled about GMOs, Zach said that for his farming family, it was a heady time full of possibility.

What Zach could not have predicted, however, was the backlash that eventually came when many Americans began protesting the use of GMOs: "I think the one thing, if all of us had to do it all over again . . . while these changes were going on, and these improvements were happening, we weren't doing a real good job at communicating that with our customers, the people who were using the things that we were raising."

The lack of communication from either the biotech industry or the farmers (or the food companies) had been described to me by the activist Lisa Stokke in my early pre-trip interviews as an initial deception that has led to a cascade of problems. She remembers being startled to learn, in the early aughts, that food could be genetically engineered. She said, "Biotechnology was thrown on us under cover of darkness . . . and it's like 'Holy shit, we've got ninety million acres of this stuff now. . . . What can we do about it?'" (Now that number topples over 170 million acres just in America.)

This attitude, that GMOs were blanketing the country "under cover of darkness," Zach says, speaks to the basic lack of trust that people seem to suddenly have in farmers like him who are working like hell to grow our food out in "flyover country."[5]

It's been unnerving, but he says he understands. He said that the lack of communication "made it all seem dark and shady like there were these scientists that were coming up with these things in labs to do harm to people, or, you know, just to make money, with no regard for the people, for the environment, for anything. And without being proactive about why we're doing these kinds of things and how a lot of these things were just a logical extension from the hybridization of crops and seed selection, it made it seem almost like we had something to hide. Obviously it's such a sensitive topic to talk about—people get all worked up about genetically modified things and farmers will get worked up about getting accused of doing harm. And I think if that communication had been handled better on the front end, we could have made this a much more reasonable discussion. Because ultimately, what you're concerned about is that you want to make sure you're feeding your kids healthy food, and that you're eating healthy food; that's ultimately what you're concerned about. And frankly that's what we're concerned about, too, you know, my kids are eating the same food as yours. We're concerned with putting out something that's safe and healthy and using our resources in a way that the next generation will be better off."

It was sunny and beautiful, and Zach was so incredibly earnest and

---

[5] A 2013 *Scientific American* piece called "It's Time to Rethink America's Corn System" by Jonathan Foley states, "Although U.S. corn is a highly productive crop, with typical yields between one-hundred-and-forty and one-hundred-and-sixty bushels per acre, the resulting delivery of food by the corn system is far lower. Today's corn crop is mainly used for biofuels (roughly 40 percent of U.S. corn is used for ethanol) and as animal feed (roughly 36 percent of U.S. corn, plus distillers grains left over from ethanol production, is fed to cattle, pigs and chickens). Much of the rest is exported. Only a tiny fraction of the national corn crop is directly used for food for Americans, much of that for high-fructose corn syrup. . . . In short, the corn crop is highly productive, but the corn system is aligned to feed cars and animals instead of feeding people."

open, and he's such a nice guy, that it was hard to not feel for him, and through him for the plight of thousands of farmers who are out there on the land, toiling to grow corn, soy, canola, and wheat, who have suddenly been caught in the uproar over GMOs. Because, let's face it, farming is not exactly a walk in the park; even if you are inside a climate-controlled tractor cab and you're spraying pesticides with a crop duster, it still is hard work.

Over the low rumble of the tractor, Zach told me that he really does believe that GMOs will protect the soil, and perhaps the future of crops on the plains, making the plains a place where he can be confident his kids have a future. And, for the record, he isn't too worried about the aquifer, either; although he does allow that the energy— from using electric or diesel motors—to get the water out of the ground and into the irrigation pivots is notable, and that the number of wells needed for farming can seem like a lot (each field needs at least one well, and one square mile would have four wells on it). Zach, however, believes that good management practices are being put into place to protect the aquifer and will keep him in water. Plus, he says, you'd see a drought coming: "It wouldn't be a thing where you turn on the faucet and nothing came out. That would be devastating. But this would be a slow development over a couple of generations. . . . We've changed our use of water even in the last ten to fifteen years. I think that we'll be able to maintain it for future generations."

And Zach's not alone in his thinking that the aquifer is doing just fine. Many farmers—and scientists—echo Zach and, further, state that the Roundup system of herbicide-resistant GMO corn and the ability to spray the herbicide to kill the weeds without having to till (or turn over) the soil is actually better, making them less vulnerable to the disasters of the past, when the topsoil got so dry it blew away. Zach said, "What happens when you till the soil is that you end up creating hardpans in the soil . . . so instead of the nice, loose soil that roots can move through easily, it gets hard and compacted down there. Our soil quality has improved quite a bit. Here we have almost no topsoil loss . . . it's improved our soil structure down there, you know. If you come out either after the irrigation system has passed or after a rain, you see wormholes everywhere. I don't remember seeing that so much as a kid—maybe I wasn't looking for it—but you can judge a lot of the health of the soil by the earthworm activity." I heard him. And as I looked at his fields, there was a part of me that was glad, at least, that I had the chance to come out here, to the epicenter of monoculture farming, to see that these may be GMOs, but at least they are grown in real dirt, for heaven's sake. It's not like these things are grown on the moon. There are dirt and worms and hawks and mice.

Some recent studies, however, have questioned whether the "no till" system of weed removal with the use of herbicides is really all that terrific. One possible downfall of this system is that because the ground is never tilled, phosphorus, a by-product from chemical fertilizers, is sitting in concentrated levels on top of the soil, so that when the rains do come, or irrigation is used, the runoff from the fields into nearby rivers contains highly concentrated phosphorous, which creates blue-green algae blooms in rivers, lakes, watershed areas, and, ultimately, in drinking water (in the summer of 2014, for instance, Toledo Ohioans could not drink the water because the algae content was so high from agricultural runoff—and in 2015, Lake Erie was found to have the same problem).

Furthermore, when you consider the herbicide (and pesticide) schedule a farmer like Zach will use on one cornfield, one wonders if tillage really has such convincing downsides. In the fall, right after harvest, Zach sprays 2,4-D,[6] an herbicide made by Dow Chemical that

---

[6] In 2014, Dow Chemical petitioned the USDA and the EPA to allow a stronger strength of the herbicide 2,4-D to be approved so that it could be released for use on fields like Zach's, where weeds are becoming resistant to the various herbicide cocktails. The new herbicide is called Enlist Duo and is a powerful combination of both glyphosate and 2,4-D. Dow also came up with corn and soybeans that are now resistant to the 2,4-D in Enlist Duo. The USDA welcomed public comment on Dow's new corn and soybeans through the spring and into part of the summer of 2014—although I think it's safe to say that most people in America had no

is an "organochlorine," made up of chlorine and carbon atoms derived from petroleum, fused together using chlorine gas, which is known to be an effective poison and was used extensively in the First World War by the Germans. 2,4-D is also one of two ingredients used, in equal parts along with 2,4,5-T, to make Agent Orange, the warfare chemical made by Monsanto and Dow and used by the U.S. military to defoliate trees and destroy crops during the Vietnam War. The health effects of Agent Orange—to U.S. military as well as the Vietnamese—have been widely reported. The statistics from the Vietnamese people alone are startling: up to 4.8 million Vietnamese were exposed to Agent Orange, and of those, the Vietnamese government has said that 500,000 babies were reportedly born with severe birth defects due to Agent Orange. Agent Orange is also linked to various B-cell lymphomas and soft tissue sarcomas, as well as a host of other cancers. Our U.S. Department of Veterans Affairs presumes that all soldiers who came to Vietnam on a boat or put boots on land were exposed to Agent Orange.

The 2,4,5-T alone contributed huge amounts of dioxin to the Vietnamese environment, causing birth defects and stillbirths at the time. High dioxin levels that tragically persist in the soil in Vietnam continue to affect the citizens, still causing birth defects and stillbirths, poisoning food, disrupting endocrine systems, and is correlated with cancers of the larynx, lungs, and prostate, to name a few.

Perhaps surprisingly, we don't have to go all the way to Vietnam to find the effects of dioxin. In Nitro, West Virginia, a Monsanto plant that made 2,4,5-T until it was shuttered in 2004 has caused massive and persistent dioxin contamination. In 2012, the biotech company finally agreed to begin relief efforts in the town, promising up to

---

idea they could comment on a 2,4-D–resistant soybean, or what 2,4-D actually was. In the fall of 2014, the USDA approved the soybeans and the EPA approved the stronger solution of 2,4-D mixed with glyphosate, despite the 500,000 comments and signatures they received asking that they not be approved. In November 2015, the EPA said it was considering withdrawing its approval of the chemical, according to the *Wall Street Journal*, "saying it has new information that suggests the weed killer is more toxic to surrounding plants than previously thought."

$84 million for medical monitoring, up to $9 million for property cleanup, and up to $29 million to cover the plaintiffs' legal fees.

Despite all this bad news about dioxin (including the depressing fact that agricultural workers from industrialized countries around the world are not only getting cancer at higher rates than the rest of us but are dying from incurable cancer more often),[7] for the farmer, the beauty of 2,4-D, Zach told me, is that it kills everything—all the plants, that is—on the field so that come springtime, he has less work to do to get his field ready for planting. When I asked him if he was at all concerned about 2,4-D, Zach said he was not. He said, "2,4-D is sprayed on every lawn in America." And it's true: your neighbor—or mine—may be using it to get rid of dandelions and clover so that they can have a monoculture of straight grass on their lawn. (Rachel Carson wrote about the emerging dangers of 2,4-D back in 1962 in *Silent Spring*. She found that plants treated with 2,4-D had sharp increases in nitrate content, killing some cattle. She hypothesized that the same danger would exist "for wild animals belonging to a group of ruminants, such as deer, antelope, sheep and goats.")

When spring does arrive, Zach will spray 2,4-D a second time in order to get the fields totally clean of weeds. He used to then apply an application of nitrogen—often in the form of anhydrous ammonia—which is a chemical fertilizer, known to be both caustic and hazardous, especially to farmers. Because of its toxicity, Zach has tried to wean his farm off it and tries to instead use some dry fertilizer, which is considered safer. After planting, Zach will spray atrazine as his "pre-emerge herbicide" so that he can get rid of any precocious early weeds. He does this, he told me, even though he is aware that atrazine

---

[7] Sandra Steingraber informs us in *Living Downstream:* "Childhood brain cancers and leukemias are consistently associated with parental exposure to paint, petroleum products, solvents and pesticides. Some exposures may occur before birth. Children can also be exposed when these materials are carried into the home on their parents' clothes and shoes, through breast milk (which can be contaminated directly or through maternal contact with father's clothing), or even through exhaled air: because solvents are, in part, cleared by lungs, parents can expose their children to carcinogens by breathing on them. In this way, a father's homecoming kiss and work-clothed embrace can contaminate his child."

gets into the groundwater, and he himself says, "I wouldn't let my kids roll around in it. It's not safe and it can and will kill you."[8]

The serious problems with atrazine—which is manufactured by the company Syngenta—are just starting to be understood from the work of Tyrone Hayes, a biologist at UC Berkeley, who has been studying frogs in sloughs and streams in Nebraska and across the United States for nearly twenty years.[9] Hayes's work has shown that atrazine use is causing endocrine disruptions, increased estrogen production, genital abnormalities, and sexual ambiguity in male frogs. And atrazine appears to be turning boy frogs into hermaphrodites, or even "gay" (meaning that male frogs are sexually confused enough to try to mate with each other). The implications to humans are not yet understood, he said, but there's no reason to think that atrazine couldn't affect human males similarly. In fact, recent studies done in Washington State and Texas have found that boys born to mothers who were exposed to atrazine were at increased risk of at least having genital abnormalities. Tyrone told me, "You know, I talk to these [farmers] in the Midwest who will say, 'Look, we don't want to use this stuff. But if my neighbor uses it and I don't, I'm going to be out of business. . . .' And farmers are like, 'Sure, anything you can do to get us free of this stuff. We know it's bad, but what are we supposed to do?'"

Although Hayes continues to look at atrazine and the effects it has on living organisms—because "the best thing about atrazine is we know what it does"—he has recently turned his focus to the chemical cocktails that are becoming more and more common in agriculture due to the weed-resistance problems farmers face. He said, "When

---

[8] Atrazine was banned in the European Union in 2004 because it was contaminating groundwater; here in America, the makers of atrazine funded a 2007 study that showed that if atrazine use was curbed, the agricultural economy would suffer.

[9] When I asked Tyrone Hayes if it was true that atrazine could kill you, he said, "Yes. But not like rat poison will kill you dead immediately. Atrazine—especially to farmworkers, through inhalation and dermal exposure—will cause health problems if you are exposed over and over, which will eventually kill you."

you mix all these chemicals together, you get these sort of emergent qualities that you can't predict from the individual chemicals." Not to mention, he said, the synergistic effect of what one farmer may be spraying that inherently mixes, to some degree, with a neighbor's combination of pesticides, which may be different. This is the new frontier of pesticide studies—a frontier the EPA hasn't yet begun to explore.

Indeed, Zach told me that he will also use a cocktail of atrazine, Roundup, 2,4-D, and some lesser-known herbicides as his pre-emerge spray to kill any errant weeds that persisted after the first application of 2,4-D and atrazine. When the plants are up, he said he sprays "side dressing," or liquid nitrogen, and he controls weeds throughout the season with one to two sprayings of the herbicide Roundup.

Let's focus for the moment on the active ingredient, glyphosate, in Monsanto's Roundup, which was first patented by Monsanto in the early '70s and put on the market in 1974. Roundup was developed to kill weeds, and today there are more than 750 products for sale in the United States that contain glyphosate. Roundup is used pervasively in industrial agriculture on GMO crops—corn, soy, and cotton—which are bred to withstand its use. However, in an evolutionary twist of fate, the weeds that glyphosate, or Roundup, is meant to kill have been evolving to tolerate it, giving way to "superweeds" that are impervious to the chemical deluge. The irony here is that when Roundup was first developed in the 1970s, there was great hope for it—some initial studies seemed to prove that weeds would never breed a resistance to it and that it was practically as safe as water. When GMOs came on the market, to be paired with the herbicide, Roundup use exploded across America—and not just on agricultural fields. You can buy bottles of Roundup at the hardware store or Walmart to get rid of undesirable weeds that might be crowding your oak trees, growing up between your bricks on your patio, or obstructing your view. (Between 2001 and 2007, as GMO products took off, glyphosate use more than doubled; 180–185 million pounds of glyphosate were used in 2007. Some researchers estimate another doubling, at least, in the last decade, but it's hard for us to know because the Bush administration, openly friendly with the chemical companies, was reportedly persuaded to stop recording glyphosate sales in 2007.)

At any rate, evolution has continued marching forward, and those pesky weeds have figured it out, making Roundup resistance a rampant problem, which has encouraged both farmers and laypeople alike to just use more of the stuff. In the meantime, Roundup isn't the only herbicide to which weeds are developing resistance: in 2013, the *New York Times* reported, "Today 217 species of weeds are resistant to at least one herbicide, according to the International Survey of Herbicide Resistant Weeds."[10] (This number had increased to 248 at the time of this writing.) We now know that it can take only a few short years for weeds to begin to develop resistances after the introduction of a new herbicide—so just turning to a new chemical, many scientists are now arguing, is not the answer.[11]

One plant that is not yet impervious to Roundup, however, is milkweed, the plant on which monarch butterflies lay their eggs and that is the larvae's only source of food until the monarch caterpillars go through metamorphosis. Milkweed, it goes without saying, is critical to monarch survival. And the milkweed population has been decimated since the introduction of GMOs and heedless spraying of Roundup, which, many researchers say, has led to an alarming decline of monarch butterflies. (There is a difference of opinion among many researchers about whether it's just the Roundup that's killing the milkweed and affecting the monarchs, or if the Bt pollen from the GMO corn is also toxic to the beloved monarch.) In recent years,

---

[10] For the record, it's not just weeds that become impervious to pesticides. As Rachel Carson wrote so deftly in *Silent Spring*, it's also insects—the same insects we strive to eradicate. She writes, "This has happened because insects, in a triumphant vindication of Darwin's principle of the survival of the fittest, have evolved super races immune to the particular insecticide used, hence a deadlier one has always to be developed—and then a deadlier one than that."

[11] The barnyardgrass weed, often found in rice paddies, has evolved so craftily to mimic the fields of rice it is so persistently contaminating that it even changes color like a chameleon from pink to a nearly identical green.

monarchs have become a very visible—to the general public—casualty, or indicator species, if you will, of planetary change brought about by the way humans are affecting the environment. In reaction to this fact, in 2014, the Natural Resources Defense Council sued the EPA for not responding to a petition the NRDC had sent decrying the EPA's allowance of the indiscriminate use of Roundup, which, the NRDC says, has not been reviewed since the 1990s, despite the incredible acreage of land being put into GMO crops. The EPA said, in response, that it's studying many causes for the decline in the monarch population and that it's conducting a "risk management approach." (At the time of the writing of this book, the monarch was under review for endangered species status and the NRDC had begun a second suit against the EPA for approving Enlist Duo, the powerful herbicide combination of glyphosate and 2,4-D made by Dow Chemical.)

And that's not all. There's more bad news coming over the wire about glyphosate: recent reports from the sugarcane fields in Central and South America point to the possibility that Roundup may be causing kidney failure in the male laborers on the plantations. In 2013, a study published in *Food and Chemical Toxicology* found that Roundup is an endocrine disruptor and increases the likelihood of hormone-dependent breast cancer. The study stated, "Our results also found that there was an additive estrogenic effect between glyphosate and genistein, a phytoestrogen in soybeans." (And you are sure to get both at once because GMO soybeans are Roundup resistant!) And, if we're still not convinced, a study released by the International Agency for Research on Cancer in early 2015 found that glyphosate (Roundup) probably causes cancer in humans, and, in particular, certainly causes non-Hodgkin's lymphoma. That same year, the World Health Organization swiftly weighed in, saying that it, too, has deduced that glyphosate is a "probable carcinogen." In response, the state of California announced in September 2015 that it was going to list glyphosate as a carcinogen.[12] Monsanto, meanwhile, is holding steady that Roundup is harmless. (Hopefully they are right, because a U.S. geological study found Roundup in 75 percent of air and rainfall test samples from the Mississippi Delta agricultural region.)

Peripherally, the controversial MIT researcher Stephanie Seneff, who looks at patterns and trends in studies but herself is neither a biologist nor an epidemiologist (and has been ridiculed for this fact), has become a new voice in the cacophony as she has begun to raise the ante with a link she's made between glyphosate and autism, which she warns may affect half the population by the year 2032. Autism is, as most of us know, on the rise, experiencing an upswing not dissimilar to the rise in asthma, which has reached epidemic proportions. Seneff's reasoning is intriguing because her basic premise is that glyphosate creates a series of deficiencies within the body by killing beneficial gut bacteria—or "microflora"—which supply our bodies with essential amino acids. She claims that glyphosate also chelates (binds and therefore makes unavailable for absorption) vitamins and minerals like manganese and iron that are necessary for healthy immune systems, which can then lead to problems in the development of our neurotransmitters. This, she says, can be linked to autism (and a variety of other transmitter conditions such as ADHD, or the newer diagnosis, "sensory development disorder").

On this last point, Seneff echoes Dr. Don Huber, emeritus professor of plant pathology at Purdue University and a former senior plant pathologist with the U.S. military who worked for the Defense Department researching chemical and biological warfare during the Vietnam War. Don has made his name lecturing on the subject of glyphosate's apparent chelation of minerals in the soil and therefore making our food plants nutritionally lacking. When I spoke to him on the phone from his

---

[12] At the time this book went to press, the state of California was still accepting comments on this proposal.

home in Idaho, he told me that his big concern is the cumulative levels of glyphosate in our soil and therefore in our food. "There are high levels of glyphosate residue in our food crops," he says. "The FDA permits this—anywhere from forty to eight hundred times higher than clinical toxicology shows can have an effect on mammalian systems."[13] Like 2,4-D, glyphosate is systemic—when it is sprayed as an herbicide, it is absorbed by the plant into every cell and the fluids of the plant. It has also been found to be more toxic when mixed into Monsanto's Roundup, because of the surfactant POEA, which is added by Monsanto to enhance efficacy, than when it is sprayed by itself.[14] In addition, it makes the soil hard and compact and affects the ecology—the bacteria, fungi, and minerals—around the root of the plant. Reporting for the *New York Times* in 2013, Stephanie Strom wrote that "Monsanto, which sells Roundup and seeds resistant to glyphosate, says 'there is no credible evidence' that the herbicide 'causes extended adverse effects to microbial processes in soil.' A team of scientists from the Agriculture Department similarly reviewed much of the research and found the herbicide to be fairly benign. In response to a request from Monsanto, the Environmental Protection Agency recently increased the amount of glyphosate that is allowed on food and feed crops." (This calls to mind a saying that my friend the environmentalist Steven Hopp likes to use: "Absence of the evidence for something is not the same as evidence for the absence of something.")

Indeed, the pervasive opinion in the farming world—out there on the plains, across the Corn Belt, and into our nation's heartland—is

---

[13] One study showed that glyphosate caused pregnancy problems in agricultural workers and affects human placental cell viability at ten times lower than what is allowed on crops.

[14] Bruce Blumberg, a scientist at UC Irvine who is studying epigenetic changes due to environmental toxins, wrote this in an email to me about POEA: "Many of these substances are used to make the chemical 'stick' to plant surfaces. Some people claim that these chemicals are more toxic than the pesticides/herbicides, which is highly dubious. What they do is increase your exposure to the chemical in question, rather than being inherently toxic (although they may be toxic). Of course, in their infinite wisdom, [the] EPA allows companies to classify all of these materials as 'inert ingredients' and not report what they are as 'trade secrets.' This is nonsense because any other company with a mass spectrometer can tell what the composition is within a day or less."

that Roundup (or glyphosate) is completely safe. Zach told me that he was at a meeting where an "EPA guy said, 'Roundup is the perfect herbicide.'" When I asked Zach if he believed this about Roundup, he said that Roundup was, comparatively, "the light touch" of all the chemical options, and he doubted it could be dangerous. Not so, says Dr. Huber. Glyphosate, he says, can persist in the soil for as many as, and sometimes more than, twenty-two years, which would affect future crops, not to mention the various organisms from butterflies up to humans that depend on the soil being healthy. Tyrone Hayes, the scientist from UC Berkeley, weighed in. When I asked him if glyphosate really could be just as safe as the EPA says it is, he looked at me like I was crazy and said, "It's designed to kill things; of course it does something." (As an aside, I need to note here that, as a small-time gardener, I understand how irritating it is to keep pests off one's plants. I struggle with cabbage moths and snails; I pick them off my plants twice a week and drown them in hot, soapy water. It's arduous. I can't even imagine doing this on a massive scale; the all-too-human desire to wage war on one's fields is, to me, understandable.)

Now, LEST YOU THINK I'm picking on Zach or any other farmers who choose to use this stuff, let me say this: the precedent for using a large amount of chemicals on our agriculture was set long before Zach was born. It began right after World War II (and was in full swing when Rachel Carson was writing *Silent Spring*) during a period called the Green Revolution, which was the brainchild of a scientist named Norman Borlaug. The Green Revolution, despite its name (which in today's parlance might suggest something more radical, involving solar panels and composting lobster shells), was actually a great push for the industrialization of agriculture—or agribusiness. Although the Green Revolution is often remembered as an initiative to stave off worldwide hunger, it was far more complicated than just altruism (and was the beginning of what the farmer George Naylor called the "military-industrial complex"). According to Peter Pringle, author of *Food, Inc.*:

Mendel to Monsanto—The Promises and Perils of the Biotech Harvest, "Toward the end of World War II, the United States decided to use its dominance in world food production to extend its global influence. . . . In a dual strategy the United States would simultaneously fight world hunger and halt the spread of communism. Population explosions in the undeveloped nations of Latin America and Asia meant there was not enough to eat. Hunger led to social upheaval that could leave nations vulnerable to communist takeover." "Green," therefore, in this case refers to large parcels of land covered with green shoots of growing wheat, corn, and rice. "Revolution," says Pringle, "referred not to the upheaval of the masses but to the combined effect of improved seeds, chemical fertilizers and pesticides, and water irrigation projects." Indeed, if there's any one moment in history we can blame for what has become our modern chemical-dependent agriculture, it would be this important period right after World War II, when we began the big business of producing synthetic chemicals from petroleum and the seed business's development of hybrids took off, "bringing corn monocultures to millions of acres," says Pringle. Also, World War II had created, Pringle writes, "a huge production capacity for nitrogen, the key ingredient of military explosives but also the main ingredient of plant fertilizer. When the war was over, factories that had produced explosives were converted; mineral fertilizer production worldwide rose from 17 million tons to today's figure of more than 150 million tons. Over three decades from 1950 to 1980, the sale of nitrogen fertilizer jumped seventeen times."[15]

---

[15] As we know by now, the runoff from chemical fertilizers creates an acid environment that lends itself to the growth of enormous toxic algae blooms, contaminating streams, ponds, and rivers. As I was writing these sentences, I was sitting in a friend's house on the ocean off the coast of Maine in a groomed seaside town. The runoff from the yards down to the ocean looked like irradiated green spiderwebs; algae snaking down the granite rocks and into the water. A likely guess is that nitrogen-rich lawn fertilizers caused what I was seeing. As we consider the incredible breadth of industrial agriculture and the chemical pesticides, herbicides, and fertilizers that go along with it, we must also consider the "shoulder problem": When chemicals are approved for Big Ag, it takes almost no time for versions of the same products to be approved for home gardeners. No longer are we just saturating the earth of the Great Plains in order to grow our food—or biodiesel—but by now we're using the very same chemicals on our lawns, affecting the flora and fauna in our own backyards. A 1994 study estimated that the average number of pesticides in the American home was between three and four. Between 2001 and

Ironically, and sadly, reports Pringle, the Green Revolution has never brought world hunger under control; instead, we will have an estimated one billion—at least—food-insecure people on the planet by 2025.

Zach tells me that as summer gets under way, if his corn plants are in good shape after everything he's sprayed up until then, he'll give them one more nitrogen spray, a "foliar feeding" spray, when the corn leaves are casting enough shade in order to control the weeds beneath them. Fungicides are introduced during the reproductive period of the plant to keep fungus diseases off because they "stress out the plant," he told me, though fungicides have been found in groundwater in many states (Maine, where I live, being one of them) and are known endocrine disruptors. After fungicides are applied, if the plants are doing well, "not too much more spray is used until after harvest," says Zach, when it begins all over again, starting with the 2,4-D that kills everything remaining on the field before winter sets in.

Perhaps remembering his audience, Zach pointed out that although this might seem like a lot of chemicals being sprayed on his plants, it's pretty much the norm of what everyone he knows does. "Chemicals aren't cheap," he says, "so we're not going to blow them for kicks and giggles." Also, he says, because the GMO corn now carries its own insecticide in the form of Bt, he applies little to no insecticide. "It's been years since I remember applying any," he says. (Later, in a phone call, Zach said that when he told me that, he wasn't thinking of the neonicotinoids—systemic pesticides that are insect neurotoxins—applied to his corn seeds as "treatments" before planting, or of the liquid insecticide that he adds to his "starter fertilizer."[16] Hearing this was complicated for me because I liked Zach—he's honest, smart, and

---

2006, it was estimated that at least 95 percent of American households stored at least one pesticide. Back in 1994, Americans spent $1.9 million on household pesticides. But in 2007, the EPA says that Americans spent over $250 million on pesticides—that's approximately 71 million pounds of the stuff! So, in 2016, if we follow the curves of increase—in homes and on agricultural fields—it is probably safe to assume that these numbers have significantly increased to dizzying proportions!

[16] You might ask, "What? Why do they need more?" Well, one answer is that the corn borer began to be resistant to Bt ten years into the planting of the first GMO corn.

an all-around nice guy. But the truth is that the pro-GMOers love to point out that less insecticide is used with the advent of GMO/Bt crops. This is just not true when you consider that each kernel of corn, each cottonseed, and each soybean is literally soaked in neonicotinoids and that neonicotinoid use has exploded worldwide to previously unheard-of levels. We will get more into this in Part 2 of this book, but I felt I had to give you a heads-up here.)

Zach told me that his father sprayed many more chemicals when he was farming when Zach was growing up. When I pushed him on this (because the numbers just don't work out in favor of this statement), he allowed that his father in fact just sprayed more insecticides and that *he* probably sprays more herbicides. Although across the country—and the globe—he's right: insecticide use—as long as we turn a blind eye to neonicotinoid use—has presumably decreased because of GMOs (which inherently carry their own insecticide), but herbicide use has skyrocketed by more than 46 percent, or 527 million pounds, since the introduction of GMO plants.[17] And it's only getting worse as more weeds become resistant to the sprays that the GMO plants are bred to withstand. Tyrone Hayes says, "My biggest concern with GMOs is that the original promise was that we're going to use a lot less pesticides . . . and it's just the opposite now. We're actually making genetically modified products that *require* pesticides, and the reason we're doing that is that the six chemical companies own about 90 percent of the seeds that we grow. So there's an inherent conflict of interest. You don't want to design something that's going to get you off the chemical; you want to design something that's going to make you *have to use* the chemical." Harvard's Dr. Eric Chivian says, point-blank, there's no gray area here: "This is a disaster for agriculture. The insecticides and herbicides that are used for growing GM plants are toxic to many

---

[17] This number is hard to track. Other reports state that as of 2013 glyphosate use had quadrupled to 250 million pounds annually. Whatever the numbers end up being, they are shocking!

organisms including pollinators like honeybees and bumblebees, other beneficial insects and birds that prey on crop pests, and earthworms and soil invertebrates that make soils fertile. So by using them we are damaging basic ecosystem functions like pollination, biological crop protection, and soil fertility. Does this make any sense at all?" (Chivian's statement made me wonder if Zach was really seeing earthworms on his fields when it rained from close to eight feet off the ground.)

As the afternoon was beginning to wane, and Zach and I had been on his tractor going back and forth across the same big square of beans for close to three hours, I began to feel that I might be overstaying my welcome.

But I did want to know one last thing: Was he—Zach Hunnicutt, the dad, husband, all-around really good-seeming guy—at all concerned that the pesticides bred into GMO foods might ultimately cause health problems? Or, for that matter, the pesticides that are sprayed on them? In response, Zach was cautiously sanguine. First, he let me know that he'd read my piece in *Elle* and he apologized for the way I was treated by some of the GMO proponents. But, he said, my story aside, "To be concerned that my diet might kill me in twenty years or fifty years or whatever . . . we need to appreciate that we have become good at making food." To illustrate this point he told me a story about how his grandparents got married in the spring of '48. That following winter was horrific—snow so high that people ran out of food. "They couldn't go to the grocery store," he said, "they couldn't go to McDonald's or Dairy Queen." He said that today "our concern isn't that my diet may kill me this week, it's that my diet may kill me in fifty years." To him, this seems a luxury, and one that is only afforded to regular Americans by people like him, working their asses off out there on the fields in flyover country. He said, "When you talk about history, we're in the one percent of the one percent."

Perhaps. But that depends on how we think about our health. Americans are actually the sickest we've ever been. Sure, most of us won't starve tomorrow or even next week, and vaccines and antibiotics have made enormous advances. But the mere fact that we won't starve—or that we can pull into the drive-through at McDonald's or Dairy Queen to make sure we don't—doesn't mean that we aren't slowly killing ourselves with what we're eating.

The stats are, frankly, terrifying: America has an obesity epidemic of epic proportions. We have the highest prevalence of diabetes in the developed world. We have one of the highest heart disease rates, and heart disease is our leading cause of death. We are in the middle of a cancer epidemic of epic proportions—one in every two men, one in every three women, not to mention children, are getting cancer. And while we're talking about inflammatory disease, let's consider allergies and autoimmune diseases for a second: currently 55 percent of American adults are deemed "allergic"—in other words, they test positive for food, skin, or inhaled allergens. This number doesn't account for the millions of people for whom testing shows nothing, as allergy testing is an inexact science. The National Health Interview Survey recently found, for instance, that since 1997 the number of children with food allergies has jumped by 50 percent, and those with skin allergies by 69 percent (and the increase isn't merely a by-product of better reporting by parents, experts say). As for autoimmune diseases like celiac, Lupus, type 1 diabetes, and eczema, it's estimated that more than 20 percent of Americans have diagnosed autoimmune disorders— to say nothing for those who live undiagnosed for years because most autoimmune diseases can take anywhere from eight to twelve years to diagnose. Celiac disease, an autoimmune condition characterized by an inability to digest gluten, is one of the hardest autoimmune disorders to diagnose—it takes an average of twelve years for most people to be diagnosed. It's also one of the fastest growing autoimmune diseases out there—currently 1 in 133 Americans is diagnosed with celiac—excluding those who are gluten sensitive or just not yet diagnosed. Some researchers have begun to trace this alarming celiac trend to GMO wheat, others to the use of glyphosate, or Roundup, which some farmers spray on wheat when it's drying down just before harvest. And, if none of the above yet warrants our attention, the *New England Journal of Medicine* released a much-publicized study in 2005 that stated that my children—and yours, if you have young ones right now—will live shorter lives than you and I will because disease rates in this country are so high. That's just not how it should be.[18]

By now, though, the back of Zach's tractor was full of cleaned, golden GMO soybeans and it seemed like it would be counterproductive to lecture him on my concerns for our global health. Besides, like with everything, there are arguments to be made on both sides of the issue. So, while his brother continued up and down the rows in the combine, Zach and I took a final trip to the eighteen-wheeler sitting and waiting along the side of the road. Zach pulled his tractor with its big grain bin up to the side of the truck and pushed some buttons. Like magic, the beans were sucked up a shoot and deposited into the back of the truck. We were able to watch the whole thing from inside the tractor on a screen. The wind stole some beans, but the majority made their way into the truck. I asked Zach if it killed him to see even a few of his beans not make it into the truck and his final tally for the day. He said "a little" but that it was such a small amount, in comparison to what he's producing, that it didn't bother him much. Abundance, it was true, seemed to surround us.

As I got down from his tractor, I thanked Zach for his time and kindness. Then, as he turned to go back to work and as I strapped myself into my Bug, I found myself thinking about the excess that farmers like Zach have become accustomed to, thanks to the Ogallala Aquifer and a farm economy that depends on government subsidies to keep going.[19] I was wondering whether people are actually better off than his grandparents were in that winter of '48 and '49, or if our

---

[18] And don't we parents have enough to freak out about with ice caps melting and disease-carrying mosquitoes and ISIS?

[19] According to Michael Pollan in *The Omnivore's Dilemma*, industrial—subsidized—corn is called by some farmers, "in disgust, a welfare queen." Zach says he understands this derogatory moniker because "there are more [government subsidy] payments to corn production

dependence on industrialized food might actually make our lives harder when a crisis hits. Not to mention the huge amount of petroleum that is used on each farm in the form of fossil fuels—to both make the pesticides and to run the machinery. Michael Pollan writes in the *The Omnivore's Dilemma* that "every bushel of industrial corn requires the equivalent of between a quarter and a third of a gallon of oil to grow it—or around fifty gallons of oil per acre of corn." Another way to say this is that around 20 percent of American's fuel goes to growing, packaging, and shipping these GMO crops. Pile onto that figure the fact that a third to a half of our food is thrown out, and that means that a lot of prairie and forest have been razed in order to make food we aren't even using. Think of the climate-changing energy going into making biodiesel, animal feed, plastics, and chemicals while still such a large percentage of the people on the planet (over half) is scrambling to eat enough to survive, even as we throw away close to half our food.

As I pointed my car east, I wondered what it would take to bring this part of the country back to something smaller, something more sustainable, something safer for both the environment and the people who inhabit it. Yet, at the same time, still keep farmers like Zach on the fields, supporting them as they attempt to feed the masses, which is one of the most honorable jobs that exists. Driving across that enormous, flat, cultivated land of the plains, the sky spread open and full of possibility above me, I was sad to realize that there may be no easy answer.

---

than to anything else. It's a staple food—or staple feed—for our food system and it's important for our security that supply stay as uninterrupted as possible."

chapter 4

As a female writer who was attacked by the pro-GMO camp after my piece came out in *Elle,* I felt a certain vulnerability when going on a road trip by myself to ask questions about Big Ag. Maybe I've just seen too many movies. Or maybe I suffered too many bad jokes from friends in the weeks leading up to this trip about going missing. Or maybe I'd taken my editor, Kerri, to heart, when, the day after she bought this book, she asked me, "Aren't you scared to go do this?" Well, not until you said that, I wasn't! In August, my friend Genevieve had told me that I was "badass" for taking on this book. "I'm not badass," I told her, anxiety starting to burble like acid reflux in the back of my throat. "Flinty, maybe. But getting less badass by the second, the more we discuss it!" So all this is to say that when I wondered whether Zach had lied to me about the location of his field, I felt exposed—and lost—on a dusty road in the middle of nowhere. And now, having left the safety of his tanklike tractor and his warm, personable, and safe presence, as I was driving across the expanse of Nebraska, a low thrum of palpable uneasiness hung tight and close.

During my reporting over the past two years, I had heard many hair-raising stories about the big biotech companies' bullying tactics. Not to mention the numerous scientists and doctors who told me that they would only talk to me off the record for fear of compromising their careers, if not their safety. Those stories had gotten under my skin. As I drove, there were three conversations in particular that I was replaying in my mind, my hands gripping the steering wheel.

Unsettling Conversation #1 with a Scientist Named Simon Hogan

Simon and I first connected in June 2012, when I flew out to Cincinnati to talk to some doctors about the allergy and autoimmune epidemic and whether GMOs could be partly to blame. He was one of many in a jam-packed day of interviews, which had been set up by Dr. Marc Rothenberg, who runs the Cincinnati Center for Eosinophilic Disorders. I arrived at Simon's office later than planned and he had somewhere else he needed to be, so we dove in immediately, sitting across from each other at his desk piled with books, medical journals, and stacks and stacks of papers. He has big, round blue eyes, short blond to gray hair, the build of a rugby player, and the confidence of good looks. He is understated, affable, articulate, and matter-of-fact.

Seven years before, while still living in his native country of Australia, Simon had coauthored a famous (or infamous, depending on whom you talked to) study on genetically modified peas, which had been engineered to contain a bit of protein from a bean. The peas in question were being developed for sub-Saharan Africa where there is a big problem with bean weevils, an old-world bruchid beetle that looks like this:

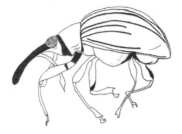

Interestingly enough, the DNA from the bean would act as a natural insecticide for the peas, keeping them safe from weevils. However, Simon's study, which was published in the *Journal of Agricultural and Food Chemistry* in 2005, indicated that the GMO peas triggered immune responses in mice when a sample of the peas was inserted into their lungs. The study became a lightning rod; Simon was both lauded and pilloried by the detractors and advocates of GMOs. *Nature Biotechnology News* magazine called his study "mush," and anti-GMO advocates called it "proof." To date, however, over a decade later, this is still the only sound study out there I know of that indicates a possible danger with GMOs. And it's a thorn in the side of the pro-GMO camp, because they've had a hell of a hard time discrediting it. And that has a lot to do with Simon, frankly, because he actually *is* badass. (Even pro-GMOers who hated his study so much it made them furious told me over and over that "Simon Hogan is an excellent scientist," which is just not praise these guys dole out super easily.)

I had read Simon's study prior to my trip but had not connected the name to the work until I sat down with him. I also didn't know anything about the controversy. A friend—also a writer—had told me that he thinks it's better to be totally ignorant as a writer because if you don't know anything, you get better stuff. In the early part of the research for this book, I was certainly testing this theory. At any rate, Simon didn't spend any time telling me about the controversy, so I was in the dark. Instead he took pains to tell me that his pea study proved nothing except that something in the modified peas "perturbed" the immune systems of mice.

He then alluded, albeit ever so cautiously, to the difficulty he had faced when the study was published. He said he'd honestly hoped to do more follow-up testing, but "we were unable to extend the study and really get down to the nuts and bolts of what was going on." Later, he gave me a tiny bit more, mentioning that it was "disappointing" that he couldn't do more follow-up studies. My interest piqued at that and I asked, "You lost funding?" He retreated. "No, no. There were a multitude of reasons—just time, place, I moved to a different institution, it wasn't carried on and so forth." When I left Cincinnati, I kept going back to that conversation in my mind. Something about it had left me slightly dissatisfied. Like something was missing. But I couldn't put my finger on what or why.

Then, one hot mid-July night, as I was lying with the then three-year-old Marsden on his twin mattress placed on the floor in our old apartment in Portland, something clicked. I had been waiting for his breath to slow and deepen so that I would know he was asleep and I could steal, like a bandit, out of the room. And as I lay there, I found my mind catching like a scratched CD on that first meeting with Simon. I was wondering why he would abandon an important study so quickly. If this is the only study out there that raises critical questions about GMOs and immunity, didn't he want to keep going on it? Was there something he just wasn't telling me? After finally slipping out of Marsy's room, I got in touch with Simon via email, telling him I had a few more questions as follow-up to our initial meeting. He agreed to talk on the phone over the weekend, when he would be away from the office on vacation.

It turned out that I, too, was taking a long weekend with Dan, Marsden, and my mother at a fishing camp on a lake in northern Maine. Every July we make the long trek to the Canadian border, our car carefully packed to the gills with field guides and food from Portland, where we know our farmers. And then we spend a few days reading, eating, catch-and-release fishing, and taking the motorboat out to zoom around the lake and visit small, sandy islands where we swim in the warm water. At night, we make feasts and laugh and play cards. It's a special summer ritual, even though every year when it arrives, it seems to have come too early and feels like too huge a push to get there. Once we pull up to the cabin, however, and see my mom's Subaru parked outside, the pine needles soft underfoot and the lake wide and shimmery black in front of us, we know we are free and unencumbered from our usual lives, and we are so grateful.

On the day Simon and I were supposed to talk, after a day of boating and swimming, Dan, Marsy, and I motored back to our cabin and decided to cook up a meal of roasted chicken, homemade potato chips, and coleslaw. Just as dinner was ready, unfortunately, it was time for me to get on the phone. Telling my family not to wait, I stole away to a small shed deemed "the office" for vacationers at the camp. I sat at a big desk, a fish chart tacked up on the wall in front of me that delineated the differences between brown trout, landlocked salmon, and white and yellow perch. Through a screen window, I could smell the chicken skin and hot, homemade potato chips in our cabin just a few hundred feet away, and I could hear my family laughing. This time, Simon seemed more comfortable and less guarded. We chatted easily about this and that, making small talk, until I brought up his pea study again. I told him I didn't feel like I'd really understood what might have happened after it was published. He was quiet for a moment. And then he began to open up.

He told me that when he first started studying the possible dangers GMOs might present if fed to animals (studies from which we might be able to subsequently extrapolate to human beings), he was doing it just out of curiosity; he said he had nothing to prove. He had funding from an Australian government agency—independent from the influence of industry, he pointed out—and he was just trying to answer some basic questions about the immune system, like, was the immune system sensitive enough that it would react to a GMO? When the study started to show some alarming results, he realized he needed to check everything about it very carefully to make sure nothing was done incorrectly. When he got the same results a second time, he tried to get it published, but no one would take it. "That was weird," he said, "because it was a really well-executed study." Then, finally, the *Journal of Agricultural and Food Chemistry* agreed to publish. He gave it a "sneaky" title, he told me, one that shouldn't have piqued any industry interest, calling it "Transgenic Expression of Bean Alpha Amylase Inhibitor in Peas Results in Altered Structure and Immunogenicity." He took pains, he told me, not to say anything in the title or study that even related to the acronym "GMO." But as soon as the study hit the press, all hell broke loose; before he knew it, the plug was pulled and he didn't have funding to do any follow-up studies.

"What happened then?" I asked.

"You know exactly what happened," he snapped.

"I actually don't," I admitted.

"I quickly recognized that if I continued the work I was doing, there would be—let's put it this way—'a lack of opportunity,' so I didn't feel I wanted to prove the point."

"In other words," I asked, "if you fought this, you wouldn't have a job?"

"Right. It was David and Goliath, really. And I thought, 'I don't need to go down that path.'"

"So you've got this huge discovery that's published in a small journal. The biotech industry gets wind of it and cracks down and you didn't fight back. Do I have that right?"

"Yes."

The line was quiet. I understood now why he'd been oblique on this subject when we first met. And I also now understood why, when the study was canceled, he'd created a silent vortex around it. There were real implications to his career. Eventually, he told me, he just dropped the subject altogether and moved to the United States. He now studies asthma and anaphylaxis in Cincinnati. "I just didn't want that to be the hill that I die on," he said. However, what Simon discovered with those peas was powerful enough that the peas never went to Africa. And this outcome, it turned out, still really irked some proponents of GMOs, so much so that even asking about his study was sure to draw fire.[1]

When I got back to our cabin, my mother was cleaning up and Dan was upstairs putting Marsy to bed. As I quickly scarfed down the food they'd left for me, I told my mother a little bit about my call with Simon. She stopped doing dishes and listened, drying her hands on her apron (which she always brings with her, even to our house). Then, unhelpfully, she told me she didn't want to hear any more, that it was scaring her and she was thinking of the movie *Silkwood*. "Fabulous, Mom," I said. "I didn't really need to sleep tonight, thanks. And plus, I was hoping for more like Julia Roberts in *Erin Brockovich*."

Stressy Story #2 Rattling Around in My Head

Tyrone Hayes, the UC Berkeley professor who has made his life's work studying atrazine, had told me that when his work on Syngenta's chemical started to show not only gender malformations but also *confusions* in frogs, he told Syngenta what he was finding and the company was not pleased. First they tried to silence him by saying he couldn't publish his work. Then, when he wouldn't back down, they went after him, discrediting his work with targeted efforts. According to a 2014 *New Yorker* piece that quoted an internal email from the company, Syngenta tried to "'purchase Tyrone Hayes as a search word on the Internet, so that anytime someone searches for Tyrone's material, the first thing they see is our material.' . . . (Searching online for 'Tyrone Hayes' now brings up an advertisement that says 'Tyrone Hayes Not Credible.')" The company went so far as to assassinate his character by

---

[1] UNL's Rick Goodman told me that the peas were eventually "ravaged by rodents" and no one could study them further.

suggesting in internal documents as well as in Internet attack campaigns that he was mentally unstable. The company also reportedly had representatives follow him to speaking engagements where the representatives would loiter menacingly, taking notes, later accosting him with foul epithets and talking to him in a manner that Tyrone felt was intended to threaten him. We will get more into his story in the last section of this book, when I go to California and meet him. But what stood out for me as I was driving across Nebraska was a story he'd told me about how the most physically vulnerable he'd felt was when he was out in the field. "I can tell you," he said, "I used to work at a little pond in Wyoming where we were doing a lot of research on atrazine in the wild. The way that you'd get there was you'd fly into Laramie . . . and it was a couple hours' drive. And the rental car place—it was a tiny airport, just a little one room—had only like three cars. And when I would drive to this spot, which is in the middle of nowhere in Wyoming, I would always get pulled over: you know, black guy driving through the middle of Wyoming—the cops always pull you over. And it occurred to me, I thought, all Syngenta would have to do was fly there, rent a car, stash some drugs in it, and I get pulled over and go to jail. So things like that. I actually stopped using that rental car place. . . . I started flying into Denver and driving five hours, you know, where I had more options. . . . [But] it did cross my mind that I could see them making somebody [like a farmer] angry who then might do violence against me." Though I'm not black and it was unlikely I would be pulled over because of my skin color, I, too, felt vulnerable as a woman trafficking in the still mostly male-dominated worlds of farming, science, and medicine.

And Tyrone's story wasn't the only thing that had set me on edge. By the time I was driving across Nebraska, I'd had more of those "off the record" phone calls than I could count and there had been a three-ring circus after the *Elle* piece went viral when some of the people I'd interviewed had recanted and stated they hadn't said the things they'd said about GMOs (despite the fact that all of the interviews were taped, transcribed, and then fact-checked by a professional fact-checker). And there was the anger, too, which had come at me in some unexpected ways.

#3: Angry Phone Call that Jangled Me Up

"Are you calling me a whore?" Bruce Chassy, a retired university scientist whose pro-GMO lobbying efforts were (or are) funded, perhaps indirectly, by Monsanto, bellowed into the phone. He was speaking to me from his home, nestled high in the mountains of Idaho.

"No, no," I said, shocked. "I wouldn't use that word. . . ." I was scrambling. The *Annie Hall*–type subtitles moving across the screen went like this: "Wow. Extreme reaction. I really pissed him off. How can I recover this? Fuck."

He went on, outraged. Soon outrage boiled down to a low simmer of indignation. But he kept talking. And I kept listening.

Earlier that spring, after someone had told me that Bruce is a retired plant biologist from the University of Illinois who had recently become a "consultant for Monsanto,"[2] I'd emailed him. (Bruce also, along the way, got a Fulbright to go to Spain, did research for the National Institutes of Health, and is now a professor emeritus of Food Safety and Nutritional Sciences at the University of Illinois—in short, this guy is no slouch.) Bruce is helping Monsanto, he told me, essentially clean up their image, because, in his words, "I think they mishandled the public relations of GM crops terribly. [They had] an arrogance about how good their product was and a total lack of

---

[2] Bruce denies emphatically in long, discursive emails that he was a consultant for Monsanto, that he worked for them or received money from them. That may be technically true, but the grants he received from the University of Illinois or its Foundation appear to have been funded by Monsanto, and Bruce's travel expenses for his pro-GMO speaking engagements appear to have been sponsored or supported, if not paid for, by Monsanto. Bruce vigorously maintains that his scientific objectivity was not compromised in any way by his Monsanto-funded grants or his Monsanto-sponsored travel. Despite his protests, it's clear that Bruce has been used as a valuable resource for Monsanto and that he was compensated for his expertise.

understanding of the concern." He says he does this not for pay but because he believes in biotechnology and what it has to offer the planet.

When I finally got Bruce on the phone, it was sometime after dinner on a cool, damp spring evening. Dan was putting Marsden to bed and it was dark out. The maple tree outside my office window—where a red-eyed vireo was making a nest with strands of dried grass, dryer lint, bits of a wasps' nest, and some of Hopper's fur from when we brushed him outside—was fluttering its leaves gently in the evening breeze. Our house, one of a handful that comprised a small village center in the quintessential New England river town of New Gloucester, Maine, was a quaint clapboard-and-stone-foundation structure with big windows (and matching drafts) that belonged to a friend who had moved down south. He had offered his house to us after the ceiling had caved in in our Portland rental apartment due to a roof leak, making it uninhabitable. In a flurry we'd put all our things in storage and landed thirty minutes north of Portland, suddenly surrounded by farms, apple trees, and pumpkin fields. The house was both hilarious in its disrepair and also wonderfully charming in certain corners where the light came in pools, illuminating old wood floors and dark molding. We loved the big yard, the three enormous sugar maples, and the snake family that lived in the old barn foundation. In March, we tapped the maples and made our own syrup, and in the spring we were ecstatic to behold each wave of blooming crocuses, daffodils, tulips, and irises.

BRUCE IS THE KIND OF GUY who jumps full throttle into a conversation, as if you've been talking for hours already, leaving little dead space, and even less space for questions. His tone isn't exactly friendly, either. Underneath the information he pelts you with is a seething quality, which is hard not to notice. First, he wanted to start with some "historical background," which he felt I needed (and I heartily agreed). According to Bruce, back when plant genetic engineering looked like it was going to be possible, the industry went to the White House (Bush Sr.) and said it might be "worthwhile to look at this new technology to see whether it would need to be regulated or not." He said that after some careful review, "The National Academy of Sciences concluded that genetic engineering was rapid, simple, and precise . . ." and therefore needed little oversight. "From a science perspective," he said, "we shouldn't even have had to talk about this." A debate wasn't necessary and the public didn't really need to be involved. So the government said, "Go for it!" Furthermore, he went on, for any GMO on the market, "[They've] probably been working on it for ten years in the lab . . ." and "from development to approval is probably ten to fifteen years." So there was ample time for the company to find any problems.

He went on to elucidate for me that any testing that's done on a GMO is done by the company themselves, never by the FDA, EPA, or USDA. This was news to me. But he said this was a good thing because it's actually safer when the developer, like Monsanto or Dow or whoever is making the product, "produces their data"—testing it for environmental and health risks from start to finish. The Feds, he told me, don't have the "facility or the scientists" to test it. When I asked him if he believes that companies are indeed transparent with their data on products they stand to make money from, or if it's really in their best interest to be transparent, he retorted, "It is a crime to withhold data" and furthermore "all those tests are available and they [the USDA/FDA/EPA] can walk in at any time to ask to see the books. . . . They do that less than one percent of the time because they don't have the staff." What did he mean, the USDA or the FDA or the EPA just simply does not have the staff to evaluate the data from the companies developing GMOs? I asked.[3] He told me that for any given product, a company would have to back up "two tractor-trailer trucks" of data and "nobody would go

---

[3] In a February 2, 2015, *New Yorker* article about food-borne pathogens called "A Bug in the System," the author, Wil S. Hylton, describes the same situation: "The F.D.A. does not have a large army of inspectors for the products under its purview. Years can elapse between official inspections at a given food producer."

through it."[4] But the salient point, he said, the one Americans need to realize, is that "no company is misrepresenting what they've done."

Bruce started to get irritated, I realize in hindsight, when, for reasons I wasn't sure about, he took a one-eighty and veered our conversation toward the anti-GMO activist groups. He especially wanted to talk about the D.C.-based watchdog group called the Center for Food Safety, whom he dismisses as a special-interest group that is "wasting our time" while they "make a lot of money" scaring the public about GMOs. Furthermore, he said, the "people opposed to GM are cheats and liars."

"Well," I asked, "can you tell me how else the regular, food-buying American people might get the right information about GMOs—if not from these special-interest groups?"

He said, "Asking the public to make judgments on things they don't know anything about [makes no sense]. [This] is highly technical stuff and really hard to understand."[5] But shouldn't people be given information in a manner they can understand? I wanted to know. Can't it be broken down so that regular parents—like me—can make an informed decision on the subject? Bruce gave a tight, annoyed chuckle. Ultimately, he said, it comes down to this: "Trust is the issue." When modified plants and animals are patented, he said, you achieve transparency. Therefore, the public should just trust the companies that have created them.

"Because they have patented the product?" I asked.

He was getting annoyed by my ignorance. He sighed. "People at the companies are the most ethical people I know," he went on. "I have less respect for university scientists than I do for industry scientists. [It's] much more important for a company scientist to be more honest than

---

[4] An added wrinkle to this: If you are searching through the Freedom of Information Act for data that has been done by a company but not reviewed or saved by the EPA, USDA, or FDA, it would not turn up in your search.

[5] University of Nebraska–Lincoln scientist Rick Goodman echoed this sentiment when he told me that "if you don't do science and don't read about science," then it's hard to exercise good, "sound judgment" with regard to any information about GMOs in the news.

a university scientist."[6] This was an odd thing to say, given he'd spent much of his own career as a university scientist. But I said "Okay" and let it drop. I didn't want to push it. We talked a little more but it didn't feel like we were getting any further, as he was kind of done with me. So I said thank you and we hung up.

I made my way downstairs to the dark kitchen at the back of the old New Gloucester house. Dan was sweeping the floor; the dishes were drying in the rack. What kind of a silly wild-goose chase was I on, anyway? If it was true that the companies were doing copious amounts of testing of their products—even though the public couldn't see any of those tests—it didn't mean they hadn't happened, right? I was suddenly inspired by Bruce's exasperated confidence, all fired up about all those hysterical watchdog groups out there screaming about the bogeyman in order to make money. "Dan," I said, "this guy I just talked to was so convincing, so assured about GMOs and their safety, I've started to really wonder . . ." "That's your story," said Dan, "the gray area, the people who are making sense on both sides, the nuance in the middle." "I suppose," I said, my mind whirling. But as I stood there, watching Dan push a small pile of dirt and dinner detritus into the dustpan with the end of the broom, I found myself going back through the conversation with Bruce. Frozen in thought while Dan cleaned, I was wondering what Bruce gained from his position, because everyone stands to gain something, I figure—even this writer—from the stance they take. Emboldened, I decided to call him back and ask him, point-blank, "What exactly is in it for you, working with Monsanto? Do you get a paycheck? Is your background in science ever compromised? How do I trust what you're telling me about the ethical actions of the people at Monsanto?"[7]

---

[6] Bruce later backpedaled on this statement, saying he believes "everyone deserves equal respect."

[7] It's not like there wasn't a precedent for my line of questions: companies like ExxonMobil and Peabody Energy were exposed for ignoring their own scientists and mounting pricey PR campaigns (replete with real scientists peddling their message) to convince the public, the government, and their own investors that climate change was a myth.

There was a second of silence and then the onslaught began: "I resent the implication that I'd lie and cheat and whore for the job. You can't buy people . . . we're university scientists!"[8]

Hoping to change the subject, I quickly asked Bruce if he was interested in talking about Simon Hogan's study, which was becoming a bellwether of sorts for those I was talking to. I was learning that it helped me root out where an interviewee's ideology on GMOs lay. Not that Bruce's ideology was unclear at this point, but I was still hungry for more information from either side that could leave me with a clear understanding I could parlay into a strong thesis statement: GMOs are bad or GMOs are okay. I felt open to inconvenient truths, even if they were just inconvenient to myself. I still wanted to vet out whether I could really pin my own health recovery on the lack of GMOs in my diet.

Bruce huffed some more but did not hang up and, though grumbly and clearly put off, he dismissed Simon's study by saying, "It was one study and most of the allergists I know were unconvinced. It was a false positive in an inappropriate study. . . . The people who used that study are not interested in science and not interested in truth." Was there any merit at all to the study? I asked. He sighed. "The pea proves

---

[8] In late 2015, the *New York Times* ran the aforementioned piece by Eric Lipton that named Bruce Chassy as one of two scientists (another was Kevin Folta, at the University of Florida) who was given an unrestricted grant of an undisclosed amount of money by Monsanto (Bruce denies the grant came directly from Monsanto) to use his mantle of "the scientist" while doing "outreach" on the ground for the company. Bruce's chief task, in 2011, it appears, was to exert pressure on the EPA to, according to the *Times*, "abandon its proposal to tighten the regulation of pesticides used on insect-resistant seeds." The Monsanto exec Eric Sachs wrote to Bruce, "It could be important to send a clear message that the scientific community is very serious about driving toward more rational, justifiable, and codified regulatory requirements that enable innovation and product development for the public good." Bruce succeeded; the EPA dropped its proposal. And clearly Bruce expected to be compensated for this work when he wrote to Sachs's assistant wondering where his check was: "A letter should be included that says the enclosed check is an unrestricted gift payable to the University of Illinois Foundation in support of the biotechnology outreach and education activities of Bruce M. Chassy." This was especially interesting to me to learn after the scientist Ignacio Chapela (see Part 3 of this book) had told me that "science is now religion" in America—instead of turning to God, we are turning to science, which he feels gives scientists an undue amount of authority and power. Others I interviewed for this book claimed that the "corporation" in America had become bigger than God, religion, or anything else. It occurred to me, reading this *Times* piece, that the marriage of science and the corporation might be the most powerful and persuasive union in our country.

that GM crops could be allergenic. Means that that particular crop was allergenic." Bingo. But he went on: "It was a lousy experiment. The animal model system had never been used [before] and wasn't accepted and it wasn't truly a food allergy, it was actually a respiratory allergy. And the scientific community was not willing to accept that conclusion." He told me about a redo of the study in Europe where they could not replicate Hogan's results.[9] What did this prove? I wondered. "The pea is a dead issue. The science is settled. . . . To the media, one paper is news. To the scientific community, one paper is nothing."

It was only later that the irony of what he said about being a university scientist occurred to me. And it was really only ironic when viewed from the safety of home, with Hopper there to protect me (we always said, to quote poet Elizabeth Bishop, that Hop was "safe as houses"). Just like when I looked up Bruce on Facebook and saw an image of a bearded guy holding a guitar and sitting in front of an impressive backdrop of shimmering mountains—distance, in this case, was everything.

But here I was, six months later, for better or for worse, right in the middle of GMO country, driving myself deeper into the story and the controversy. If off-the-record conversations, some unpleasant

---

[9] I did speak with the scientist, Michelle Epstein, who conducted the study that tried to replicate Simon's study. She was soft-spoken, thoughtful, and extremely open-minded. She told me, "In our hands [the mice] had no response." Her conclusion is that the animal models Simon used must have been different somehow. What she came down to, she told me, was that the study should be done more places "with different mice" because her experience shows her that "the animal model is clearly not predictive for people." More studies, she said, would start to get us more answers. As an aside, she said, in regard to GMOs, "I just hope they're safe because they're sure out there." She said, "I have a high regard for Hogan. He does excellent work." But, she said, her differing results still trouble her. "This is something I have dreams about," she said. (And, when I went back to Simon to tell him about my conversation with Epstein, he took some time to read through her study. He then told me, essentially, that her study "doesn't prove anything by the looks of it," and that "they're just muddying the waters." He broke it down for me this way: "All that they're saying is that 'because we saw response in *all* proteins, then that doesn't mean that the transgenic [GMO] ones are more allergenic.'" I asked him what this meant in regular language and he said, essentially, that "they can't disprove [my] paper, but they are casting doubts on it." At the end of the day, he said, "I could sit down for four days and provide a thousand explanations for the data they got. . . ." But, he said, "I'm at peace with my study and we performed it with the necessary scientific rigor.")

phone calls, and a handful of scary anecdotes had put me over the edge back home in Maine, why in the world had I stupidly gotten on a plane to ask for more? Should I really dance in the eye of this hurricane? I wondered. To keep going—rather than turn my car around and just head back to Denver, which seemed like a really nice town right about now—I had to put my head down and suspend all thought. I tuned the iPod to Ryan Adams and let him carry me for the next eighty-something miles.

chapter 5

When I began seeing signs for Lincoln, Nebraska, I decided to call Richard Goodman, the former Monsanto researcher, seed scientist, and project manager now at the University of Nebraska–Lincoln. I had first connected with Rick back in August 2012 and had stayed in touch with him throughout the writing of my *Elle* piece. I remembered my first conversation with him as I was driving: it was hot and muggy at home in Portland and I had stacks of notebooks and notes on loose pieces of paper piled all around me with a magazine deadline looming. Needing to work somewhere quiet, I was at our friends Dan and Joan Amory's house while they were out at their summer place on North Haven. I had taken over the glass dining table in their sunroom, a plush pink carpet under my bare feet. Sitting in their house, my chaos surrounding me, I was starting to feel that I didn't have any idea how to compile all the disparate pieces of information I was getting. Every so often, I would seek refuge from the disorder by looking out the window at Joan's garden, a secret masterpiece of trees, flowers, wooden benches, and tempting hiding places. It occurred to me as I was sitting there that someone had told me about a former Monsanto employee who had endless energy for the subject of GMOs. I needed "endless energy" right then. So I picked up my cell phone. On the second ring, Rick picked up: "Rick Goodman speaking."

Rick told me that he'd grown up in Spokane, Washington. He went to college at Eastern Washington University, where he received a BS, then on to Ohio State University, where he received a PhD in dairy science, and finally to Cornell, where he did a postdoc in immunology. He first began working for Monsanto in 1997. By then, this was years after the discovery in the 1980s that you could move DNA from one species—a bacterium or a fish, for example—and shoot it from a gun into a plant. What drew him to biotechnology, he told me, was the ability to harness "the potential to make products that are more successful." When I hesitated at the idea that a person in the lab could somehow "make" plants more successfully than ten thousand years of farmers who have known how to select for genetic strengths, cross-breed, graft, or hybridize within species, while paying attention to the needs of crops in their environments, Rick told me that "when you make a GM plant, you have to do years of testing [in the lab and then the greenhouse] and work with farmers." For him, this indicated that farmers were still in the mix, and therefore it wasn't like some crazy scientists were out there "under cover of darkness" making dangerous things in labs. Also, he told me, the makers of GMOs are doing this *for* farmers.

With farmers and the history of the arid Great Plains in mind, while at Monsanto, Rick's "baby" was a GMO wheat that he helped develop in the early 2000s to be pest- and drought-resistant. His GMO wheat never went to market, however, because the Europeans and the Japanese proclaimed that they would not buy it—and they still won't—effectively killing the project. Shortly thereafter, Rick left Monsanto. According to him, it had nothing to do with the failed wheat (which is still a sore subject) but everything to do with a boss who started to ride him in a manner he didn't like.

Today, Rick runs the allergy database out of Lincoln. This is the database used worldwide to determine what proteins are considered allergens; it contains no proteins that are inserted into or generated from GMO foods—in other words, it cannot be used to determine whether GMO foods could, perhaps, be increasing allergenicity. The database is funded primarily by the six major biotech companies: Dow, DuPont, Monsanto, Syngenta, BASF, and Bayer. "Where are you going to get the money otherwise?" Rick prodded me—asking what is really the million-dollar question in science today, as biotech companies give more generously than any other industry to the science departments of most colleges and universities in America. He punctuated this thought by saying, "It depends on the eye of the beholder whether there's a conflict."

Currently, the only way for a doctor, or a scientist, or even the FDA to ascertain whether a pesticide bred into GMO crops (and its resultant proteins) could possibly disrupt the immune system, or cause an allergy, is to use Rick's database. If they don't find it on that database (which they won't), then, if they're really high-tech, they need to make a comparison between the amino acid sequence of a known allergen—like peanuts, wheat, or milk—to the amino acid sequence of the protein being inserted into the host plant (so they will compare, for instance, the sequence of Bt to the sequence of walnuts). If there is a DNA match to a known allergen, then allergenicity can be established. But you still won't find it on the database because usually such a product—one that does have an amino acid sequence similar to a known allergen—is never allowed to go to market, so therefore the logic goes that it need not be recorded on the database.

There are many scientists who say this is a system that makes no sense—that it doesn't allow us to know anything about the products we are modifying except that they don't contain a milk- or peanut-like allergen.[1] Simon Hogan said, "Some of the questions that are being

---

[1] There is a theory floating around that GMO corn contains some peanut genes to enhance growth. I was never able to verify this, though I did find quite a bit of "anecdotal" commentary on the Internet from people who are peanut allergic and claim to be allergic to GMO corn. I wasn't sure what to make of this information one way or the other, since it seemed unlikely to me that peanut anything would be used by the makers of GM because of the risk.

asked aren't relevant; 'the amino acid sequence doesn't match a known allergen'—not a relevant question! It may not have a homologous sequence [but would still be an allergen]." At any rate, Rick is a fierce, loyal, and enthusiastic defender of his list—the allergen database—and of biotechnology in general. He believes the list makes perfect sense and the way it works is entirely efficient. He bristles when it's suggested that there might be more questions to ask.

In this same vein, Rick has been known to criticize opinions on GMOs that he disagrees with, and he brings an unrestricted vigor to the pursuit. He is, frankly, a bit like a homing missile, somehow finding anything that hits the airwaves—or Internet—that is anti-GMO. It was in this way that he gained some international attention when he denounced a 2012 study done by a French scientist by the name of Gilles-Eric Séralini that posited that Monsanto's GMO (MON863) corn, when fed to rats, left them with enormous, cancerous tumors. Séralini fed the rats the corn for two years—a huge chunk of their estimated life span, which is usually between two and a half and three and a half years. Monsanto, on the other hand, has done feeding trials with their GMO foods for only ninety days; they claim this is enough time to establish risk.

The Séralini study was criticized by many as having some flaws—the primary flaw being that the kind of rats used, the Sprague Dawley, tend, apparently, to get tumors as they age into their twilight years of two or three, regardless of feed. And Goodman made the amusing and pointed comment that using those rats for that long was like using a ninety-year-old man to study cancer outcomes. Touché! But, to be fair, Séralini's was the first study that seemed to make a convincing—and understandable-to-the-mainstream (the photos alone of the rats with enormous tumors were electrifying!)—link between cancer and

---

I asked Rick to clarify whether peanut genes would ever be used in GM corn or soy. He said he didn't know of any but that it was possible. Even if they were used, he said, "Remember that 99.5 percent (or more) of the peanut genes do not encode an allergen and would be perfectly safe for peanut-allergic subjects." But Simon Hogan told me he thought it was very unlikely. He wrote in an email to me: "There is just so much baggage that comes with this concept that it would probably be the very last option." I guess the way I come down on this is that anything is possible and we just don't know.

GMO corn. It's notable, also, that the National Toxicology Program in the United States uses the same rat for studying carcinogens and has found that this kind of rat develops tumors at about the same rate as most people do in industrialized nations. Where that leaves us with Séralini's study, I'm not sure, but it doesn't seem to obviate it. To date, there hasn't been a second study that I know of that feeds rats organic feed and compares the two.

Outraged by Séralini's study, Rick took it upon himself to write to the editor of the journal *Food and Chemical Toxicology* and decry their publication of a bogus study. Whether he then began pressuring *Food and Chemical Toxicology* to rescind their publication is up for debate; he says he did not, others say he did. At any rate, he did suddenly find a place on the editorial board of the journal. (He has since resigned.) And the study was then retracted and the press reported that the study had been widely discredited. (It was republished in *Environmental Sciences Europe* in June 2014.) The uproar over Séralini's study was remarkable in two respects: the study itself was sensationalistic and scary; and the controversy was so huge that it made it so that no one who wanted real answers (like a mom shopping at the grocery store) knew what the hell to think. And Rick seemed to be at the epicenter of the hoopla.

The scientist Belinda Martineau, who was on the California-based team that developed the first GMO food—a tomato called the Flavr Savr, which was bred to not go soft as it sat on supermarket shelves— told me that in the midst of the Séralini craziness, she emailed some scientists she knew at Monsanto and said, "'Look . . . They've outlined the experiment for you. All you guys have to do is repeat that experiment and put this thing to rest one way or the other.' They won't do it. And like I say, I think the FDA should make them do it. The FDA sends them a letter saying, 'We accept your conclusion that this is as safe as any other corn product. But we remind you that'—you can go on the FDA website and see these letters—'we remind you that it's your responsibility, Monsanto, to make sure that what you're selling is safe and wholesome' and whatnot. So, you know, here there's a question about whether it's safe and wholesome, and they should have to repeat that study." The American scientist Michelle Epstein, who lives in Europe (and whom I interviewed about Simon Hogan's pea study), told me that the EU, at least, intends to repeat the study. "The EU feels it's necessary to spend a lot of money to figure out whether there's an ounce of truth in this," she said.[2] She seemed to think this was an incredible waste of time—and that, essentially, Séralini's study, which, she said, "was poorly done," was robbing money from more important scientific projects that needed funding.

Séralini notwithstanding, although Rick and I had gotten along just fine for almost a year's worth of conversations—and I'd really enjoyed many of our chats because he is so thorough, suffers questions with aplomb, and will go to great lengths to make sure one understands a concept—he took issue with my piece in *Elle*. He believed it would play into the hands of the anti-GMO people and that for all the time he had spent with me, he had been reduced to tiny sound bites that didn't cover every angle of the science of GMOs. (He was right about this; it's really, really hard to write about science in the same amount of detail as a scientist, who knows the terrain, can explain science, and can make sure we understand every deviance and possibility.) Subsequently, Rick began to make some noise about my piece after it was published. First with a deluge of emails to me:

"What drives you?"

"What do you eat?"

"My first thought was to invite you to come to Lincoln and spend one or two days learning more about food safety. . . . You don't seem to listen regarding the ability of this technology to ensure food security for those who need it most, and with fewer chemicals, fewer risks,

---

[2] I was not able to verify with another source that the EU is engaged in such trials. But I did find that the EFSA—the European Food Safety Authority—is now recommending feeding trials that span two years, as opposed to the ninety days recommended here in the United States and thought to be enough time by industry.

greater safety. You don't seem to listen to the scientists who have done the work. Who understand food safety testing and have a background to be able to explain the safety evaluation limitations and process. I was looking forward to a well-written balanced piece." (Ouch!) And that wasn't all. Soon a journalist by the name of Jon Entine went after me with Rick as his source. (Entine was reported by *Mother Jones* magazine to be a "hired gun" for Big Ag and, at one point, Entine listed Monsanto as a "select client" of his. Even so, Entine disputes the connection to Monsanto, saying he never "consulted or worked for the company." That may be technically true, as it appears that the money he made working for a public relations company, which had been hired by Monsanto, was paid to him by the PR company itself. But one has to wonder about his continued support of Monsanto when the *Chicago Tribune* publishes an article in fall 2015 that exposes, through emails obtained under the Freedom of Information Act by the nonprofit group U.S. Right to Know, that Entine's website, the Genetic Literacy Project, published a series of pro-GMO articles, which were prompted by the Monsanto executive Eric Sachs. Unsurprisingly, the articles— all written by scientists from highbrow institutions like Harvard and Cornell—smack of rigged science, no matter how much the authors themselves protest this assignation.) After a deluge of aggressive calls to my agent, Entine and *Slate*, the online magazine, went ahead with a piece that indicated that some of my sources—including Rick—had recanted their interviews. It was a peculiar time in my life. In many ways I had expected something like this, but even when you're expecting the worst, it's bizarre when it happens. Suddenly the team at *Elle* and I were sifting through interviews and checking their transcripts against the printed piece (which had been thoroughly fact-checked once before). The only thing we could figure had transpired was that the same fear I'd witnessed throughout my reporting had resurfaced, and some subjects must have felt pressured. About what and by whom, we didn't know. We guessed in the end that it would be easier for them to say they'd never said what they were recorded as having said than to face pro-GMO wrath. *Elle* went public with a letter that stood by my piece and Entine fired off a second article railing against their defense. The Internet blogosphere was in full-tilt spin, reacting to the drama.

Now, for some, this would have been incidence enough to steer clear of Rick. But as I was driving across Nebraska and on my way to Iowa, despite the hovering and perhaps ridiculous Karen Silkwood–cum–Julia Roberts concerns I harbored, a certain courage welled up in me. And, also, honestly, before his attacks in the wake of the *Elle* piece, he had given endless amounts of time to me on the phone, assiduously going detail by detail over everything I wanted to learn about GMOs. So, hoping for the best, I decided to call Rick and tell him I was in Nebraska and driving toward Lincoln. Did he have time to meet with me? He said he did—and he was actually warm and kind sounding, even eager to meet in person. We made a plan for me to come to his office building so that we could have tea outside a snack bar on the UNL campus called the Dairy Store.

When I pulled up, like a bad penny rolling back into his life, he was waiting for me with a white UNL mug full of tea. In person, Rick is more wiry and pale than I had imagined; his arms look like tightly wound rope, springing fully loaded out of his collared T-shirt. In his midsixties, he has a brown handlebar mustache and brown hair and there's a toughness to him, the aspect of, to borrow from Winston Churchill, a tough chicken with a tough neck.

We sat down and immediately started talking about agriculture—big versus small. This was clearly on my mind as I had just come from Zach's farm and had been witnessing Big Ag everywhere out the car window. It took only about five minutes before we were deeply engrossed once again, like no time had passed since our very first conversations two years earlier. Rick heartily believes that if we did away with Big Ag and went back to more localized, small-scale, and biodiverse farming, we'd never be able to grow enough food in and around Lincoln, Nebraska, to feed even the people living in the immediate vicinity, let alone the world. It's too cold and too dry, he says. I wondered, though, what the water output would be to grow a variety of vegetables on the same land—and some, indeed, in greenhouses as we've gotten very good at doing in my home state of Maine—and if it would be anything comparable to the water needed for large industrial crops like corn, which is widely understood to be the biggest water hog in farming. He was unmoved by this idea and didn't feel that it would achieve the larger goal, which, he states, is to combat worldwide hunger. I asked, But what if we took that corn and used it—or the land it's on—to just feed the people in a hundred-mile radius, making the goal smaller and more localized? Wouldn't that be more efficient? He gave me a withering look, like that wasn't really the point and that he recognized, now, the same annoying questions he'd suffered from me before.

I told him that I was thinking about Michael Pollan's description, in *The Omnivore's Dilemma*, of our corn system: "So the mountain [of corn] grows, from four billion bushels in 1970 to ten billion bushels today. Moving that mountain of cheap corn—finding the people and animals to consume it, the cars to burn it, the new products to absorb it, and the nations to import it—has become the principal task of the industrial food system, since the supply of corn vastly exceeds the demand." The name Michael Pollan did little to help me; Rick has little love for Pollan, it turns out.

As a last-ditch effort to try to get Rick to consider my position on small-scale agriculture, I reached for another big name in the book world (sure to impress him) and summarized a story from Barbara Kingsolver's *Animal, Vegetable, Miracle: A Year of Food Life,* when her friends David and Elsie, longtime Iowan farmers, visit her in Virginia and give an organic dairy workshop to farmers "who were looking for new answers." She writes, "It was a discouraged lot who attended the meeting, most of them nearly bankrupt, who'd spent their careers following modern dairy methods to the letter: growth hormones, antibiotics, mechanization. David is a deeply modest man, but the irony of the situation could not have been lost on him. There sat a group of hardworking farmers who'd watched their animals, land, and accounts slide into ruin during the half-century since the USDA declared as its official policy, 'Get big or get out.'" To this, Rick pointed out that, ultimately, if we changed tack and lean in favor of more diverse crops on smaller farms, then there's still the problem of labor, which would ruin the whole prospect. "You need cheap labor," he said. When I suggested that so many people in America still need jobs, ever since the recession, he scoffed. Americans aren't going to do those jobs, he said. He suggested using "Mexicans . . . but then the whole system would need to change." So we are left, to his mind, with huge monocropping farms of soy and corn with only one guy out there on his huge tractor— his only employee—because it's just way easier and, perhaps, cheaper (if you disregard for the moment the astronomical costs of pesticides and fuel) than growing a variety of foods and hiring actual human beings to shepherd them from the ground to our plates.

Rick made a segue here to an issue that is dear to his heart, which is the need for "sustainable" agriculture in third world countries where hunger, poverty, crop diseases, and pests are rampant. He feels that GMOs are the answer to many ills—especially hunger—in arid, poor places like sub-Saharan Africa and India. He says that we need a combination of the United States growing food and those countries themselves supplying their own food to stave off starvation. So it really gets his goat when he learns that Indian farmers have begun to resist GMOs—led by the Indian activist Vandana Shiva. Shiva, now practically a household name in some circles, believes that the large multinational companies such as Monsanto are imposing a "food totalitarianism" on the world.

As a backdrop, the situation in India is particularly interesting because Indian farmers have been planting GMO cotton—Bt cotton, which is developed and marketed by Monsanto—since it was first introduced in farm trials in India in 2001. Some say, however, that it has made the already dire situation of Indian cotton farmers that much more perilous because they have to buy the more expensive and patented seeds, which require that the farmers also buy the necessary pesticides and fertilizers to make these crops succeed. Technically, Monsanto and others do not allow seeds to be saved—by breeders or researchers—without paying a fee to use the technology. For a time they tried to regulate this by including a "terminator" gene in their seeds that makes the seeds infertile, but this was extremely unpopular and presented a public relations challenge to the company. These days, in North America, most of their seeds do not contain the terminator gene. Instead, it's said that they monitor the farms that buy their seeds and will test the seeds growing on any farm that they deem suspicious.

However, in India, thanks to the Farmer's Rights Act of 2001, which was penned with Shiva's help, farmers are allowed to save their seeds, though they still need to pay that "royalty" or technology fee. The Farmer's Rights Act notwithstanding, cotton farmers in India are in a constant cycle of borrowing to buy new seeds or pay the technology fees, borrowing to buy pesticides and fertilizers that are the necessary accompaniments to the seeds, and then, when anything like a drought or monsoon compromises their yield, they have to borrow to buy new seeds again the next season, impoverishing them in perpetuity. Some, like Shiva, have blamed this punishing system for the high suicide rate among India's farmers. In her blog, Shiva says, "The suicides have further intensified after the introduction of GMO Bt cotton. . . . As a human being, it concerns me deeply that 284,694 small farmers of India, the most resilient and courageous people I have known, have in recent times been driven to the desperation of taking their lives because of a debt trap created by a corporate-driven economy of greed that profits from selling them costly chemicals and nonrenewable seeds. And we must not forget that the agrochemical industry is the biotechnology industry is the global seed industry." A 2014 article by the journalist Michael Specter in the *New Yorker* took issue with Shiva and her assessment of the situation in India (not to mention her entire position on GMOs, which clearly didn't hold much weight for him); regarding his trip to India, he wrote that "I neither saw nor heard anything that supported Vandana Shiva's theory that Bt cotton has caused an 'epidemic' of suicides."

Whether or not Bt cotton has contributed to the suicides, what's clear is that there is a definite movement of Indian farmers who are resisting Big Ag. Rick finds this enormously frustrating. He said, when you "go to India and people say, 'Oh my gosh, we need to make sure we keep the manual labor job; we don't want big agriculture; we don't want genetically modified stuff; we don't want chemical fertilizers and pesticides,' uh, well, if you look at the people who are doing the manual labor agriculture, you know, they live a pretty poor life. The only way they send their kids to school is because the government subsidizes them."[3]

A MONTH AND A HALF LATER, when I was in Belgium following around some beekeepers, I hired a cab to take me from a honey conference back to my hotel so that I could eat lunch and write down my notes before an evening of presentations. My cabdriver was from Cape Verde. We got to talking about what I was doing in Belgium, why I'd come, and then, like everyone I've met while researching this book, he, too, had something to say about GMOs. He explained that the Africans for the most part are resisting GMOs because "in Africa, a whole row of Africans will be working a field. If you replace them with GMO crops—crops that need chemicals and tractors—you replace a whole row, if not a whole farm, or a whole town of workers."

This sentiment is one that I had a cursory familiarity with because I knew something of Africa's rejection of GMOs, partially for the same reason my cabdriver gave but also because back in 2002, during the African famine, Zimbabwe, Mozambique, and Zambia refused food aid

---

[3] The government subsidies in the United States pay farmers to grow much more food than we can ever use, and the waste this generates, including piles and piles of corn and soy that sit in storage bins, sometimes for years at a time, or never to be used at all, is incredible. So we shouldn't necessarily throw stones in glass houses!

from the United States because they did not want genetically modified corn. (Zambia's President Mwanawasa said, famously, "Simply because my people are hungry, that is no justification to give them poison.") As Peter Pringle writes in *Food, Inc.*, "How did the fear of GM foods rise to this tragic level? . . . [B]iotech companies had failed to convince the international community outside the United States—even nations in Africa on the brink of starvation—that these novel crops were safe for humans and the environment." Furthermore, the United States could not guarantee that any bag of corn sent to Africa was GMO-free because corn hasn't, historically, been carefully separated in the American grain system. Eventually Mozambique and Zimbabwe accepted *ground* U.S. corn, which could not affect their own crops, but Zambia held steady to their original position. Although the Americans accused the Zambian government of putting their people at risk of dying of starvation, the Zambians believed that there was plenty of non-GMO corn still growing in the world, so they would simply procure that. They felt that if they brought GMO corn into the country—even as food aid—there would be no protecting against some of the seed being planted and eventually contaminating their own crops, which they feared might lead to unexpected health problems in the future. Furthermore, the Zambians exported their corn to Europe and the Europeans wanted GMO-free food. They were concerned that their acceptance of American aid would compromise this economic necessity. Both anti-biotech and pro-biotech interest groups pounced on this story, spinning it whichever way benefited them most. Interestingly, these days, despite what appears to still be a general African skepticism that GMOs will be good for the African nations, Big Ag and the multinationals have their sights set on Africa and have named the continent "the breadbasket for the world." Currently GMO bananas and cassava are being introduced in Africa, and other crops are being tested for wide release.

As evening started to fall, creating long shadows along the hedgerow outside the Dairy Store, I realized that Rick and I had made some relatively discursive forays into debating what one could actually grow in Nebraska and feeding the world. So I circled back to my essential question: Could GMOs make any of us sick? According to Rick, Monsanto takes pains to investigate every claim of possible harm—and that they're good sports about it, too. He likes to use the example of animal feed to show how silly and misinformed the people who make the claims are: "I mean, quite often, when I worked at Monsanto, some farmer—maybe in Iowa, maybe in Europe or whatever—would say 'I had pigs dying and I think it's because they ate MON810 corn' [a popular Monsanto corn product used for animal feed, and similar to the one Séralini used in his study]." Rick started laughing here because he found this so ludicrous. "So when you go—I mean, I shouldn't laugh— so when you go and you have a nutritionist—whether it's someone from the USDA or whether it's an animal scientist from Monsanto, that goes and investigates, and goes, 'Okay, what are you feeding the animals, blah blah blah' . . . well, if you have veterinarians look at the animals, they say, 'Well, you weren't giving them any iron or calcium or water. . . .' It's usually stuff like that. And then there are the cases where people are putting pesticides out on their plants and then they let their animals graze soon afterward. And then, oh well, they die. . . . You know, guess what? You're not supposed to spray pesticides and then let your animals graze on that. That has happened a number of times in India. That has nothing to do with GM. That has to do with bad animal practices and bad farming techniques, right?"

Of course, he's right. How can you possibly blame such situations— if indeed farmers aren't giving their animals water, or are turning their animals out on freshly sprayed pasture—on GMO foods, or the industry itself? (Later, Dave Murphy, from Food Democracy Now!, would tell me that this is an old trick, one that farmers across the middle of the country are hip to. When they complain about the feed, he said, they are told they are bad farmers, which, according to Dave, is rarely the case.) However, if we stop and think for a second about what Rick is saying, there's something else about his line of thinking that sticks: over time a pesticide will be mitigated some by rain and drift, and the soil will absorb some and pollinators will take some away. But how can we be sure that a chemical sprayed on our food that will kill an animal that eats it won't have more subtle long-term effects on humans who are undoubtedly being exposed to smaller amounts of the pesticide with every bite they take? Samuel Epstein, MD, a professor in the School of Environmentalism at the University of Illinois, puts it this way in the documentary *The Corporation,* a film about corporate corruption: "If I take a gun and shoot you, that's criminal. If I expose you to some chemicals which knowingly are going to kill you, what difference does it make if it takes longer?"

Rick stands by the premise that Monsanto—and, by extension, all biotech companies—exhaustively test their products. He likes to tell the story of a time when he was working at Monsanto and a product was introduced that they realized might cause problems. The product, he told me (though he was purposely vague), had IgE binding capacity, meaning that a protein that had been bred into it was allergenic and had a similar amino acid sequence to a food with an allergic profile (though, in this case, it wasn't something obvious like peanuts— it was something people are apparently very rarely allergic to; again, he wouldn't tell me what it was). According to Rick, the company tried to figure out exactly what was happening—why would the introduction of the DNA from "a food product that's commonly consumed and that's rarely had any allergies associated with it" have an IgE-binding capacity when meshed into their desired product? How was the protein staying intact? he wanted to know. Even in stomach acid? They tried to figure it out—investigating everything they could think of, but nothing seemed to lessen the IgE binding of the inserted protein. Eventually, Rick said he thought the protein was cross-reacting with a carbohydrate, which was unusual. Whatever the reason really was, at that point, even though they had quite a few million dollars invested in it, he told me, Monsanto did not go ahead with the product. (A few million might be a lot to you or me, but to Monsanto, which is valued at close to $60 billion and profits $16 billion per year, this is not necessarily a lot of money to lose sleep over.) Subsequently, they halted its production. To Rick, however, this is the kind of incident that should allay fears that Big Biotech might be careless in its testing and evaluation of products: "I think it speaks pretty responsibly," he told me.

Rick (and others) also often speak of the experience of Steve Taylor, a scientist at Lincoln and a colleague of Rick's. I had called Steve in the summer of 2012, before I had ever spoken with Rick. Steve's name had come up because I heard he'd done work on the allergenicity of some soybeans for Pioneer, the seed division of DuPont (best known as the makers of Teflon).⁴ At the time, I was mulling over Simon Hogan's pea study, and I thought that Steve might be able to help me understand the importance (or lack thereof) of Simon's work.

When I got on the phone with Steve, I asked him whether Simon's study might indicate that all GMO crops in general could increase allergenicity, even though the protein that was inserted might, in and of itself, seem harmless. He immediately bristled. Instead of talking about Simon's study, Steve wanted to turn my attention to a study he himself had done in 1992 on the allergenicity of soybeans. Back then, Pioneer approached Taylor about a crop of genetically modified soybeans that contained a gene from a Brazil nut, an undisputedly allergenic food. According to Taylor, in the creation of the new soybean, no one (at Pioneer) had bothered "to find out what protein in the Brazil nut was carrying the allergen." They had just inserted some Brazil nut protein and hoped it would be okay. So Steve then began testing the product and found that the allergenic part of the Brazil nut protein had been transferred. "When I gave them the results," he said, "they killed the project and they let me publish it. Those are the kinds of studies that are done all the time. That study documented that risk existed. [Since then] the companies have been very vigilant about it. If they make a product that makes people sick, they will destroy their own industry."

When I turned our conversation to Bt, he told me that "[the Bt

---

⁴ DuPont was in the process, at the time of this writing, of a proposed merger with Dow Chemical to make an even bigger biotech giant.

pesticide is] expressed at extremely low levels in GMO crops. So there's almost none of it there. Secondly, it's digested in the gastro-intestinal tract. And we know that it doesn't have an amino acid sequence similar to known allergens." Although pushing Steve too much seemed inadvisable, I pointed out to him that I thought I'd learned that even low levels of something could make people sick and, furthermore, that the only real tests for digestibility of the inserted Cryproteins that industry has done to date have been done in a test tube with an acidic base meant to simulate stomach acid. This does not take into account a variety of factors, including the widespread use of PPIs, or proton pump inhibitors (like Nexium or Prilosec, used to treat ulcers, GERD [gastro esophageal reflux disease], and *H. pylori*), which would affect the pH of the gut, making it less acidic and there-fore less likely to destroy any foreign proteins before they could become allergens.[5] I mentioned that Simon had told me that "there are enough situations where the Bt would never get broken down" in our stomachs to make allergenicity possible. And also, I said, Simon had told me about the "leaky gut," which is defined by Dr. Andrew Weil, the Amer-ican holistic medicine guru and author of numerous health-related books, as follows: "Leaky gut syndrome is not generally recognized by conventional physicians, but evidence is accumulating that it is a real condition that affects the lining of the intestines. The theory is that leaky gut syndrome (also called increased intestinal permeability) is the result of damage to the intestinal lining, making it less able to protect the internal environment as well as to filter needed nutrients and other biological substances. As a consequence, some bacteria and their toxins, incompletely digested proteins and fats, and waste not normally absorbed may 'leak' out of the intestines into the blood-stream. This triggers an autoimmune reaction, which can lead to gas-trointestinal problems such as abdominal bloating, excessive gas, and cramps, fatigue, food sensitivities, joint pain, skin rashes, and auto-

---

[5] This is an important point to break down for the layperson: If you take a lot of PPIs, you may be a more allergic person. Period.

immunity." Anything from toxins to overuse of anti-inflammatories to chronic inflammation or chronic use of PPIs can cause this condition (and there is some evidence that antibiotic overuse, which damages the microbes in the gut, also plays a part).

Steve wasn't interested in this line of thinking. "PPIs wouldn't get in the way," he said, briskly moving on to my use of the word "epidemic" when describing the uptick in allergies in America.[6] "I think epidemic is a strong word," he said. Do you think more studies like Simon Hogan's should be done? I asked. To find out whether small, seemingly benign changes to DNA could possibly perturb the immune system? Steve cut me off: "I don't want to comment on it," he said. "You're on a glorified fishing expedition and I just don't want to go with you." Then he hung up, and the line went dead.

The point at which Simon's study seems to really rankle many of the GMO proponents is not that dissimilar from the Séralini battlegrounds in that the issue at hand seems to be the animal models. Rick told me, "No animal model will predict what happens in humans," and Steve Taylor said essentially the same thing, that Simon Hogan's study would not "be considered a reliable approach to evaluating all GMO crops" because it used animals. When I later mentioned this to Simon Hogan, he warned me of this refrain: "They will argue that animal studies are not valid. How come drugs used by the FDA are tested on animal studies? . . . If you had a GM that was tested like a drug . . . I think that would alleviate a significant amount of concern

---

[6] In a confusing moment that seemed to me to be the kind of doublespeak that has rattled all of us regular nonscience folks out there just trying to understand whether GMOs are indeed okay for us to eat, I have included here a moment from an interview of mine with Rick. Rick: "People did experiments that were kind of wacky and they put tons of Cry 1Ab [Bt protein] down mice, right? And the only time they saw an effect was when you put a ton of Maalox into the mice." Caitlin: "Maalox?" Rick: "It's an antacid." Caitlin: "So what's the relationship between Maalox and the Cry?" Rick: "It prevents digestion. . . ." Caitlin: "So it slows everything down?" Rick: "Well, beyond slowing it down. I mean, if you eat enough antacid, you don't digest food very well—there are in humans, in human studies there are data that says if you take a lot of the antacid—the little purple pill—you have increased probability of becoming allergic. That's a fact of life, you know. . . ." Caitlin: "So you don't think there could be a correlation here, though?" Rick: "No, I don't."

from the public."[7] But without animal tests, we have no idea what to think, says Simon. "To me that just seems like it's an excellent business: if you can't pin them down, you can't accuse them of anything." Later, Simon said ruefully, "*We* are the ultimate animal study."

Other than the animal study issue, Rick told me that his biggest beef with Simon's study is more of an ethical one. He said he felt that impoverished sub-Saharan farmers desperately needed an insecticidal cowpea because they store their peas in sacks under their beds and one or two weevils can ruin an entire stockpile. Furthermore, he said, "If it wasn't related to GM, no one would even have paid attention to it and it wouldn't have been in the *Journal of Ag and Food Chem*. This isn't a big company that is making it. It's really intended to provide farmers in sub-Saharan Africa with good insect control. . . . That possibility is gone because of Hogan's test."

In both Rick Goodman's and Steve Taylor's examples of the times that Big Biotech was savvy enough to take a product off the market, known allergens were used. But Simon's study gets closer to theorizing something more nuanced: What happens when you insert the DNA of an *unknown* allergen, like from a bacterium, or Bt, which no one has spent much time researching as an allergen, into a plant? And what about those resultant proteins that are created each time an insertion is made? Sometimes as many as eight different proteins can be made with each insertion, "besides the protein which is desired," according to the plant pathologist Don Huber. How does the immune system react to those? If they are not on Rick's Allergy Database list, will we ever know?

These questions, alone, Simon Hogan says, are enough to say, "Halt. We need to define this, we need to understand this." However, he told me, in his travels to various conferences where allergenicity is discussed, there is often a big and powerful cadre of industry scientists as

---

[7] Maine congresswoman Chellie Pingree spoke to this dearth in testing in an interview with me in fall 2014: "With drugs, we say, 'You've got to prove that on every possible mouse in the world it's fine,' whereas with most chemicals in the environment, you've got to have enough studies that show without a doubt that you're going to fall down with cancer tomorrow."

well as academics. He said there had been, for years, really, a feeling that "we were in a time-standing-still type thing" in answering some basic questions about GMOs. (He challenged me then: "Who funds those meetings?" alluding to the idea that Biotech funded most of them. A little research on my part showed that that was often the case.) The research and conversation on GMOs was not progressing, he told me, and the same questions were forever being asked and the same answers being generated by the industry, like some kind of kaleidoscopic closed loop. "When we go to these meetings," Hogan said, "and have these discussions, we're in flat-out neutral in that nothing moves, and that's because it gets bogged down in this whole thing. No one's taken, I feel, the time and effort to sit down and say: these are the testing criteria." What about the companies themselves, I wondered out loud, aren't they testing the products for safety or allergenicity or at least evaluating the tests, as Bruce Chassy had said they were? Hogan said flatly, "I don't believe the right test or protocols are in place to specifically answer those questions." And later he said, "You would think that the American government or the EPA or the FDA would demand that [the studies] be given to independent scientists."[8]

What does that mean, I wanted to know, for the rest of us, those of us who have no way to do clinical tests on anyone other than ourselves? Must we wait for the mills of the industry and academic gods to grind fine enough that there are answers, despite the rapidity with which we are modifying not only our environment but also ourselves? It seems that the slow pace at which we're actually understanding what we're doing to our food, water, and planet is so far behind our changes; we will never catch up. I can't help but think of Rachel Carson's warning in *Silent Spring*: "Given time—time not in years but in

---

[8] When I asked Congresswoman Pingree about this, she said that in Washington, "the federal government is in the same sort of shape as the research universities. The EPA is probably two-thirds the size it was ten years ago. There's staff cuts, there's science cuts, there's rooms full of paper that they can't begin to read . . . there's not enough people to do their own research in pure science. You get these big chunks of science nobody's responsible for. . . . We've built these regulatory silos that don't look at the bigger picture."

millennia—life adjusts, and a balance has been reached. For time is the essential ingredient; but in the modern world there is no time. The rapidity of change and the speed with which new situations are created follow the impetuous and heedless pace of man rather than the deliberate pace of nature." Or, to put it another way, in Simon's words: "Once you get past an approval setting and the plant goes into the big, wide world, it's never coming back."

"Especially in the case of corn?" I asked.

"It doesn't matter that it's corn or pea. It could be fish or anything along those lines . . . once it gets past [government approval], there's no return because you don't actually know, we don't definitively know what these proteins could do." He went on to explain that we're just starting to learn about things like "mitochondrial stress" or "unfolded protein response," inflammatory responses that occur within our cells when they are stressed by, for instance, novel proteins (perhaps the proteins bred into GMO plants) that influence their structure and how they function. So, he said, not for the first time, "We need to define this, we need to understand this."

And we need to consider possible changes in our epigenetics, another thing I learned about in Cincinnati, which is the teeny-tiny writing that is coded on the top of our DNA and tells our DNA what information to turn off or on. Our epigenetics, scientists are learning, are being changed by environmental toxins. These are invisible changes, ones we don't even know are happening but which will affect not only our cells' health but also, in the bigger picture, our own health and then also that of our progeny, and theirs in turn, forever changing what we pass down in our bloodline.

Simon said he was pessimistic, in general, that the kind of money that was needed ($500 thousand to $1 million, for a good, deep initial study) would be made available to scientists like himself from any of the big funding agencies such as the NIH, for instance, to really look into these issues. Here, he echoed many scientists I spoke with while researching this book—I was told repeatedly that the money just isn't there for research on GMOs. Tyrone Hayes, on the other hand, told me that the money *is* actually out there, if you can get it from industry. But industry doesn't, in general, want an author or scientist to publish data that will hurt its product. Not to mention the risk any scientist feels he or she might be taking by wading into the murky pool of GMOs, especially if they want to preserve their reputation.

As Rick and I continued to talk, the Dairy Store, which had supplied our tea, was emptying out. A light wind was picking up and rustling the bushes, so I pulled on my coat. It started to feel odd, all of a sudden, to be face-to-face with this man who had really gone for my jugular after the piece in *Elle* came out, and yet I was still hopeful (this is a flaw of mine, this tendency) that somehow we might connect some dots between us. I realized what made it hard for me to really understand this guy was that I did not know what makes him so positive of the good GMOs can do, despite all the evidence I was gathering that seemed to indicate that there was more that could go wrong than could go right with GMOs if we weren't careful. I wanted to know why he takes it so personally when GMOs are criticized. I asked him what, ultimately, this was about for him. He leaned in across the table, smiled at me a flat and confident grimace, and confided, "It's kind of like a religion."

I found this, on the surface, a peculiar admission because he no longer directly works within Biotech (though, I guess, some people might claim he's just as entrenched in Biotech under the auspices of UNL as he ever was). When I asked him why he would leave a company he was so obviously proud to work for and so invested in, he began telling me a story about how, toward the end of his time at Monsanto, around the time his wheat "baby" was canceled, some scientists, whom he would not name, came to Monsanto concerned about a soybean Monsanto had engineered, and told the company they'd found something potentially unsafe with the soybean. These scientists, Rick told me, told Monsanto they were going to publish their data. According to Rick, the study was "bad science"—"they didn't have appropriate methods of detecting things"—so he became the lead person working on a new study, which Monsanto set up to disprove their claims. In the meantime, the original scientists decided not to publish what they had found and instead signed on as coauthors of the study Rick was now heading up. During his work, already feeling defeated by the killed wheat project, Rick told me he began to have a conflict with his boss, who, he said, was trying to control him. Here he gestured with his thumb on the table, as if he were squishing a bug. "I mean, I was running programs that were pretty big, and all of a sudden he became my boss and he wanted to control everything, and he wouldn't give me any information but I had to give him every bit of information [about the safety study we were conducting on the soybeans]." He suspected that his boss was trying to take credit for Rick's hard work. Rick couldn't take it anymore, he told me, and left Monsanto in 2004 because "I'm not the kind of person who has somebody pushing down on my head all the time and gets along."

What ever became of that wheat, though? I wanted to know. It was on my mind because in the summer of 2013, just before I began my odyssey in search for answers about GMOs, some of that very same wheat showed up in a farmer's field in Oregon, raising questions about whether Rick's wheat could still be growing somewhere, and therefore was mixed in with regular wheat a decade later, even though Rick (and Monsanto) claim that all wheat endeavors had been effectively halted. I told Rick that some people think the wheat mystery points to the possibility that Monsanto may still be tinkering with their wheat products in the open air with the hopes of bringing them back to market. Monsanto, for their part, says they have no idea how the wheat ended up in Oregon and that their best guess is that someone who is anti-biotech "intentionally introduced" the wheat in that farmer's field in order to "create problems." Still others have posited that another likely scenario is that a bag of this GMO wheat somehow sat around (for ten years or so?) and got mixed in with conventional wheat seed until it was planted in Oregon and discovered by the farmer. Some cry that GMO wheat has already been mixed in with the wheat we are currently consuming but that the public just has no idea. "God knows how it got there," says Rick.

I was tired and hungry and it was getting dark and downright windy by now. My mind was spinning with images of rogue Franken-wheat that was looming as big as scarecrows in my imagination and secret Monsanto studies aimed at discrediting concerned scientists. And, for some reason, something about Rick and his anger—at me, at anyone who tried to take on Biotech, at his old boss at Monsanto—began to feel perilous. I was far from my family and home and I was realizing that I had many more miles to go on this journey before I figured out anything that was more informational than just a whole lot of controversy. The thought of it seemed exhausting.

I told Rick I needed to go and followed him inside the bright lights of the Dairy Store to throw out my cup and say good-bye. As we stood talking next to a trash can before I got ready to leave, he admitted that he didn't understand why I'd gotten so sick a few years earlier, and he allowed that there might have been "something else" about corn, not the genetic engineering of it, that could have bothered me. "You could have an allergic reaction to something in corn, but I don't believe it was the [GM] protein." That was as close as he was going to get, I realized, to acknowledging that something could have been wrong with me at all, let alone something that was solved when I stopped eating corn. And there was a part of me that wondered if he was absolutely right: I had learned during my research that corn is an inflammatory food; also, I learned that corn can get mold on it in the co-op bins and some people can be sensitive to that mold. And there were probably other possibilities, too, ones I hadn't thought of and he hadn't either.

Just then my phone pinged with a text message, interrupting my thoughts about corn and what about it had made me sick. I looked at it, thinking it might be Dan and Marsy calling to say good night, since it was bedtime back east. Rick then made what I think he thought was a joke. He said that it was probably my husband wondering whether

I'd been "kidnapped." Something inside me froze. When I looked up at him with a smile, hoping for one back, he didn't reciprocate. It was awkward and quiet for a moment. Then I said thank you and made my way out to my car to leave.

About a mile away I stopped at a Cumberland Farms to fill up with gas. When I got back in the car, there was a message on my phone from Rick: "I came back out and saw your car is still here. Are you okay?" In my anxious state, I was confused by his text. Why was he checking on me? *This project is just making you jumpy*, I told myself. Disregarding the burbling panic in my stomach for the moment, I fired up the Internet on the iPhone and found a Hampton Inn in Omaha, an hour east. Even though I was exhausted, I wanted to put some miles down before I rested.

Later, after driving in the dark along highways full of tractor-trailers, I came into Omaha, a bigger, denser city than I had anticipated. Big gray stone-and-steel office buildings and monolithic hotels, their lights illuminating the dark, Midwestern night, were surrounded by a handful of spaghetti-like roads and highways, roping their way in and out of the city. It was very late and I was tired when I pulled into the Hampton Inn. I parked and checked in. The receptionist told me that they had a pool and, though it was about to close, she could ask to have it kept open a bit longer for me. In my room, I unpacked my bags and as I was changing into my bathing suit, I got another text from Rick that said, "Sorry. I thought you were still there because a little silver car was where yours was. It was a Fiat 500 though. Thanks for the chat. Have a safe trip." Relieved that he just seemed to be genuinely concerned for my welfare, I texted him back: "Thank you for looking out for me. I was already on my way and couldn't text and drive. Thank you for taking the time. I look forward to more conversations. C." Mollified, I made my way to the pool and, alone in the blue water, I swam back and forth, unwinding the anxiety that had coursed through me in front of that gas station in Lincoln. Finally ready to sleep, I got into bed with Ian Frazier's *Great Plains* and read until my eyes closed.

chapter 6

When I awoke to a gray, humid day in Omaha, my brain was slow and foggy. I made three cups of green tea at the downstairs coffee bar and brought them back up to my room. I sat on my rumpled bed and drank them slowly and meditatively, one at a time. I was trying to sift through everything I'd learned from Zach and Rick, everything I'd seen and heard as I drove from Denver to Omaha.

And I was trying to get up the energy for my next push of driving across Iowa to the home of Lisa Stokke and Dave Murphy, the founders of the activist group Food Democracy Now!, whose goal, according to their website, is to bring awareness to the following issues: "From rising childhood and adult obesity to issues of food safety, air and water pollution, worker's rights and global warming, our current food system is leading our nation to an unsustainable future. Food Democracy Now! members have a different vision. We know we can build a food system that gives our communities equal access to healthy food, and respects the dignity of the farmers who produce it." Since 2008 when they started, Food Democracy Now! has become, arguably, the loudest and most influential organization in the food movement—in addition to the usual social media and online presence, they also have a targeted email list of more than 650,000 subscribers. And lately their focus has become almost unilaterally to take down GMOs and the companies that make them.

When I started putting together my trip to the Corn Belt, I had added Lisa and Dave to my itinerary because I wanted to try to understand what they were actually against—what concrete objections they had to Big Ag—and what they stood for. I needed to prepare my questions that morning in Omaha, but as I sat and sipped my tea, I found that, for some reason, all I was doing was thinking about Rachel Carson, the mother of all environmental activism (you've probably already caught on to that).

In 1960, when Carson was writing *Silent Spring*, she was dying from breast cancer. The treatments were exhausting and painful, leaving her debilitated. Her hands ached. She developed phlebitis—a condition that causes the veins to become painfully inflamed— in her legs. At one point she lost her sight. But she continued to press forward, determined to finish *Silent Spring* before she died. In 1962, it was published, and it became an immediate best seller. Despite her worsening condition, Carson went on the road to talk about the book, appearing on CBS and before Congress to offer testimony on pesticides. President John F. Kennedy, inspired by the book, appointed a committee to study pesticide use.

But not everyone celebrated her work: the chemical industry attacked her, identifying her as a left-wing fearmonger with cultish "nature" tendencies, and accused her of trying to undermine the American effort to supply adequate food to combat world hunger. By the time of her death in 1964, however, the effect of *Silent Spring* had begun the modern environmental movement: In 1970, the first Earth Day was celebrated and the EPA was formed. In 1972, DDT—the insecticide that she had scrutinized and maligned—was banned from use in the United States. The Clean Water Act and the Endangered

Species Act were subsequently passed. It seemed as though America was on its way to becoming a world leader in eradicating the dangerous and toxic chemicals we had spent the last thirty years, in a post–World War II frenzy, creating and pumping into the environment. Even though the world had lost Carson, she had contributed to changing it for the better.

Then something happened: even as public knowledge increased, and despite her dire warnings in *Silent Spring* ("For the first time in the history of the world, every human being is now subjected to contact with dangerous chemicals, from the moment of conception until death"), chemical production, somehow, continued to march forward at an unprecedented pace. Business was always finding more ways to create industries that churned out more toxic products. As the years passed, products made from and with toxic chemicals would eventually flood our lives with a dizzying preponderance. Instead of trying to find ways to work with nature, the goal of the corporation became a single-minded and ruthless pillaging from nature in order to make products and stuff, while at the same time finding more and more ways to eradicate certain aspects of nature—weeds, rodents, insects—that humans found displeasing. And yet by eradicating that which has displeased us, we've been blazing a long and destructive warpath into our ecosystem, destroying organisms that are necessary—in ways we might never have thought of—to our own survival.

Today there are hundreds of thousands of chemicals in the environment—most of them unregulated and untested. When Carson was writing *Silent Spring*, she said that "almost five hundred" new chemicals "find their way into actual use in the United States" annually, "500 new chemicals to which the bodies of men and animals are required somehow to adapt each year, chemicals totally outside the limit of biologic experience." Today that number is 700. And, as of today, nearly 85,000 chemicals are commercially used by industry—and over four billion tons of toxic chemicals are released into the U.S. environment—air, water, soil—every year. Seventy-two million pounds of those four billion are known carcinogens. Most of those 85,000 chemicals have been "grandfathered"—meaning they do not need to be tested for safety by our government or by the industry creating them. Under the Toxic Substances Control Act of 1976, the EPA can't order a company to test a substance unless the agency has been provided enough evidence that it's dangerous. Because of this modus vivendi, the companies get to regulate themselves; the EPA has only been able to test two hundred of those 85,000 chemicals, and only five have ever been banned. This is how we do "risk assessment" in this country, rather than using what the EU calls the "precautionary principle," which sets the responsibility squarely on the shoulders of the company. Here, the consumer must fight for her own life. As Mount Sinai Hospital in New York City states on its website, "today's children face hazards that were neither known nor imagined a few decades ago. Children are at risk of exposure to thousands of new synthetic chemicals. . . . Many of these chemicals have been dispersed widely into the environment. Some will persist in the environment for decades and even centuries. Most of these chemicals did not previously exist in nature. Of the top 20 chemicals discharged to the environment, nearly 75% are known or suspected to be toxic to the developing human brain." And, terrifyingly, many of these toxins that come to us and our children are coating and also inside our food—the basic thing we are providing to keep them not only alive, but also well.

And then there's our water. A 2007 study on ground and drinking water contamination from pesticides in the Great Plains found results that were shocking: Reservoir water was contaminated with at least twenty-seven herbicides and two insecticides. Twenty-one herbicides were found in twenty-eight drinking water samples. And much of the water was contaminated not only from pesticide sprays leaching into the ground but also from rain and snow. In other words, the pesticides had *vaporized* and gone into clouds and then been deposited back down on Earth. Until I read this, I honestly hadn't stopped to think before about rain and snow carrying pesticides. So does this mean that even if I'm buying exclusively organic, I am not safe? That there is nowhere to hide, even for the clouds? Tyrone Hayes's words were starting to haunt me: "We can invent new chemicals much faster than we can evolve."

By now, we are seeing the disastrous effects: Our planet—the waters, earth, and air (and therefore ourselves)—is saturated with chemicals and toxins. We have permanently altered the climate. And we have changed tack so blindly in favor of monocultures of a few key crops—corn, soy, and cotton, predominantly—in a hungry thirst to produce more, always more, that we are losing the precious biodiversity our planet needs. In my son's lifetime, countless prairie grasses, milkweed, ash trees, emperor penguins, moose, polar bears, monarch butterflies, bees, and many other species may disappear for good. This is a tragedy. Carson wrote, "All this has been risked—for what?"

It was not until I began my odyssey across our breadbasket that I realized how prescient Carson's question was. And how disturbing it is that we failed to hear the larger meaning of what she was crying out a half century ago—enough time has passed that we could have actually started to undo the damage we had already done. And, if this is any kind of coda at all, it is worth mentioning that in 2007, Senator Benjamin Cardin from Maryland intended to submit a resolution celebrating the centennial of Rachel Carson's birth, but it was blocked by Senator Tom Coburn from Oklahoma (known to have biotech industry ties), who had said a year earlier, "The junk science and stigma surrounding DDT—the cheapest and most effective insecticide on the planet—have finally been jettisoned."

That morning in Omaha, in the way that brains can go tangential, I found myself focusing on one simple, imperative question: *What happened?* And what came to me, somehow, was the image of an errant milkweed plant I'd seen at the edge of Zach's field. There was something courageous and moving about that one plant, the plant I thought I'd never witness since I assumed—and had been told by the media—that all milkweed would be lost to the sea of GMO corn and soy and the glyphosate they come with. But that one plant was there, waggling in the breeze, a testament to the fact that Nature, when given half a chance, may be more resilient than we think.

Energized by the thought of that hopeful plant, I gathered my things, packed them, and got ready to check out and start driving again. The fatigue, and a kind of hopelessness that was clouding my morning, started to part. I wheeled my bag out to the parking lot to find my car. Under the left tire, I saw a large green sticklike thing. What is that? I wondered out loud. A piece of plastic? I set down my bags and bent over to look. There, still as Stonehenge, was a huge praying mantis. It looked like this:

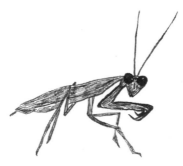

Wondering what in the world it was doing in the middle of the Corn Belt, I looked it up on my iPhone and found that you can buy praying mantis eggs and hatch them to use on your fields for insect control instead of pesticides (you can buy green ones that are native, or brown ones from China). I read that some farmers across the Midwest are trying them out because of the increasing resistances some pests are developing to pesticides. I took a picture of my green, long-legged buddy and sent it to Marsden via Dan's email. Then I picked him up—spiny and light like a feather—and moved him to the side of the parking lot.

I returned to the hotel to get as big a cup of coffee as I could find for that day's push and, back in the car, I continued my drive east.

. . .

AT THE BORDER between Nebraska and Iowa, the landscape out my car window looked, to me, as if the glacier that came over this part of the world was given specific instructions: "You go flat back there and hilly here." And the land had said, "Roger that!" (In reality, the hills along the Missouri River on the Iowa side are mostly the result of wind-blown dusty dirt. My friend Steve Hopp, who grew up in that part of the country, wrote me, "The Missouri used to be ankle deep and a mile wide. The wind, mostly from the West, hit the moist air and dropped the dust, making the hills. Cool, huh?")

After the stark land of the plains, Iowa undulates with a big-hipped and bucolic voluptuousness. Although the land is less dry and dusty than just a few miles to the west, Iowa is less green; instead it is so densely planted with corn, it makes Nebraska look biodiverse! Michael Pollan writes in *The Omnivore's Dilemma*, "Iowa begins to look a little different when you think of its sprawling fields as cities of corn, the land in its own way settled as densely as Manhattan for the very same purpose: to maximize real estate values. There may be little pavement out here, but this is no middle landscape."

Iowa smells different from Nebraska, too: instead of the dusty harvest smell, I was confronted by a much stronger smell of manure (from hog confinements or CAFOs?) for most of my drive. Where Nebraska is flat and wide and doesn't seem to have towns, really, instead being more tied to the geography of far-flung homesteads and then Walmarts serving as some kind of village center point, Iowa has little towns that you reach via *Bridges of Madison County*–type covered bridges that rise above golden waves of corn and are marked by innocent-looking white storybook farm buildings. These are the last vestiges of the kind of family farming that made Iowa Iowa—the poster child for American farming.

About 2,500 years ago, nomadic peoples began settling along the Iowan rivers, and were learning farming techniques, which began the agricultural tradition of the state. Iowa, historically, has some of the most fertile soil in the world, which eventually attracted European settlers to the state, after the U.S. government allowed settlers to begin populating the region in 1833. (Iowa, named for the Iowa River, which was named for the Ioway Indian tribe, joined the Union in 1846.) Those settlers began raising diversified crops of corn, oats, beans, squash, wheat, pumpkins, and fruits and also raised cows, pigs, and chickens on their family farms. In just a few years, in response to the gold mine in rich, dark soil and ideal farming conditions, much of the prairie and forests were plowed up for agricultural use. During the Civil War, wheat prices went so far down that the bottom dropped out of the market, which prompted Iowan farmers to turn to corn—this was the very beginning of Iowa becoming "the corn state." In those early years, farmers rotated corn with oats to keep the soil fertile and prevent crop diseases and insects. Eventually they began feeding corn to their pigs and cattle and the state started to turn much of its corn production to animal, rather than human, feed. By the start of the twentieth century, corn was a major Iowan crop; it was king.

At first, I admit, the corn cities in Iowa are mesmerizing. I found myself awed by the beauty of them, the tall, golden, fertile plants with their shaggy tassels, browning leaves, and planty aspirations to reach for the sky and grow taller and fuller with each rainfall (or irrigation). There's an innocence and hopefulness to corn—as if it has its own naïve selfhood—which is distinctly American, it seems to me, despite the telling fact that the EPA registers GMO corn as a "pesticide" rather than a food. Just seeing that much of it growing across the land makes one think of Thanksgiving, new growth, fertility, corn on the cob, the girl next door, apple pie, and, ultimately, Americana. As I drove, I heard Greg Brown singing his song "The Iowa Waltz": "Home in the midst of the corn, / The middle of the U.S.A. / Here's where I was born, / And here's where I'm goin' to stay."

A long time ago my dad gave Dan a postcard book (you know, the kind of book that's postcard shaped and every entry in it *is* an actual postcard you can mail, with a little outlined box for a stamp?) called

From the Heartland. It's filled with photographs of Iowa by a guy named Pete Wettach, an amateur, or hobbyist, photographer who also worked as a county supervisor for the Farm Security Administration during the 1930s and '40s. As he made his rounds, he lugged with him a 12-pound Graflex camera and took photographs of farmers, their families, and their farms. What he created, while Dorothea Lange and Walker Evans were showing us the desperation of the Depression and Dust Bowl just a little farther west and to the south, was, instead, a beautiful, hopeful, and nostalgic representation of the times as seen through a different lens. Instead of abject poverty, through his eyes, we see family farms where people are hanging on and the land is still rich and giving.

When I left for my flight from Portland, Maine, to Denver, Colorado, I had brought this pocket-sized book with me, throwing it into my bag, kind of as a sentimental afterthought. But an hour into Iowa, I remembered I had it, and when I pulled over at a rest area to use the bathroom and get a coffee, I fished it out of my backpack. Sitting there at that gray, concrete rest stop, a little rain smattering my windshield and the smell of weak coffee filling the car, I was transported: A woman standing in the middle of prairie covered with clover. She wears a white dress, over which she's pulled on a white, patterned smock. She has a bandanna in her hair and there's a big metal bucket near her bare legs. Surrounding her, like the train of an enormous white wedding dress, is her flock of chickens, hustling toward her and squawking to be fed. Behind her sits a small barn, a windmill, a bunch of trees (!), some fencing, and what looks like part of a tractor. In another, two men are threshing (removing the grain from the plant) what looks like wheat. One man sits atop a big wooden wagon, filled with the unthreshed plants, and his two enormous and magnificent dark horses stand patiently waiting. Another man sits atop the threshing machine, which is another large and sprawling wooden structure. This apparatus shoots the wheat stalks out a big pipe into a huge mountain of haylike odds and ends beside them. More images: two men standing on top of a hay bale that's as big as an ocean liner, the land below them flat and long until it hits a tree line; in another, corn stacked in tasseled pyramids all over a field while it dries down. Or this one: an early factory farm (today it would be called free-range) of 4,800 tom turkeys, congregating in the middle of a huge swath of open field. And, finally, one of my favorites: a farmer and his wife lugging a huge basket of tomatoes out of their field while their two towheaded kids stand by, the little girl looking quizzically at the camera and the boy patting their fluffy white dog, while an old and faithful tractor sits behind them.

As I was looking at these photos, especially one of a father and son on a tractor pulled by two horses that the son is minding while the dad fills a seeder, I remembered a trip I took in early September up to northern Maine in order to spend a day gleaning corn on an organic farm. (Remember the famous Millet painting called *The Gleaners* of the three peasant women who are picking up—gleaning—stray grains of wheat after a harvest? That's what I did; it's hard work, by the way.) The farmer's name was Jim Gerritsen and on his Wood Prairie Farm he grows mostly an impressive selection of organic potatoes—many I'd never heard of, such as Sunshine, Huckleberry Gold, Prairie Blush, and Cranberry Red. His potatoes are mostly grown for seed, which he sells through a mail-order business to just about every organic farmer in Maine—and beyond—along with a few other vegetable crops, which he also grows for seeds. Jim—a tall, pageboy-haired and angular-faced man—has become a loud, oppositional voice working against Biotech from within organic farming in Maine, his voice reaching farmers across the country. (Jim told me it was he whom Pollan quotes in *Botany of Desire*, after a lengthy phone interview late one night with the author. Pollan writes, "'If there's a source of evil in agriculture,' an organic farmer from Maine had told me, 'its name is Monsanto.'")

I had spoken with Jim several times about GMOs and corn, and then one day he called me up and told me that his corn was ready. He asked if I wanted to come harvest with his family. I said yes and packed my car for an overnight trip up to *the* County (as we call Aroostook here in Maine, because it is so big, covering most of the top of the state). I left Portland at night, driving and driving farther and farther north, as the last vestiges of urban and suburban sprawl peeled away from the roads. By the time I got near Baxter State Park, U2 blasting on the radio to keep me awake, I was navigating a shiny black macadam that cut through huge swaths of trees as a golden harvest moon hung in the pink-fading-to-a-dark-midnight-blue sky. The moon followed me like the moon that follows Owl in one of Marsy's favorite stories, "Owl and the Moon," in the collection *Owl at Home* by Arnold Lobel.

Jim had told me that I should keep my lights on high beams as I drove and that I should swing my eyes from side to side like a search-and-rescue beacon, looking for moose crossing the road. I did as he said; I didn't see any moose, but I did see a coyote off to the side eating roadkill. That night, I slept in a cheap motel, six miles from the Canadian border, then got up early the next day to meet Jim and his family—two daughters, named Sarah and Amy, a son named Caleb, and his wife, Megan (his son Peter has flown the coop and moved to Portland where he works as a carpenter)—in the potato fields. All morning we harvested small purple Caribe taters that were slightly bigger than large radishes. While we worked, Jim and I talked.

Jim's main concern is the long-term effect of taking the fate of seeds—and, therefore, life on the planet as we know it—out of the hands of farmers who have been working with seeds and crops for ten thousand years. For generations, the farmer's job has been to save his seeds and select for the best traits for his climate, soil, and community, becoming a steward of not only the current generation's food but also the food of our future. Now, Jim says, the seed companies are essentially "patenting life" with their genetically engineered seeds that are bred within the lab to express insect resistance, pesticide resistance, and drought tolerance. None of this is necessary, he told me. And all those claims of needing to feed the world are, essentially, bogus, he said. He told me that the Rodale Institute did a thirty-year study that proved that organic agriculture can produce just as much, or more, yield over a period of time as industrial agriculture. And that, furthermore, it's been proven that organic crops actually do better in drought conditions than industrial and GMO crops—even those that have been bred to be drought-resistant—because organic crops are better at retaining moisture and are more resilient to water stress.[1]

For skeptics who say, "Well, that's all well and good, but isn't organic more expensive?" Jim is prepared. In an email to me, he itemized, in bold, six legitimate reasons organic is more expensive:

1. **THE VALUE OF QUALITY.** Everyone understands Cadillacs cost more than VWs.

2. **ORGANIC IS QUALITY.** Since nutrient-dense certified-organic food is nutritionally superior, tastes better than chemical food, and is virtually free of pesticide residues, it is reasonable to expect to have to pay more for quality.

3. **FEDERAL SUBSIDY.** Processed food which relies on commodity crops [that] are heavily subsidized by the federal government (like GE corn, GE soy, and GE canola) do not reflect the real cost of growing the food.

4. **HUMAN LOSS.** Additionally, many of the true costs created by chemical crops have been externalized. For example, every farmer using the insecticide "Sevin" (carbaryl) bears some moral responsibility (which economists would translate into numerical currency) for the 1984 Union Carbide accident which killed at least 2,259 people in India.

5. **ENVIRONMENTAL LOSS.** Additionally, environmental damage is customarily externalized because Nature does not retain a legal team. As one example, the environmental loss—foisted on Nature as a debit—of volatilizing carbon from the soil (humus) where it belongs, and industrial ag pushing it into the atmosphere as

---

[1] Some people say soil without pesticides in it retains moisture better.

climate-warming carbon dioxide, is leading to expanding catastrophic harm, yet those real costs have been externalized.

6. **SUBSIDIZED ENERGY.** Another subsidized and externalized cost which tremendously benefits conventional chemical agriculture is its addiction to cheap energy. For generations we have maintained an expensive worldwide military presence which insures oil will keep flowing at low cost to power industrialized farm equipment and to manufacture fertilizers.

Even more damning than all of the above, Jim told me that because Biotech has, essentially, constructed a monopoly on the seed business (looped in with its chemical pesticide business) and therefore taken over farming, there is a widespread and legitimate fear of contamination for farmers like Jim. He said that his question is, how can we keep seeds that are free of genetic engineering pure? "My perspective as a farmer is that I have a right to farm on my farm the way I want to farm and Monsanto does not have the right to contaminate my farm," he said.

Jim, along with seventy-three other farmers across New England and the United States, have tried—mostly unsuccessfully—to bring a lawsuit against Monsanto (Organic Seed Growers & Trade Association v. Monsanto) for preemptive contamination of their crops. (Although OSGATA was not completely successful in its suit, they did get the court to hold Monsanto at its word that it would not sue for patent infringement for inadvertent trace amounts—less than 1 percent—of contamination. And they got the district court to agree that "some unlicensed—and unintended—use of transgenic seeds is inevitable.") Jim told me that what spurred the suit was the fact that "there is rampant contamination in corn and canola," speaking to the fact that both corn and canola wind pollinate (some call this "volunteerism"), making it extremely hard to viably separate organic farms from inorganic unless you have a large distance, far enough that wind, bees, and birds cannot go back and forth. We're talking miles, here—preferably with something in between like woods and mountains to act as a natural barrier. Simon Hogan had mentioned the impossibility of good separation between crops when I visited him in Cincinnati: "If you drive down Highway 83 in Nebraska, you will see volunteerism of corn in the ditches," he said. At the time when I was visiting Simon, I had not yet been to Nebraska, so I had not seen it for my own eyes. But when I finally made it out there and felt that wind, saw that corn grown from fence to fence, roadside to roadside, and saw the harvest dust everywhere—in the air, in ditches, on cars—I knew that pollination time would be something to behold, and that nothing could stop it.

Jim went on, "So it angers me when I hear that a biotech rep at a USDA meeting is asserting that there has been no economic impact on organic crops—it ignores the fact that they have destroyed the [long-term] viability of our crops. If we're at risk as organic seed growers . . . You have eliminated the ability for American growers to provide GMO-free crops. And this suffocates your right in the marketplace. That's why we've gone to court: preeminently because not only can they contaminate us, but they can claim that we are in possession of their patent and they can sue us for patent infringement of their crops." Jim ruefully said that our government could have done this differently, more respectfully. He said, "The USDA had choices. They could have required Monsanto to only grow blue corn so that GMO corn would be visibly distinct from what other farmers have grown. That would have been one solution [to contamination]. Another would have been for them to allow Monsanto to only grow corn that could not pollinate. But they chose not to do that." Since that never happened and contamination is by now a fait accompli, Jim believes that Monsanto must be stopped, or else they will achieve a worldwide dominion of our seed and, ultimately, our food supply. This is a powerfully potent image. What will our world look like when a handful of multinational companies, rather than our farmers, control all our food?

Just before lunchtime, we made our way to the corn patch where I was, ostensibly, meant to walk behind the tractor and pick up corn that the tractor left behind. But the old, antique tractor—the kind you remember from your childhood, with big wheels and a small seat kind of like the tractor in the *Otis the Tractor* children's books—was not working properly. And so Jim, Megan, Sarah, Amy, and I all walked along the rows and literally hand-harvested the corn—shucked it—while Caleb drove the tractor, pulling the wagon behind him, into which we lobbed our cobs as we went along. Thinking back to that moment as I was driving across Iowa, I almost laughed at the difference between Jim's "put-put-puttety chuffing" tractor and the enormous and powerful computerized control room of Zach's operation. What stopped my guffaw was the realization that there is nothing in the way that Jim and his family live that is not completely tied to their piece of earth. And there's a temerity and also a dignity to that.

In the end, the corn on Jim's farm wasn't very plentiful—only a few rows (and I'm not really sure we even needed a tractor at all), as it had been an extremely wet summer and the corn hadn't done particularly well. The corn we harvested would be saved almost exclusively for seed, Jim told me. Each cob that I held felt alive, and when I peeled off the green husk, it emitted a musky, sweet, grassy, milky perfume that made my mouth water even though it was only nine in the morning. I suddenly ached for corn on the cob—but more than that, for an agrarian life where I was sure that everything that was pulled out of the ground for me or my child to eat was pure and not contaminated by even an errant thought of chemicals. Sourcing food has become so complicated, it occurred to me—there are so many variables to think about and juggle in one's head.

After working, Jim brought me to his house, a sprawling, two-floor construction built above a potato shed. Off the kitchen, where a pan of brownies sat on a small table, the sink full of the morning's breakfast dishes, was Jim's office, from which he runs not only his business but also his anti-Monsanto campaign. Piles and piles of papers and folders covered every surface, and an ancient, stained computer was crammed in the corner. Jim told me that it's from that computer that he writes his long, late-night anti-GMO manifestos that he emails in a newsletter. Upstairs, he showed me a warren of rooms—kids' bedrooms, seed catalog offices, etc.—and led me to the bedroom he shares with Megan. On top of a bureau I saw a tall pile of his pants, all the exact same kind of tan Carhartt work pants, folded so neatly they almost looked pressed. Next to them was a pile of his collared shirts, many of them dungaree, neatly folded like in a clothing store. This was where he kept his uniform.

He led me downstairs and I said good-bye, getting back into my car. As I drove out his long driveway, the sun was hot and steaming up the damp potato fields. Jim had suggested I stop and pick a few Yukon Golds for my dinner that night, so I parked and got out with a sweatshirt to wrap them in, given that I didn't have a spare bag. I found the loamy ground littered with huge, yellow potatoes, freshly turned over by the tractor. I easily picked up eight perfect beauties and I called Dan to tell him I was bringing home some part of dinner. He told me that was great because my aunt Sally and uncle Tom were visiting; they'd just gone out to Frith Farm together, an organic farm not far from us, where the Wesleyan-graduate farmer, Daniel, was raising chickens on pasture with very little grain (what they got was organic and Maine grown). My Dan told me they'd picked up a beautiful, freshly slaughtered chicken for our dinner. That night, after my long drive home, we ate the potatoes mashed with butter and Maine sea salt along with our chicken, which was roasted with olive oil, salt, pepper, and crushed coriander seeds until the skin was crackling. We all agreed we'd never tasted potatoes so sweet, so fresh, so soft, or so silken on the tongue.

As I pushed on across Iowa to meet Lisa and Dave, I saw billboards along the side of the road like this one: "I'm an organic farmer. I pull weeds." I saw one farm with cows and llamas in the same pen, which was a funny—and wonderful—sight. Along the edges of the cornfields I saw big tractor-trailer trucks hovering on the sides, poised and ready to cart away mountains of grain. For a little while as I drove, despite everything I knew about the corn I was witnessing, I was lulled into a lush feeling of security: this is food, this is our heart-land, and this is our breadbasket—we will not go hungry with all this food right here, this incredible, generous abundance.

chapter 7

Outside of Des Moines I headed north for Clear Lake, a small Iowan town where Lisa and Dave were based. As I drove, I began to weary a bit of corn—Pablo Neruda writes in his poem "A Certain Weariness": "I am weary of chickens—we never know what they think, and they look at us with dry eyes as though we were unimportant." Greg Brown adapts this poem during the patter in his album *The Live One* in his song "Canned Goods." This is one of my family's most favorite songs. It's about his grandmother canning vegetables and fruit and capturing "a little of the summer" by "putting it all in jars." Every summer when Dan and I are in the canning frenzy that has become de rigueur to our lives, Dan sings this song while he halves peaches and stews tomatoes: "Peaches on the shelf, potatoes in the bin, supper ready everybody come on in, taste a little of the summer, taste a little of the summer, my grandma put it all in jars." Anyway, during the talky part, Greg says of Neruda's chickens: "It's true . . . they do . . . and we are. But it's hard to take that from a damn chicken."

As I drove I noticed how little natural land had been left—read: none. On the 114-mile route from Des Moines to Clear Lake, I saw only one tiny patch of ground that was not monocropped in the middle of a cornfield. This one little sliver had a fence with a metal sign affixed to it that boasted that it was a "wetland mitigation area." It was probably one acre of land, if that. Susan Sontag wrote in her 1965 essay "The Imagination of Disaster": "For we live under continual threat of two equally fearful, but seemingly opposed, destinies: unremitting banality and inconceivable terror." And it occurred to me as I felt my heart sinking further and further into my sneakers, the more corn I saw and the less natural land, that, in a way, this GMO issue achieves the pinnacle of her statement. Somehow, in all those acres of land, there's the incredible banality of a monoculture in our agriculture, which translates into a monoculture in our food, our landscape, and our imaginations, even. And, at the same time, I think that we all feel somewhere inside us a deep, intrinsic, and incredibly human terror that as we snuff out the last wild places and grab more and more of what vestiges of Nature remain, all the while getting more out of touch with how our food is grown (and, I might venture to say, what makes food nourishment), we aren't sure we will ever be able to find a way back.

SOON I WAS ABLE to turn from "unremitting banality" and make my way to Clear Lake, Iowa, an all-American town. It's got your quintessential suburban sprawl, a big, gray grain elevator in the center of town, which looms, tall and instructive—"This is what we stand for," kind of like a New England church on a town common—and leafy streets that end in cornfields. Following Lisa's directions, I made my way to their rental house, on a small cul-de-sac in a development. On the back side of the development, corn grew up to the back doors of the houses. At first I did a little double take: this is where these two renegades who are trying to kill Monsanto live? Outside sat two silver Mercedes SUVs.[1]

Inside, the house is like a lot of low, suburban houses I see along

---

[1] Bought used, from a local dealer, they later told me.

the road in the evenings as I drive along and hope for an Edward Hopper peek into private lives—it's much more airy and light than you think it may be from the outside. When I walked in, I found Dave sitting at the dining room table on a phone call. He held his iPhone away from his head and motioned for me to come in while the conversation continued on speakerphone. In a time-bending déjà vu, I heard a voice I recognized: it was Jim Gerritsen, the potato farmer from up in the County back home. There appeared to be three or four people on the line and the topic was the 2013 initiative on the ballot in Washington State to get GMOs labeled.

Dave was wearing a black John Deere trucker hat (the kind with the netting on the back), jeans, a navy blue "You Have a Right to Know" T-shirt under a plaid collared shirt, which was untucked and unbuttoned, and snazzy sneakers. Dave is a fortysomething, big, heavyset guy. A former football player, he went to Exeter and was recruited by Nebraska, Iowa State, Northwestern, and all the Ivies. He ended up at Dartmouth, where he played offensive tackle. "I'm very good. I mean, I like to hit people," he told me. His senior year, Dartmouth won the Ivies, beating Princeton, something Dave is still rather proud of. At Dartmouth, Dave was an editor of *The Dartmouth Review* and was in the fraternity Alpha Delta, "where the beer was." Alpha Delta, incidentally, was also the frat that the guy who co-wrote *Animal House*, Chris Miller, belonged to. He based his short stories, which eventually became the movie, on his experiences there. And, even though the president of Dartmouth is an Alpha Delta alum, the frat was recently derecognized because of "branding" during initiation rituals. Dave has brown hair, a cropped, brown beard with the tiniest sprinkle of gray, and baleful hazel eyes that are big and watery and look right into yours with a bracing openness.

While he talked on the phone, Dave pulled out a glass, got me some water, and started making me a cup of coffee. I went out to the car and brought in a plastic container of salad greens I'd bought in Denver a couple of days earlier and some jarred salad dressing (depressing in its austerity, as I was trying to stay as clean as possible) and sat down at the table to eat my snack. While I ate, I listened to Dave's call, which seemed to be meandering around the issue of funding and how much was needed to defeat the opposition—Monsanto and the other Big Biotech companies, coalesced together under the auspices of the Grocery Manufacturers Association, or the GMA. The Biotech campaign platform was that labeling would drive up the cost of food. This was getting to voters, understandably. There's enough in the world that costs too much right now, and feeding our families is already hard enough. But before making my trip I had heard this argument and had called up Severin Beliveau, a former Monsanto lawyer and lobbyist based in Maine. Sev had eventually decided that he did not like Monsanto's business practices and stopped working with them, and now he is a vocal, and acerbic, opponent, even working with MOFGA, the Maine Organic Farmers and Gardeners Association, against Monsanto to secure GMO labeling in Maine in 2014. I asked him if food would really become more expensive if it were labeled. He said, "That's absolute myth. That is a classic argument, [that] the consumer suffers. It's absolute baloney. It's not gonna cost more money." Furthermore, said Beliveau, Americans recognize that many other countries—including all of Europe—manage to label, so the consumer will wonder, why can't we?

As I was listening to Dave's phone call, I heard the participants mention California's 2012 Prop 37, the first and very high-profile "right to know" campaign, which stated that consumers had the right to know if GMOs were in their food. Like in California, the opposition—the GMA and biotech companies—in Washington was far outspending the activists. It was clear just from listening to Dave and the others that finding the funding to even come close to the money Biotech had doubled down was going to be impossible. So the question became, what is the least possible amount we need to do some serious damage? As a litmus test, the people on the phone call were discussing Prop 37, and how it failed despite widespread public discomfort with GMOs.

The numbers they threw around from the California initiative were shocking: Monsanto gave more than $8 million; DuPont contributed more than $5 million; Pepsi, more than $2 million; BASF, Dow, Syngenta, and Bayer each another $2 million; Coca-Cola, over $1.5 million; and ConAgra Foods and Nestlé both contributed over a million. Morton Salt contributed close to $15,000.[2] This time, however, the individual companies weren't coming in under their own names. They had learned from that. Instead, they had a cover.

Sev told me this is a strategy. "They [Monsanto] don't appear individually as a corporation. They hide through . . . they function through a trade association."

"Like the GMA?" I asked.

"Yeah, yeah. GMA, that's right," he said. "If they went up before a hearing . . . and identified themselves as Monsanto . . . they immediately would alienate half the committee just by virtue of the company itself."

"Why is that?" I asked.

"Because I just think they've developed a reputation of not being truthful."

"Even in Washington, D.C., or just at the state level?"

"I think generally," he said. In Washington State, Sev told me, Monsanto knew this time not to put off voters this way. No one would think anything, he said, of something called, benignly, the Grocery Manufacturers Association.

When Dave was done with his phone call, he got himself some water and sat down with a harrumph at the dining table. He looked exhausted and already battle weary.

Soon Lisa emerged from their bedroom. In her late forties, blonde, of medium height, with quick, restless cornflower-blue eyes, she is unpretentious in a classically Midwestern way—her manner is unadorned, her haircut is a practical bob, her clothes are functional. She

---

[2] You might ask, Morton Salt? Why do they have skin in the game? Your common iodized table salt has dextrose, made from corn, added to it that acts as a "free-flowing agent."

was wearing a clean T-shirt, jeans, and sneakers and was warm and welcoming. However, I sensed immediately from both of them a slight discomfort with what to do with me; a writer was in their house. Now what?

When writing about people and their lives, there's always a funny balance to strike between being friendly and warm, someone your subject trusts and wants to talk to, and establishing and reestablishing the obvious, which is that you are there because you will be writing about them. This can be tough because, sometimes, like with Zach or Jim, there's a real pull, as a human being, to just want to "hang out" a bit. Luckily, Lisa had a plan for my first evening, which took some of the pressure off. We were going to go together—just the two of us, as neither Dave, who wanted to work on a press release, nor her twelve-year-old, Sam, who wanted to hang out at home, seemed keen on joining—to her son Gabe's high school football game. I saw this as a good way to ease into my time with them, by getting a quintessential Midwestern experience and some girl time.

Lisa and I got into her silver SUV and took off toward the game. As we drove, the sky got gray and rainy and the ubiquitous corn glowed against the darkness as if lighted from within. I asked Lisa if this was the landscape she remembered from her childhood—corn, corn everywhere. She said that she did remember lots of corn waving across the landscape but that there was one big difference: there were more breaks in the monotony of it. She remembers when the farms had animals, too—pigs and horses and cows and chickens. And fruit trees, gardens, and a dog or two loitering outside as well because somebody actually *lived* there. She said there used to be large areas of grass and prairie in between the farms. And she remembers more birds and many more butterflies. "I was just telling David the other day that I never see caterpillars. Like, when I was a kid I was always collecting caterpillars on my grandma's farm." Now all those trees, gardens, and farm animals are gone and, instead, most Iowan farms are just corn from property line to property line. And, often, no farmer actually

owns that land—it's all owned by the biotech companies. (Coincidentally, when I was rewatching one of my favorite old movies, *Rain Man,*
later in the fall, I was amazed when I caught a glimpse of the middle of
America in the 1980s, when Tom Cruise and Dustin Hoffman were
passing through on their iconic road trip; instead of the monolithic
GMO corn planted everywhere, the farmland captured by the camera
is diverse: grass, hay, ruminating cows, trees.)

As we drove, Lisa told me about growing up in Clear Lake, Iowa.
She was born, she said, to conservative evangelicals, and she had always
wanted a way out. (Dave and Lisa share the evangelical background
and both told me that if they were sick on a Sunday and they had to
stay home from Sunday School, they were prescribed with the same
tonic: watching Jerry Falwell.) Lisa went to Buena Vista University in
the next town over, Mason City, and soon after had her first child, a
son named Ethan. She went on to have three more children, Lydia,
Gabe, and Sam. Despite her bigger dreams, she somehow never managed to leave Clear Lake.

After having her kids, she said, living in Clear Lake began to feel
oppressive. "That's another reason I think I'm crazy to live here. If I
didn't have a car or a plane or a means for getting outside of this, I
mean I literally could not eat here. There's nothing, you know. There
are no farmers in a ten- or twenty-mile radius that are creating organic
food. There's no stores, no shops, there's no restaurant. It's really a
desert." When Ethan was a baby, Lisa was renting a small house near
the Clear Lake (itself an agricultural saga of blue/green algae blooms
caused by chemical fertilizer runoff, which have made the water un-
drinkable, unswimmable, and unfishable at times) where she ripped
up the backyard and started planting a garden. "I would grow herbs
and I would grow amaranth and beets and peas and all kind of things,"
she said. As Ethan grew up and she began adding her second and third
children to her small family, she was becoming increasingly conscious
of what she was feeding them because "You know, once I knew that all
of these pesticides and genetically engineered ingredients were in [our]

food, I just couldn't in good conscience be feeding them to my kids." So she began driving two hours to Minnesota to frequent an organic market and started working with various grassroots organizations to try to bring an awareness of food to her local community. With Phyllis and Paul Willis, the founders of Niman Ranch Pork, she started a slow food group, of which she was the leader. In that position she began organizing luncheons that celebrated local and organic foods. At first, she says, this felt good to her—she was actively working against the food paradigm that had been handed to her, growing up in the middle of Iowa, as if it were the only option.

But then, as organic became regulated by the USDA in 2002, organic went from, Lisa said, "the people's label, the farmer's label, to being a corporate label, and it became an opportunity for moneymaking." (In 2009, under Obama, the eventual tagline for the USDA farmers market initiative was "Know your farmer, know your food.") When the USDA came into the picture, she said it suddenly wasn't the same experience to buy organic. Organic now had many different meanings: there was "100 percent organic," which meant that all ingredients were organic; there was "95 percent organic," which still got the USDA seal of "organic" but of which 5 percent of the ingredients might not be organic; then there was "made with organic ingredients," which meant that at least 70 percent of the ingredients were organic; and then there was "less than 70 percent organic," which just said "specific organic ingredients" and three of the organic ingredients needed to be listed on the label. "All natural" didn't mean anything because it was not necessarily organic. This new rubric for deciding what was natural and organic enraged Lisa. She said she went through a six-month slump. "I mean, I wasn't *depressed* depressed, but it was really confusing." She says that on top of the clean food she was trying to buy, she came to the realization that living in Iowa, in the middle of cornfields sprayed with pesticides, she couldn't even take matters into her own hands. She said, "I could grow this, I could grow that. But there's always going to be something blowing around.

There's always going to be drift." And that made her feel like a "kicked animal."

That feeling, in many ways, was the seed from which Food Democracy Now! was born. "It was like, no matter what, I absolutely cannot fully protect my children or myself. . . ." She says she realized, on a fundamental level, that "There really isn't any democracy in this [food system]. I really do not have a voice." When she and Dave started Food Democracy Now!, it became the voice she had always longed for.

Soon, with donations pouring in, it became clear to her and Dave that other people wanted a voice, too, in a food system that was becoming more and more industrialized. What they never could have anticipated, she told me, was both how all-encompassing Food Democracy Now! would become and how influential. Dave likes to joke about FDN!'s uncanny power. "It's two people; it's a laptop in Iowa," he says. "No one in the world ever thought there'd be a movement in the United States that was this close, that was on fire across twenty-six states. It's a huge national conversation. . . . I mean it's shaking the foundations of our political system."

By the time Lisa and I pulled up at the football field, it was getting dark and spitting rain. The game was already under way. Her eldest son, Ethan, a tall, thin, blond guy, met us as we walked to the metal bleachers. He told us that Gabe seemed to be benched. Lisa's father, a gray-haired man with a diminutive stature, was already sitting, and we climbed up to him, our feet clanging, and sat down. People around us ate popcorn out of little red, white, and blue paper boxes and the Friday-night lights glittered on the field. Save for the flat farmland covered with corn that stretched out and away from the football field, we could have been anywhere in America that evening. It was hard for me not to see Kyle Chandler and his team from the now iconic television series or to hear Bruce Springsteen in the background, ". . . son take a good look around: this is your hometown, this is your hometown, this is your hometown, this is your hometown . . ." *This is your heartland; this is our heartland*, I said to myself.

As we took in the sunset and the game, Lisa wanted to talk about Percy Schmeiser, the Canadian canola farmer whose 1,030 acres of conventional canola fields were contaminated in 1997 by Monsanto's Roundup Ready canola and who was then sued by the biotech giant for $195,000 for using the seed from plants that resulted from the contamination. (Schmeiser then countersued them for the original contamination!)

In many ways the story of Percy Schmeiser has become one of apocryphal lore in the anti-GMO movement. Schmeiser's story is essentially this: Schmeiser had been saving his canola seeds, every harvest, for fifty years and had never, he claimed, bought Monsanto's product. He claims that in the late nineties Monsanto reps came to his area and conducted secret meetings in the evenings with small groups of farmers—meetings to which he says he was never invited. The goal of these meetings, he says, was to tell farmers about their new Roundup Ready canola, which would enable them to spray Roundup all over their canola crops and not kill the canola itself. The seeds, with the Roundup-resistant gene, were patented. Actually, Monsanto went a step further than that: the gene itself is patented, which is the really interesting—and wacky—wrinkle to the patenting of GMO foods (it's this fact that caused Jim Gerritsen to say that Monsanto is trying to "patent life" itself). However, because canola pollen can travel via wind and insects, one possible scenario was that Schmeiser's canola had been contaminated from pollinating GMO canola on neighboring farms. (Canola, a brassica in the same family as mustard, kale, and broccoli, has, scientist Belinda Martineau told me, "weedy characteristics" and will pollinate "all over the place.") Another possible scenario is the one that Schmeiser claims: some seed must have been dropped from a truck carrying GMO canola onto his field where it grew. (Schmeiser himself did a little research and a neighbor who was growing GMO seed told Schmeiser that he was transporting some of his seed past Schmeiser's farm, right where the contamination happened, and did indeed lose some seed, which blew off his truck because he had a ripped tarp covering the seed.) Schmeiser does not appear to have been entirely blameless, however; the seeds he harvested and replanted actually came from plants that had survived his application of Roundup, which killed all but the Roundup-resistant plants. It therefore seems plausible to suggest that perhaps Schmeiser was indeed attempting to use Monsanto's technology to enhance the qualities of his own breeding program. At any rate, Monsanto sued Schmeiser for patent infringement based on Schmeiser's gathering and planting of those seeds from the Roundup-resistant plants that grew on his property. Because the laws protect the property itself (here, Monsanto's patented cells and genes[3]) and not the way the genes got into the property, Schmeiser was found guilty in the Federal Court of Canada. However, in a follow-up verdict from the Canadian Supreme Court, he was not required to pay any money (because he made no profit from this situation and because he had not caused the initial contamination) though the "guilty" part—for replanting the Monsanto seeds—stuck, which outraged Schmeiser. He has been railing against the "guilty" verdict ever since, becoming a folk hero to many.

In the meantime, it's become so common for Roundup Ready canola genes to be found in organic canola that contamination has become unavoidable, making it almost impossible for canola farmers in Canada and the United States to claim their canola is clean (and, as many farmers with whom I spoke for this book mentioned, they find it laughable when they see a "non-GMO" label on anything to do with canola—canola oil will always be contaminated, they said). What the rest of us going about our lives shopping for food, cooking, eating, and trying to stay afloat may not realize is that non-GMO farmers (of all ilk—corn, soy, cotton, and canola) can be forced, I was told by both Lisa and Dave, to pay large fines to Monsanto for seed contamination— farmers as young, promising, and sophisticated as Zach Hunnicutt but who have been brazen enough to try to grow organic or non-GMO in

---

[3] Though some courts have ruled that you cannot patent "a higher life-form."

the middle of flyover country. (Farmers have also been sued by Monsanto for reusing seed and not paying the patent fees, and seed cleaners—people hired to clean seeds of debris for replanting—have been sued for cleaning patented seeds that the farmer intends to replant.) More often than not, the popular wisdom goes, the farmers and cleaners often go ahead and pay up, rather than fight a corporation with endlessly deep pockets.[4] To ensure that they are able to monitor any contamination, Monsanto has a hotline that neighbors can call to report their fellow farmers who they believe may be using the company's patented seed without paying the licensing fees. These stories— which can smack sometimes of more fable than real—outrage non-GMO and organic farmers because they feel Monsanto's practices are divisive to farmers. I was told that as consumers push for GMO-free products or ask for more labeling, farmers who have been contaminated through no fault of their own are stuck, unable to get out of the GMO loop. Severin Beliveau, the former Monsanto lobbyist, spoke to this cycle, saying, "What they're [Monsanto] doing now is absolutely outrageous. What they're attempting to do against farmers and suing the farmers and all these other things that you read about. I think it's outrageous!" For what it's worth, I did ask Zach Hunnicutt if he knew of this happening to any farmers he knew or anyone friends of his knew. He said no. He did say, however, that he's heard the stories, and where he comes down is: "I don't doubt that a handful of things like that have happened. I don't think people are makin' this up. But I don't think it's widespread or even frequent."

Figuring I knew most of Schmeiser's story, Lisa brushed over the details quickly and then turned to what she really wanted to talk about, which was the intimidation of Schmeiser. She told me that she and Dave know Schmeiser well and that his story had stuck with her. She said that Schmeiser was stalked and intimidated for years during his legal battles and that still today Monsanto has their "goons" park in

---

[4] A seed cleaner named Mo Parr was sued by Monsanto for "aiding and abetting" farmers who were reusing seeds. Monsanto won that case.

a truck across the road from Schmeiser's farm (Schmeiser has said publicly that Monsanto reps have threatened both him and his wife). These kinds of stories, she said, can make you paranoid doing the kind of work she does—you start to see Monsanto danger lurking in all corners. Lisa told me that she herself recently thought a car hovering outside their house could be someone from Monsanto and has claimed that someone loosened all the lug nuts on her car and even broke a tie rod, putting her and Dave in danger while driving (though upon further research, I honestly wasn't sure anyone could actually have broken her tie rod—the pivot point between the steering system, steering arm, and wheel—as this would have rendered her car not at all drivable). However, it wasn't logical for me to completely shrug off Lisa's fears because I knew that my panic in Lincoln wasn't born out of nothing. I, too, had heard the stories. Like the one published in *The Nation* magazine in 2010 that claimed that Monsanto hired Blackwater for "security" against activist groups—this story has been subject to the Internet rumor mills, so it's hard at this point to say what really happened. For the record, Monsanto refutes the *Nation* piece, stating on its website, "Monsanto did not hire Blackwater, nor did we approve the firm infiltrating any groups as was suggested in the *Nation* article. In 2008, 2009 and early 2010 a firm called Total Intelligence Solutions (TIS) provided Monsanto's security group with reports about activities or groups that could pose a risk to the company, its personnel, or its global operations." A little over a year later, Lisa texted me that she was looking to find some way to get more security around FDN!'s communiqués. She had seen Laura Poitras's film *Citizenfour* about NSA surveillance and knew from a casual conversation we'd had about the film that I used to be, long ago, when I was young and seeking in New York City, Poitras's dog walker and sitter. Lisa wrote, "I'm working on a new project and see little point if everything I communicate is monitored. Ugh." And that "tech people and even other activists are so slow to this reality. Denial, maybe. I need help." She wanted to know if I could put her in touch with Poitras. I could not, having no idea how to get in touch with her myself since she's patently hard to reach (given the incredible surveillance on her ever since she started telling Edward Snowden's [the former National Security Agency contractor who became a whistle-blower about the NSA's surveillance of regular Americans] story in 2013).

That night, as Lisa and I drove back to her and Dave's home, the cornfields blanketed in velvety darkness, it occurred to me that this fear about the Goliath of Big Ag might be part of the reason Lisa and Dave are together. There is something about Dave's physical presence—that former-offensive-tackle body—coupled with his political surety, his quick and ironic mind, and his go-for-broke-come-hell-or-high-water attitude that could make a person hanging out with him feel emboldened to take on any behemoth.

chapter 8

When Lisa met Dave, he was working in politics in D.C. By then he had graduated Dartmouth and come back home to Iowa City for a spell, where he tried to be a writer of fiction but, by his own admission, mostly drank for three years. Of that time, Dave said, "I love Iowa but for someone who's nineteen, twenty years old—I wanted to be a writer." With writing as his goal, he managed to get into the MFA program in creative writing at Columbia. His adviser was Michael Cunningham, author of the Pulitzer Prize–winning novel *The Hours*. Somehow, despite this pedigree (one that many writers would give their eyeteeth for), Dave ended up eventually ditching writing and taking a left turn, moving from New York City to Washington, D.C., where he worked on Virginia senator Jim Webb's primary race. He told me that he felt sure he'd found his calling in D.C. and that his destiny was politics on a national level.

But then his sister, Chris, who stayed in Iowa and lived near their parents' land on the Okoboji lakes, called him one night saying she needed his help. "My sister's farm was under threat of having a factory farm built next to it. It's a beautiful piece of land, you know. . . .

There's some original untouched prairie in that area, and it's really rare to have virgin prairie. I've been really blessed with knowing how beautiful this land is and can be. And I felt outraged that they were going to build this near my sister's farm . . . next to a very sensitive watershed area." At first Dave resisted. "I said, no, no one's going to pay me to fight factory farms in Iowa." He was worried about his student debt and he thought coming home to Iowa would prove to be a dead end.

And not only that, there was family baggage. As a child, growing up in a family of Evangelical Christians, Dave said his father's favorite line in the Bible is "a rod is for the fool's back." Dave and I were sitting in his dining room when he started opening up to me about his childhood. It was Saturday afternoon and the screen door was open and a faintly cool breeze was coming in, belying the closed-in feeling of being landlocked in the middle of America. Lisa had gone off to bring Ethan, who lives on his own in downtown Clear Lake, some Benadryl because he'd broken out in hives after eating some fish sticks. Downstairs her two youngest children, Gabe and Sam, were playing video games. Lydia, her seventeen-year-old daughter, was with a friend. There was a quiet to the afternoon, in that way that everything can stop on a Saturday and there's a deeply comforting feeling that everyone in a family is off tending to various parts of their lives but that they will come back again and gather. Lisa had made some cream of squash soup that was bubbling away on the stove for our lunch; we were just waiting for her to come back.

Dave continued to share with me a portrait of a home atmosphere that was highly charged and violent at times. Dave told me that he ended up taking his physical rage from his childhood and funneling it into football, where he excelled. From his descriptions it seemed almost impossible that he would come out as well as he did, going to Dartmouth and eventually founding a powerful nonprofit. And even more uncanny that he would emerge so full of love and compassion for not only his family, whom he says he is still close to, but for his home state that, despite some rough memories, will always be a sacred place for him.

Suddenly reticent to say any more, Dave turned back to the story of his sister, Chris. He said that she began calling him regularly, in tears, fearful that the farmers who wanted the factory farms would hurt her or her kids. "They kind of felt that if I was there, they wouldn't fuck with her," he said. He agreed to come back for two months and "help run a state senate race" for the Democrat Mel Berryhill, because politics seemed like the logical place from which to fight this issue. He said he figured they'd get local control (political control of the local authorities) on this issue—"because factory farms was really a hot issue . . . here in Iowa at that time"—and then he'd go back to D.C., where he had a girlfriend and a life. But while there, he got more and more involved with his home state and with farmers who were trying to stand up to Big Ag. "People asked me, you know, 'Can you stay here and work during the legislative session? We could use you to push the local control bill forward.' And I said, 'Well, I don't know.'" Then, finally, he got talked into it and he began traveling between Iowa and D.C. on a weekly basis. He kept figuring, still, that it would be easy for the Democrats to establish local control. "It was the bedrock of their rural platform, to support local farms," he said. Once accomplished, he'd head back to D.C. But, unfortunately, on that first senate race, they didn't win. (Even so, he and his family were able to defeat the proposed factory farm near their land.) This was the first indication to him that Iowan politics around food needed more attention than he had anticipated.

Eventually, Dave was hired by the Farmers Union to put on the 2007 Food and Family Farm Presidential Summit in Iowa, with the idea that he would try to get candidates in the upcoming Iowa caucus to understand and promote policies that would support family farms and farmers markets and, he said, "ultimately to try to get regulations to stop federal funding going to factory farms." In the early months of this work he was still going back and forth to D.C., still trying to keep some vestiges of his personal life there afloat. Then, in 2007, on Earth Day, he met Lisa at a Slow Food sustainable luncheon she had organized, where he happened to appear as a guest of Phyllis and Paul Willis.

Everything changed for him that afternoon: He went back to D.C. and packed up to move home to Iowa. It seems as though he fell as much for the woman as for the idea of what they could accomplish together: "We didn't actually start talking until I packed up my stuff in D.C. and was on the drive home. You know, that's when we first connected. I thought we could get change. I really felt like if people want this, if people believe it, yeah, we're going to get change." Dave says that Lisa's integrity and her passion for changing the system as a mother made him feel deeply connected to her. He said, "It takes real strength and real courage and integrity to be in a small town and say, 'You know what? I'm not going to participate in this system. This is a really harmful system not only to my health but to my children's health. . . . I mean, she's really had to fight to overcome a lot of hurdles and obstacles to do that as a single mother in a small town where, I mean, taking your kids to day care and having someone who's in charge of day care say, 'You can't bring organic milk in here' . . . that's unconscionable." Dave's eyes well with tears and his voice falters when he tells this story.

Together, in the coming months, they began to form Food Democracy Now! while Dave continued to work for the Farmers Union. As they got closer to the Presidential Summit, Dave became concerned that most of the political staffers he was talking to "didn't know what GMOs were, they didn't know what genetic engineering was, no one had any idea about it." Dave says he met with the head of Obama's campaign, who "was asking me all these questions about, 'How could farmers support Obama?' 'Would they support Obama?' and then we tried to pitch some ideas to him. And then I think a couple of days later Lisa and I went into this restaurant, Centro, which serves local food, and he [the campaign manager] was there with a couple other staffers and we were talking and he wanted to ask me if I thought the Obama campaign should run negative ads and I said, 'Sure, I think you should run negative ads.' He said, 'No one thinks they really work.' I said, 'Anyone who tells you that hasn't won an election. People respond really well to negative ads.' A lot of dirty campaigns have been run here [in Iowa] and everyone talks about how 'Oh, we shouldn't run negative ads.' Anyway, I told him that he would have to beat the Clintons. And then he goes to Lisa, 'What do you think, do you think we should run negative ads?' And Lisa's like, 'I don't really care; I just want to know about what your candidate thinks about GMOs?' And he goes, 'GM *what?*' This guy was the head of the Democratic Senatorial Campaign Committee for several years. . . . He didn't even know what a GMO was. And Lisa and I looked at each other and I think we just shook our heads like, 'I can't believe these guys don't know what any of this stuff is.'"

Later, when Obama came to Iowa for the summit, his campaign began to get hip to the idea that GMOs might be a topic they should pay attention to. They were guessing that it could be an issue some farmers might want discussed in a political forum. According to Dave, he was responsible for crafting the following language that made it into Obama's speech at the summit: "Here's what I'll do as president. I'll immediately implement Country of Origin Labeling because Americans should know where their food comes from. And we'll let folks know whether their food has been genetically modified because Americans should know what they're buying." Dave is quick to point out how disappointed he is that Obama did not make good on this promise; and that, in his opinion, Obama has ties to industry, ties that neither he nor Lisa anticipated back in those heady, hopeful days of 2007. Dr. Eric Chivian, Harvard University professor and founder of the Center for Health and the Global Environment, parroted their disappointment and went a step further: "It's no secret that Monsanto and the other GM crop and chemical companies are enormously powerful politically in Iowa, where the first presidential caucus is held." It's notable to me that, in 2009, Obama appointed Tom Vilsack, the former Iowan governor (1999–2007) who has widely been criticized by activists as an advocate and even a "shill" for Monsanto, as the head of the USDA.

When Lisa got back, she served us the creamy soup she'd thrown together—just grass-fed cream, pureed roasted squash, salt, pepper, and some paprika—and we all sat down together. I was hungry, and Dave and I had been talking for a bit by then about how he got into activism, rather than sticking with the more straightforward political trajectory he seemed initially destined for. I asked him to elaborate on why he thinks the topic of GMOs has become such a lightning rod in American politics. He said, "I think when people, when the American public sees things being done behind closed doors and in secrecy, it frightens them because they know democracy is being manipulated. I just think there have been so many examples in the last decade with Bush going to war, lying about weapons of mass destruction, the collapse of Wall Street, the Internet bubble . . . People are absolutely losing faith [in their] experts and elected officials. . . . People are just like, 'For God sakes, they're right, this is exactly how they operate and our elected officials are in collusion with Monsanto, one of the worst corporations on the planet.'"

Lisa chimed in, "It was never put to your basic Iowan: 'Is this how you want your agriculture to look? Do you want to become home to industrialized agriculture? Do you want to have all your land razed [and turned into] a monocropping system? Do you want to have very little biodiversity? Do you want to have dead soil? Do you want to have . . . very little mineral content in your soil and consequently your food? Do you want us not to grow food here? We're just going to grow corn and soybeans, it's going to go into gas tanks and livestock and high-fructose corn syrup for corporations.' That was not put to the people of Iowa. They were never asked that." Lisa continued, "When we started five years ago, hardly anyone knew what GMOs were, and now the whole country is waking up to what these are. It's just this incredible movement. And I like to think we had a significant role."

One of Dave's particular talents is coming up with wording that is sure to get attention—both negative and positive. His most successful example of this, he says, is the "Monsanto Protection Act," which was the moniker he gave Section 735, an appropriations bill, brought before President Obama in the spring of 2013. Section 735 was penned, at least in part, by Senator Roy Blunt from Missouri, who reportedly worked with Monsanto on the language of the rider. Essentially, Section 735 protects biotech companies like Monsanto from litigation if their GMO seeds are deemed dangerous (or make people sick). According to supporters of the bill, the goal was simply to protect the biotech companies from activists who might use the court system to force farmers to destroy their genetically modified crops. In other words, Biotech said, "Hey, we're protecting farmers here!" When the environmental and food movement groups caught wind that Section 735 was going to be signed into law by Obama, they began to mobilize to try to get it stopped. According to Dave, "the Center for Food Safety and other nonprofits were calling it 'The Biotech Rider,' 'The Monsanto Rider,' and I looked at Lisa and I'm like, 'What is this? A Steely Dan song?' I said, 'This is terrible, you're not going to win talking about a "Biotech Rider" . . .' I'm like, 'Fuck that. This is the Monsanto Protection Act.'" Well, that name stuck and it really took off. And it outraged people enough, according to Dave, that a firestorm was started: Dave said that 100,000 phone calls were made to the White House and FDN! was able to garner 300,000 signatures to their initiative asking that Section 735 be revoked. In response to the deluge, a staffer from the White House called, Dave says, and said, "'The way you guys have framed this . . . my own mother won't understand why Obama's not a bad guy when he signs this' . . . I said, 'Obama is a constitutional law attorney. If anyone understands . . .

something that's a potential threat to judicial review or separation of powers, he should say something.'" In the end, the Monsanto Protection Act was signed and stayed. But it was only to last six months and at least one senator, Barbara Mikulski, a Democrat from Maryland, publicly apologized for its existence. As *Politico* magazine wrote of the bill, "Indeed the collapse of the traditional appropriations process in Congress may magnify the power of single-interest lobbies that have the money and skill to stay focused on their goals." But the incident galvanized the food movement and injected energy into the labeling campaigns, mostly because of the language he used, Dave said.

To illustrate his point that President Obama never had any real interest in having GMOs labeled, or supporting the food movement and organics, Dave likes to tell a story he says he was told when Obama first got elected. "During the transition period, apparently some famous chef cooked him a private meal. And the chef asked him, you know, he said, 'Well, what are you going to do to promote organics, are you going to label genetically engineered foods, take care of the farms, etc.?' And [Obama] goes, 'Show me the movement' . . ." Dave says that, although disappointing, this story was a call to action for both him and Lisa: "That's what we've been working to do ever since, when we started Food Democracy Now!"

In the meantime, though, their traction in D.C. with the Obama administration has eroded, Dave says. "So we're the schmucks who do all the work to get Obama elected during the Iowa caucus. I mean, I organized farmers for him! And not only will they not see us, but they treat us like lepers. They treat us like lepers." He continues, "So it appalls me that Obama sits there in the White House, I mean, he has a quote unquote 'organic garden'—you know his wife planted that— and I think it's a great thing, but then they're just rubber-stamping these GMO crops and they're ignoring all possible harm. . . . They're just burying their heads in the sand intentionally." With an eye on the future, I asked Dave what he anticipated when Obama was gone. Couldn't it get worse? I asked. His answer was pessimistic. "It almost doesn't matter who's in the White House because it's been a corporate takeover of our government," he said. "This is gangster capitalism." And then he elaborated further, "There are six hundred corporate lobbyists controlling America. No one in the White House does."

But his pessimism, Dave says, does little to dampen the vigor with which he's attacked this subject. In a moment of heartfelt candidness, he told me that he's driven mostly by his desire to save his home state. He told me that he finds the Iowan cornfields hypnotic and he's always thinking about growing up near Okoboji Lake and what Iowa was like for him as a child. For him, the recent transformation of Iowa—and by "recent" we're only talking in the last fifty years or so—is just heartbreaking. "Iowa is the most transformed landscape of any state on the planet. Ninety-three percent of our land is in agricultural production. It is single-handedly the most human engineered landscape. Ninety-three percent. Over thirty one million acres of cropland in Iowa. They did that by . . . first plowing over the prairies, cutting 'em down and plowing them over, and draining the swamps. In one hundred and fifty years they've basically wiped out ninety-nine percent of virgin prairie." Since the advent of genetically engineered crops and the continued push for more and more production of corn in order to meet federal ethanol mandates, in the last thirty years the landscape has changed even more, Dave told me. There was a wistful sadness to Dave's tone that afternoon when he said he almost never sees butterflies anymore. "I just had a monarch flying above the porch this morning"—he turned at that moment to Lisa—"when you were—I can't remember what you were doing. And I was like, 'Oh my God, that's amazing, that's so beautiful.' You know, 'cause if you really pay attention, you know industrial agriculture and specifically seed treatments and neonicotinoids and the Bt [corn] are impacting biodiversity in a really harmful way. And just to see butterflies is just, um, magical because you're like, 'How much longer can they sustain this assault on their ability to reproduce?'"

chapter 9

On my last evening with Lisa and Dave, I offered to cook dinner—not only as a way of busying myself doing something a tad more useful than standing around asking them questions but also to allay the general fatigue in their house. It seemed like they needed a break from talk and talk about work.

Like the homes of many American middle-class to affluent families, Dave and Lisa's is abundant with food—all organic, but much of it premade. Cupboards overflow with crackers and snacks; the fridge nearly groans under the weight of cheeses and vegetables, juices, organic grass–fed cream and milk from a nearby dairy, and meats. The spice drawer bulges with everything a cook could ever want. Lisa mentioned to me in passing that it was hard for her that she and Dave spent as much time as they did working on food issues but that, at home, they didn't have time to invest in cleaner homemade food for themselves. The irony did not seem lost on her. The best she could do, she said, was to hit Whole Foods, over an hour away in Des Moines, every couple of weeks when they are flying home from yet another business trip and stock up. Recently, because she was concerned about her youngest son, Sam, and some health issues he was having, Lisa had been buying more gluten-free foods, hoping they might help him. Many of these contained corn products, I pointed out. Lisa looked alarmed, then just exhausted. Those labels had eluded her.

While Lisa decanted a French red wine for us to sip, I started rooting around in Dave and Lisa's fridge and cupboards. Soon, I pulled out a jar of red quinoa, two big, beautiful bunches of lacinato kale, and a jar of tahini. As I set to work browning the quinoa in olive oil and salt, adding water only when it was nice and toasty smelling, Lisa told me that she often wished she lived in France, where the discussion about GMOs is much more open because the Europeans, in general, are not as influenced by the industry. Do you think that's true or just what we think from over here? Like a "grass is greener" kind of thing? I asked. She said, "Well, take this wine, for instance." She showed me the label, which depicted a figure wielding a large scythe, and said it was made to support the *faucheurs volontaires*—or volunteer reapers—who are a group of "6,700 activists," she said, who "engage in crop pulls of genetically engineered crops growing in open-air field trials throughout France and other European countries." When sixty or so *volontaires* were arrested and then fined in 2010 for destroying field trials in France of GMO grapes, Lisa told me that "people in France came together and held concerts, sold special beer and wine and even potato chips to be sold for proceeds, and they were able to raise all the money they needed. So different than what would happen here in the U.S., eh?"[1] Although I'd heard some stories like this already, this kind of widespread public support of activists certainly intrigued me, and I made a mental note to learn more about GMO resistance in Europe.

After I had the quinoa going, I cleaned and chopped the kale. Then

---

[1] From the department of things we didn't know: A GMO yeast was approved for use in the United States in 2003 and has been used ever since in this country's winemaking. (So those GMO-free labels on organic wine I used to scoff at really are true!) And traces of glyphosate have been found in U.S.-grown wine!

I scooped some tahini into a medium-size bowl and added a little water to thin it, and some salt, olive oil, maple syrup, black pepper, paprika, and crushed garlic, making a savory/sweet sesame sauce. When the quinoa was almost done, I steamed the kale. I found a handmade pottery platter on a shelf piled with beautiful plates, bowls, and serving dishes and arranged the red quinoa on one half and the kale on the other side. I sprinkled toasted sesame seeds all over the meal and put the bowl of sauce next to it. Lisa, Dave, and I sat down to eat. Lisa's kids had all dispersed—her daughter, Lydia, was out with her boyfriend, Gabe was at football, and Sam had eaten earlier and was in the basement playing video games. After one bite, Dave looked at me and said, "This is really delicious. Thank you. It's so wonderful to have something so clean and simple. I wish we ate like this all the time." Lisa assented with an "Mmmm" and dug in herself.

The next morning, on Sunday, I woke up early enough to swim in the pool at the Holiday Inn where I was staying. The pool was full of families and kids splashing and cavorting in the water. As much as I love my own children, there's a funny thing that happens when I'm out in my job life and have to interact with other people's kids making noise and mess: I totally don't want to deal with it. I'm the grumpy crank who does not want to sit next to a screaming baby on the plane. I don't find kids cannonballing in and out of the pool at all fun. And yet, here's my contradiction: if someone gives *my* kids the hairy eyeball, the mother lion in me roars. That morning, finding the pool not at all restful, I went back to my room, dressed, packed my bags, and drove back to Dave and Lisa's to take a walk with them before leaving for the airport.

We meandered together with their black Lab, Cash, through their development and along the perimeter lined with cornfields. They both told me that, on some level, they're ready for new chapters in their lives: The work has been hard, relentless, and punishing at times. It has been a strain on their relationship. They spend an inordinate amount of time indoors, staring at their computers, managing crises, and dealing with what Dave calls "the box of chocolates" of the Internet. "There's a lot of great things out there, but *boy*, be careful what you ask for."

These days, when she has free time, Lisa dreams of working more with plant medicine—something she told me she is passionate about. That morning in Clear Lake, as we walked, she picked up various wild herbs growing on the sides of the lawns and told me what they could do—"Plantain," she said, referring to a thick, ear-shaped leaf from a clump along the edge of a lawn, for instance, "is a great anti-inflammatory and draining agent," she said. "You just macerate it in your mouth and put it on a sting or a bug bite," she instructed. And Dave still wants to be a writer. "I'm meant to be a writer. And I think if I can get this work done, I'll go back to writing fiction, finish a novel. . . ." But Dave says the only way he'll quit is when he's succeeded at slinging a mortal rock from his slingshot: "I want to destroy our opponent. That's what I want to do."

"You want to destroy Monsanto?" I asked.

"And the others. Monsanto is just one company. Give me ten million dollars, it'll be over in three years."

"That's all you'd need is ten million dollars?"

"And three years. . . . I think if you give me ten million dollars, I'll put a spear through their heart. . . . We get labeling, it's the beginning of the end for them."

When I got into the car that afternoon, the sun was still high and golden over the cornfields and the wind felt fresh and, somehow, clean. I drove the straight shot, down the center of the state from Clear Lake to Des Moines where I would catch my plane to Atlanta and from Atlanta home to Maine. Even though it was Sunday, farmers were out harvesting corn with their huge green combines and tractors. Corn poured like golden coins into rumbling container trucks with ball-capped men sitting in the driver's seats. I did not see any birds or animals on my drive, just corn and more corn and, occasionally, a large swath of soybean fields.

In the airport, after surveying all the possibilities, the furry corn-cob key chains and I ♥ IOWA stickers, I bought Marsden a navy blue John Deere hat and went to sit at the gate. While sitting there, I started remembering my first night in Clear Lake, when I had checked into the local Holiday Inn Express. In the lobby there was a fake fireplace around which three older couples sat, talking like it was old times. The boy behind the desk, who couldn't have been any older than twenty-three, was reading a book of poems by Charles Bukowski; he had carefully stuck Post-its throughout the book. I asked him why and he said because it was a library book and he wanted to photocopy the poems he liked. I asked him if he liked writing and he said he did. In an unusual moment of openness, I told him I was a writer. He asked what I was writing and I told him a book about GMOs. "Oh, like Monsanto?" he asked, and gestured to the cornfields behind the hotel.

"Maybe," I said. "Don't tell anyone." I winked.

"I've got your back," he said.

Sitting at my gate, I wondered at the cultural significance of a corporation that has become such a legendary giant that even in casual conversations it is recognized as an entity to be feared. How does that looming fear control people's actions? Control farmers? Control our food?

When the plane took off in the late afternoon, the sun was slant-ing horizontally across the farmland below, making it shimmer. The roads that cut through the fields were dusty and the acres and acres of amber waves of grain looked so neatly tended, without weeds or mess of any kind, that I found myself wondering where the hand of the farmer was. If pesticides and machines and corporations can do this work with so little actual input from the farmer himself, then is he still needed? Looking out my airplane window, as we turned and veered east, I found myself sad to leave this complicated terrain. I would miss those chopped-up prairies, big combines, cornfields standing straight and tall, and the complicated issues surrounding farming, pesticides, food, power, and just being an American.

In a bag at my feet were two zip-locked bags of talismans I was bringing home: one held some dried GMO soybean pods and a GMO corncob from Zach's fields in Nebraska; the other, a handful of dried sagebrush from eastern Colorado, a dried purple coneflower I'd found on my walk with Lisa and Dave that morning, and a nut that fell from a yellow buckeye tree near Clear Lake when Lisa and I had walked along its shores. These were real, tangible artifacts of our changing world—the one bag held our imminent future and the other the diversity of the natural world that doggedly tries to hold on, even so.

I took one last look at Iowa through the fading light out my window. Below, spreading as far as I could see, a long chain of interconnected sloughs shone like a trail of diamonds through the fields. They reached westward and disappeared in a gleam of light.

PART 2

Honey: The Other Side of the Atlantic

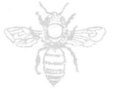

"He will eat curds and honey when he knows enough
to reject the wrong and choose the right."

—Isaiah 7:15

"If the bee disappears from the surface of the earth,
man would have no more than four years to live."

—attributed (perhaps falsely) to Albert Einstein[1]

---

[1] I use this quote here—which was supposedly first used by some beekeepers at a rally in Brussels in 1994 and has been discredited from having anything to do with Einstein—only to underline the desperate situation we may, globally, be facing if the honeybees are destroyed. Also, I think it's interesting to debate how this statement makes us feel when we read it, rather than whether Einstein, who was neither an etymologist nor a botanist, said it, which he very well likely didn't.

chapter 10

Three weeks later, I stood beside the train tracks in Cologne, Germany. It was dark. My contact—and companion for the last three days—a tall, blue-eyed, more-salt-than-pepper-haired German beekeeper named Walter Haefeker, stood next to me. A huge billboard perched overhead was made up of green and yellow lights and shone the number "4711" for the limey, fresh, and slightly antiseptic cologne.[1] Finding my gaze on the sign, Walter told me that that exact billboard had been there, in the same place, since he was a small child visiting his grandmother in Cologne.

We were tiddly from our stop around the corner in a cavernous pub filled with long wooden tables where we'd eaten blood sausage with applesauce and mashed potatoes; Walter had drunk a large stein of beer while I'd had some wine from the Rhine Valley. For the last four days, ever since I'd met up with him at a beekeeping convention outside of Brussels, I'd been trailing Walter in that annoying way

---

[1] I knew it well, and just looking at the sign I could smell the cologne, because my mother, who spent some of her girlhood in Spain, had grown up using it. There is always an errant bottle of it somewhere in her bathroom, more for nostalgia than anything else.

documentary writers have, the constant devil on the subject's back, never disappearing, always hovering. From the convention we'd gone on to Brussels, the seat of the European Union, where he'd had meetings in the Parliament and European Commission. Then we'd taken a commuter train north to Cologne, where we'd met his friend Wolfgang at his favorite pub. Wolfgang, in the early 2000s, oversaw the initial labeling of GMOs for the German government. We would soon be on our way to Munich via the overnight train to meet a beekeeper named Karl Heinz Bablok, whose honey had caused a kerfuffle because he'd said it was contaminated with GMO pollen.

In a few moments, our iron horse came screeching into the station and, lumping our bags behind us, Walter and I boarded the train and gave our tickets to a dark-haired, smoldering-eyed, muscular man who reminded me of Vronsky in *Anna Karenina*. After depositing Walter at his berth, Vronsky helped me to mine, placing my bag for me on the small cot. He opened the doors wide enough so that I could peer in and see my accommodations. Having already pegged me for a damsel out of her element—which I surely was—he showed me how to work the lights, and then asked me in a thick accent what time I'd like to be awoken for breakfast and whether he should bring me tea or coffee. For a moment I could only stammer a bit, as I couldn't quite pull myself from the pages of my Russian novel. "Tea," I squeaked. Then, with a glint in his eye and a flourish of his arms, he closed the door and I was left in my boxlike room to figure out how to wash my face and brush my teeth.

As I was lying in the dark on my surprisingly soft and comfortable bed, warm under a comforter made up of a thick wool blanket buttoned into a clean, crisp cotton duvet cover, the train rocked and clacked along. I snuggled in, feeling cozy, and studied the safety card that described the many ways I could get off the train in tunnels and on bridges and what kinds of alarms would sound if my dark-eyed hero failed to come save me.

Then, using the flashlight on my phone, I turned to Ian Frazier's

Great Plains, the final pages of which I'd been meting out on this trip—hoping, as we all do with books that tether us—that I could stretch it a couple more nights. As I closed the back cover and turned off the light, I suddenly missed the big, complicated country I call home. I missed those plains I'd stood on not even a month ago in Nebraska; I missed our expansive vistas. And I missed Dan and Marsden, who were waiting for me in Italy while I zigzagged across central Europe with Walter.

Nestled into that narrow mattress and staring at the ceiling, I found my mind drop down in a freefall to land, uncomfortably, at the beginning of my journey. I was remembering a Tuesday morning in the fall of 2010. Dan and I were driving down the highway and away from our apartment in Portland toward Maine Medical's imaging center in Scarborough, where I was scheduled for a brain scan. By then I'd been sick for the better part of three years and we were scared. Conditions like multiple sclerosis and brain tumors were on the table. The results were supposed to be forwarded to my neurologist in Boston, who had ordered a second nerve test to be done at Mass General the following week.

It was just getting light out that Tuesday morning and shards of sun were hitting the colored leaves of the trees along the highway. The fact that we were driving somewhere alone, without Marsden, initially stirred in us the anticipation of an adventure, which was usually exciting. But I didn't want us to have to go on this particular journey. We'd already done enough hard journeys: one out west to California to start our newly married lives in the land of milk and honey, then another during the recession that brought us back home to Maine to move in with my mother. We'd gone through the journey of writing my memoir and Dan's first year in graduate school. And we'd begun the journey of becoming parents to Marsden.

Twenty minutes later, I was lying strapped to a table as the MRI machine groaned, shuddered, and then made tap-tap-tap sounds as it moved me, slowly, into the tube. My eyes were on Dan, who stood at my ankles. Then I disappeared from him, but I could feel his warm hands on my feet, and through the use of a little mirror above my face, I could see his eyes. He was looking *right* at me, wherever I was. The last time he had looked at me this way, I was giving birth to Marsden in Santa Monica, California.

The machine cranked and creaked and moved me to the next position and then Marcy, the technician, spoke through the earphones. "How are you doing in there?" she asked.

And I said the most honest thing I could think of: "I don't understand how I got here."

She was quiet for a full beat. "I'm sorry," she said. And then, almost like it was an afterthought, she muttered to herself, "I don't know how anyone gets here."

The brain scan brought no answers and by Christmas of 2010, I had gotten worse. I was so feeble I had to stay in bed most of the time. My son and husband went out into the world without me, snowshoeing, doing the shopping, and going to parties and playdates. We celebrated a grim holiday that year with me on the couch, my legs propped up with pillows under my achy knees.

Now, MILES FROM HOME on a train bulleting down the center of Germany, I felt a kind of relief wash over me that that was a long time ago, and that I was finally better, that all indications seemed to prove that whatever it was, it would never come back. Comforted by these thoughts, and that I was safe now in the, to borrow from Dylan Thomas, "close and holy darkness," I finally fell asleep.

In the morning, Vronsky banged on my door and handed me a cup of hot tea. "Hurry," he said. "We are arriving in Munich." I downed the tea in three gulps, washed my face, and got dressed in some cleanish clothes just as the train careened to a halt. I could hear people descending out of their berths.

When I emerged from my own, Walter was waiting, wearing a clean, pressed collared shirt. He looked like he'd just spent the night in a five-star hotel, not on the same train with me. He laughed when he saw me and said, "You realize they had to knock a bunch of times for you—they couldn't wake you up!" I was tired. This journey had been a lot, both physically and emotionally. And the train had become my womb for a few hours. I gave him a wry smile and followed him off the train into the bustle of Munich.

chapter 11

Walter and I had originally connected through a scientist at the University of California at Berkeley named Ignacio Chapela. I'd come to Ignacio through Tyrone Hayes, the herpetologist at UC Berkeley who studied frogs and atrazine. Tyrone had told me that Ignacio had had a huge ordeal—a lawsuit, threats, you name it—after he published a paper in *Nature* that showed that the United States' GMO corn was contaminating Mexican landrace corn. Since our initial connection, I'd been interviewing Ignacio on and off, trying to get his story down, because it fascinated me.

On this day, it was mid-September and boiling—a real Indian summer—and I was on the phone with Ignacio. In my upstairs writing room, even with a fan on full blast, I was dripping with sweat. He and I were talking about the fallout from my *Elle* magazine piece. Suddenly, he took a left turn to tell me about a GMO-testing device he had been designing for European beekeepers. He said something about a guy named Walter and threw out some rambling words about honey. I remember that I was scribbling notes and when he started on this honey tangent, I paused and thought, *What the hell are we doing now? Gosh, these scientists are nuts!*

Instead, I said, "Uh-huh." Ever the good reporter. "Tell me more."

Ignacio told me that this gadget he was making was inspired by a "need," he said, of beekeepers and honey importers for an inexpensive and effective way to test honey for GMO pollen or crop residues before their honey went to market. The Germans, Ignacio told me, were becoming particularly sensitive about GMOs—they did not want GMO pollen in their honey, and if they had to have it, they wanted it labeled.

This was—call me stupid—a revelatory thought. I had never considered the pollen in my honey (to put a finer point on it, I had no idea there *was* pollen in my honey). Or that I could reject one kind of pollen over another. Or where the bees that made my honey had been foraging. In fact, I'd never even spent much time considering the bee itself. The honey I thought about was something I imbibed in hot water with lemon for colds, drizzled on cereal and yogurt at breakfast time, and recalled my mother using in place of sugar for most of my crunchy childhood, claiming that it was "healthier." I thought about honey when I read *Winnie-the-Pooh* out loud to Marsden, and when spring came and the ants took up residence under the toaster in order to make their sticky journey to the honey jar. I loved to use honey in a recipe I'd originally found in an old *Martha Stewart Living* magazine for gingered honey carrots. To make them, you simply julienne the carrots and throw them in a pan with some ginger, honey, sea salt, and butter and cook until they are toothsome. I like to make this recipe for Thanksgiving along with the standard turkey, stuffing, Swiss chard gratin, homemade pickles, and chutneys I serve. Also, my good friend Jodi was getting really into bees and had recently started her own hives in her double-lot backyard in Portland. She sometimes gave us jars of her thick, amber honey in the fall. When she starts handing out Ball jars, I'll make a fresh plum, honey, and cinnamon tart with a simple oat flour and butter crust. But, to be frank, until Ignacio started yammering on about honey, the *what* of honey or even the *how* of it, hadn't really crossed my mind.

Ignacio elucidated more: He said that the Germans are truly crazy about honey. It's practically been a food group in some parts of Europe, he said, since 7000 BC. The Romans used to offer it to their gods, he said, and Napoleon carried a flag decorated with three bees—the flag of Elba—and had bees embroidered on his robes. Honeybees didn't make it to America until the seventeenth century, and by then the Europeans had built entire parts of their culture around honey. In Germany, in particular, a traditional breakfast across all regions of the country, he said, is bread with honey, often served with some muesli, yogurt, and fruit. Children are given bread with honey as an afternoon snack the way some French kids are given baguette smeared with butter and filled with a hunk of dark chocolate when they get home from school. And, he said, honey is considered by many Germans to be medicinal. In recent years, in fact, because of the incredible demand for honey—and the decreasing bee populations worldwide—the Germans are now importing honey from places as far-flung as Brazil, Africa, Canada, Argentina, India, and, sometimes, China. He said that he'd learned honey comes packed in big drums—or barrels—and that each drum is the result of sometimes "hundreds of families," all of whom have a few beehives each. By the time it's in the drum, it's been moved from its local providence—wherever that is—to a co-op to a middleman to a huge drum and eventually to Germany, where it will be bottled and labeled.

Ignacio said that a German importer had told him that he had hit a stumbling block in his importation business: In order to make sure his honey is GMO-free, he has to run some expensive PCR testing (testing for GMO DNA) to be sure the "GMO-free" label is accurate. And the problem was that his drums are often contaminated. He told Ignacio that even a small amount of GMO DNA from just one family's operation could ruin a whole drum, in which he's already invested quite a bit of time and money. So Ignacio had asked the guy, "Well, what do you do with it if it does have GMO DNA? Do you dump the honey into the sea or what?" And the guy says to Ignacio, "Oh no. We just send it to the U.S. where people don't care."

I remember writing in my notebook that hot day: "Wow, Americans don't care? Do the people not care? Or do the people just not know enough? Caitlin, learn more about honey and bees and Germans and labeling." Before we hung up, I asked Ignacio if he had a contact in Germany who could explain the honey situation to me. He said, "Sure. I'll email you."

I got off the phone and decided, while I waited for Ignacio's email, that I'd do some cursory research on honey. There was a lot to learn.

Honey, it turns out, really is the product of a Herculean amount of dedicated work foraging for nectar on the part of the bee. A single bee will travel up to four miles to source good nectar (sometimes going as far as seven miles to find it if conditions are not favorable) and will pollinate, in the process, a hundred thousand different plants (a single bee colony can pollinate 300 million flowers a day), making bees, some say, the "angels of agriculture," because without them, a third of our crops would cease to exist. After nectar foraging, in a complicated process of regurgitation, evaporation (using their wings to fan the nectar), and storage in the honeycomb, they make the final product, which we humans enjoy. (Lest we be worried about this, the bees usually make much more honey than they need to survive, so if we are conscientious in how we do it, we can take their honey and not harm the hive at all.)

I learned that each single worker bee lives, in the summer months, only six weeks, unbelievably, to create this sublime and complicated sweetness humans have craved for millennia. Indeed, honey appears in cave drawings that depict people hunting honey from wild bees as far back as 1500 BC, which seems to indicate that honey was the first "sweet" people tasted. (The early honey hunters in Germany, or

Zeidlerei, as they were called, carried crossbows in order to shoot ropes around tall tree branches so that they could hoist themselves up to wild hives to gather honey—this was before bees were domesticated with wood box hives, as they are now. In Germany, being a *Zeidler* was such a revered job that the city of Feucht took the image of the town *Zeidlerei* as its insignia.)

There is a myriad of uses for the wax, propolis (a resinous mixture bees collect from pine tree buds and sap), and pollen collected from a hive. Propolis can be used as an immune booster and can be an effective treatment of cold sores, wounds, and burns, and bee pollen has been touted as a natural remedy for seasonal allergies, lethargy, and eczema. In World War II beeswax was used as a sealant to coat tents, belts, and the metal casings of bullets. And, recently, the military has been attempting to use bees along with dogs to track land mines because of their incredible ability to smell.

Furthermore, all honey is not created equal: There's the superpure stuff you can buy at your local farmers market, which, if you're a discerning customer, you might be sure to purchase "antibiotic and treatment free."[1] Then, on the other side, there's the stuff that's been illegally imported from China—cheap honey often found in plastic bears on diner counters and in packets in fast-food restaurants all over the United States. This honey has arrived in huge barrels that are often not actually full of real honey; instead, the honey itself has been diluted with high-fructose corn syrup, rice syrup, or other nonhoney sweeteners, and it can have traces of an antibiotic called chloramphenicol, which is very toxic and illegal to give to food-producing animals in the United States yet somehow sometimes makes it through our screening process. Chloramphenicol can be dangerous, even fatal, to a small percentage of the population. (Even

---

[1] Ask your beekeeper where they place their hives. (Next to organic farms or the highway, for instance, might be the right question . . . though keep in mind it's pretty hard to control bees, since they forage and will, very likely, get chemical exposure, making this writer wonder whether it's possible to get truly "clean" honey.)

more scandalous, honey has often been found to be intentionally mis-labeled so that impurities are harder to trace. A 2013 investigative piece in *Bloomberg Businessweek* found that some importers of honey have intentionally "laundered" or changed the country of origin labels, claiming their honey comes from India when it actually came from China and then was shipped to India, where it was relabeled before it was imported into the United States.) You know the bears, they're everywhere:

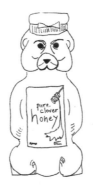

Before long, I was at once excited and concerned about honey. It appeared to be this incredible substance that held deep cultural and agricultural significance and was, clearly, for so many, more compli-cated than just a simple pleasure.

A few minutes later, I was shaken out of sweet honey reveries by the computer ping of an email coming in. Ignacio had sent an email introducing me to Walter.

> Dear Caitlin, Dear Walter,
>
> It remains, to complete an introduction, to say to Walter that Caitlin is a thoughtful, careful and persistent journalist, a very good writer and someone who will not back down from a story even under heavy fire. She wrote the very good and careful piece in *Elle* magazine, which attracted the

blood-hound/pit-bull pack led by Jon Entine, and from there
a whole storm-in-a-teacup.

Caitlin has been talking to me for some months about her
project for a book . . . I think she will discover and write
a wonderful story, especially by talking to people like
you, Walter.

I do trust that you both will find the contact of use and
interest.

My best,
Ignacio

After that (flattering) intro, Walter and I exchanged a flurry of emails
and then finally got on the phone to talk. I told him that before we
went too far, I wanted to know more about who he was and why I
needed to even think about honey as it pertained to GMOs.

Walter Haefeker told me that he grew up in the intellectually and
culturally vibrant city of Munich and that he is the elder son of two
college professors. When he was in high school, he left home and
moved into an apartment on his own because he was "having trouble
with authority." His grandfather, he said, was an officer in World
War II, in the Wehrmacht, an occupying force that was stationed in
Bretagne, until he was killed in a sneak attack by French partisans.
Walter's mother, he said, had never questioned the story she was told
as a child: that her father had been a war hero. Coming from the
postwar generation, Walter chafed at this. He saw his grandfather as
someone who, if not a Nazi, was a "useful tool for the Nazis." He said
in a later email, "In my mind, he allowed himself to be sucked into
the Nazi war machine and seemed to feel pretty good about it while
he was on the winning team." To him, he said, heroism is something
else altogether. He wrote, "The real heroes are probably the ones who
deserted or leaked information to allow the public to see the truth.

This is what I would have seen as a hero. My mother is more like many military family members in the U.S. who see their father or mother as a war hero and do not question the legality of the missions."

Walter matriculated early to the University of Munich, where he further outraged his parents by switching from a focus on mechanical engineering to the study of philosophy, which they thought would be useless. They subsequently stopped paying for his education.

However, while still studying engineering, he had begun working on math problems on one of the first personal computers that had become available, something called a Video Genie, which was a Radio Shack TRS-80 clone with a Z80 processor. It looked like this:

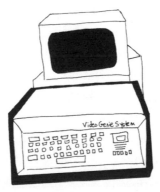

Yes, this looked more like a typewriter than what we think of as computers today!

Walter found this Video Genie computer fascinating. After dropping his engineering degree work, with more spare time, he taught himself how to program. Soon he set up a little company called Merkle Microcomputer, on the side of his schooling, which developed software for doctors. He used the proceeds, he told me, "to finance my philosophy education." This worked for a while. But as he continued to work on the software company, it got "bigger and bigger" and he had "less and less time for philosophy."

Very quickly, his company began to compete relatively successfully with Siemens, the large multinational company that builds computer applications for the medical field. Siemens took notice, swooped in, and made Walter an offer he "couldn't refuse." Still only in his early twenties, he decided to ditch college altogether and began to rise quickly as an employee of Siemens. "Among the blind, the one-eyed is king," he says of his unusual ascendance in the brand-new tech industry. Siemens decided they wanted to move Walter to California, where they offered to put him in charge of running a division in the Silicon Valley office. He quickly married his girlfriend, Angelika, whom he'd met in college, and together they packed up and moved to San Francisco, where they had two sons. Shortly thereafter, he became disenchanted with Siemens and quit.

But by then he had the entrepreneurial bug. He started setting up one company after another, he told me. "I somehow figured out relatively early in life that if I'm bored at something, I'm not good at it. I need to be involved in something fascinating; otherwise, I suck. My game plan was 'Make yourself obsolete as quickly as possible. Go in, set something up, hire the right people, give them the right plan, and then get the hell out of the way and be free to do something new,'" he said. Eventually Walter ended up as the COO (chief operating officer) of a company named Mediaplex, which was an Internet advertising technology company that helped companies achieve things such as advertising banners on their websites. (An example might be something like if Tickets.com were selling tickets to a Jason Isbell concert, Mediaplex would help Tickets.com build a banner that showed how many tickets were left and what the cost of the remaining tickets was, and this information would be updating continually.) Mediaplex was incredibly successful and eventually had its IPO with Lehman Brothers. On that one day, Walter made enough money to retire, even though by then he was only in his early forties. A self-made American Dream at that point, he could have gone anywhere, done anything. Walter, however, was losing his interest in America. It was early 2001 and he had watched George W. Bush's election and "just anticipated incredibly stupid choices," he said.

So he and Angelika decided that it was time to "sell everything and get out." She and their sons flew ahead to Germany; that May, Walter set sail for Europe on a yacht that he had harbored in San Francisco Bay. On the journey he removed the American flag and chose, instead, to fly the Maltese flag because, he said, "This is a small country nobody has a beef with."

Back in Germany, Walter and Angelika bought an old house in the town of Seeshaupt, one of the most exclusive and tony towns outside of Munich, situated on Lake Starnberg. They remodeled it so that they could heat it effectively with firewood and wood pellets. (Walter eventually put in an "automatic heating" unit that burns wood pellets, for which he developed his own software to control and monitor it.) They bought a large parcel of forest nearby to provide enough wood to heat with and an old farm tractor to haul the wood. The tractor piqued his interest in old farm equipment, so he began perusing eBay regularly. In an auction comprising various items, he won two old-fashioned basket beehives that arrived sealed with cow dung. He said that when they were dropped off at his farm with all the other equipment, he decided that he "didn't want them as a museum," so he set them up in his garden. Walter then went out and bought two artificial swarms. When he got them home, he brought his sons, Marc and Tommy, outside to look. His youngest, Tommy, then six, ran inside and got some sunflowers in a vase and brought them out to feed the bees. When he saw that his boys were "just drawn in" by the bees, something emotional happened to Walter. He said that for some people "it's not that you're choosing bees; bees choose you. There's certain people where something happens and you're a beekeeper." For Walter, this was that something.

Walter and his family jumped into the beekeeping enterprise with the same energy he had used to establish all his businesses in the past.

Walter studied beekeeping intensely; he wanted to become an expert at it. Soon he and his family went from two beehives to more than a hundred. In short order, however, both Tommy and Angelika developed serious allergies to beestings. This was very upsetting to both of them because the family had fallen in love with beekeeping and bees. Also, Angelika had just completed a bumblebee-breeding course in Bonn; and all of a sudden she could not continue with this newfound passion. In response, Walter and Angelika enrolled Tommy in a desensitization program at a local university clinic while Walter, undeterred, forged ahead with the bees. He moved the boxes away from their home to their forest property and carried on alone, now solely in charge of the bees. But together, the whole family found some connection by designing the honey labels together and marketing the honey at holiday markets where they made beeswax candles with children. They invested as a family in growing their brand and educating people about honey and bees. Never leaving his tech background behind, Walter eventually developed an iPhone app called iQueen, which helps people plan out queen breeding schedules. He was all in.

One gets the sense that the pastoral life, even with the serious intensity with which he approached beekeeping, and though seductive after years in Silicon Valley, was not going to totally satisfy Walter's incredible energy and drive for larger success. He started to get involved in local beekeeping associations, and back in 2003, when he was the "new kid on the block" in the German wing of the European Professional Beekeepers Association, he was assigned, he said, "the new problem that no one else had time for": GMOs.

At that time, the general idea in Europe was that eventually "Europe would go whole hog for the GMOs just like Canada and the U.S.," he said. Walter was tasked to figure out what that would mean for beekeepers, because "beekeeping is an open system—it's not a barn. In other words, we don't decide what we're feeding our animals. Any change in agriculture would affect bees."

At first, he said, he thought this would be an interesting project but not necessarily life altering: "I wasn't an anti-GMO activist looking for a fight, you know, picking up some bees to do it." But he dove in anyway: "Together with some colleagues I went out to figure out the properties of the crops and what the legal situation was and relatively quickly I realized that this was going to be a huge problem for us . . . [and] that there was no intention [on the EU level] to do anything to protect our products or our bees from the impact of GMOs." Walter threw himself into understanding everything he possibly could about GMOs—from the science to the political climate—and the possible risks to bees. What he learned made him fearful that what was coming down the pike would be, he said, a "disaster" for bees and beekeepers. And to put a finer point on it, if it was a disaster for the bees' health, then what did that mean about the effects on humans?

Then, as if by divine intervention, he found Karl Heinz Bablok—the "hero" of this story, he told me. Bablok was a beekeeper whose honey had apparently been contaminated with GMO pollen. And it was at that moment that Walter realized he'd hit a fork in the road of his life. Suddenly, bees, beekeeping, honey, and the agricultural policies that surrounded apiculture would become his raison d'être.

chapter 12

Okay, so I was hooked. We had honey (arguably one of the purest, most iconic food substances out there), a hero, mysterious GMO contaminations, Europeans grappling with their GMO-labeling issues, and the fate of bees (apparently as hot an issue in Europe as here at home in America, which I understood in only the vaguest terms so far). And I had a completely bilingual tour guide who, incidentally, had just said, "If you want to learn more about honey and meet Karl Heinz Bablok, I will be at a bee conference outside of Brussels in November. You can meet me there."

That night, after putting Marsy to bed, I asked Dan how crazy he thought it would be for me to go all the way to Europe to hang out with a handful of German beekeepers whose honey had *maybe* been contaminated with GMOs. I was freighted, it sometimes felt, with an awesome task: to shed some light on the GMO issue as it stands today; to open the door for a better, more informed national debate in America; to write the primer for all those parents out there who didn't understand (like I didn't) what the hell this GMO discussion was all about, and, at the same time, to not turn into some crazy siren on the subject. I told Dan about how, through my initial phone call with Walter, I'd come to believe that honey was the perfect lens through which to examine the European policies on GMOs, and by doing so, I'd learn what was different in our country.

To make sure I wasn't presenting Dan with a very expensive but totally half-baked plan for spending our money and gallivanting around the globe, I had given myself a second short crash course that afternoon before coming home. This one was on the GMO discussion across the pond. I can't tell you how many times I'd heard from Americans, whenever I told them that I was working on this book, "They do it so much better in Europe." This was always delivered to me as such an incontrovertible fact. I wanted to know, do they really do it better there? What's different? Should I go all the way over there to find out?

When GMOs were first in development in the United States in the late eighties and early nineties, the Reagan-Bush administration, instead of taking a critical and scientific approach to the new products, was "inclined," writes Peter Pringle in *Food, Inc.*, as a result of some heavy lobbying from Monsanto, "to give U.S. companies every opportunity to exploit the new technology without being weighed down by burdensome rules." He goes on to write, "Despite persuasive scientific arguments that biotech engineering was more than just an extension of traditional breeding, and despite a general acknowledgment that the nation's laws governing food safety were not equipped to take care of the new science, the administration decided to treat the new foods as no different from the old ones. It was the product that mattered, not the process." This position was further adopted with the appointment of David Kessler as commissioner to the FDA in 1990. He, according to Pringle, "gave his full support to the Reagan-Bush stance, overruling scientists in his office who warned that genetic engineering was unknown territory that might create unexpected risks in plants and even people." According to a 1999 piece in the *New York Times* by Marian Burros, which covered the public hearings that were convened because of the FDA's apparent siding with industry, the FDA biotechnology coordinator, Dr. James Maryanski, was informed at least twice in private memorandums, once by an FDA compliance officer, Dr. Linda Kahl, and then by an FDA microbiologist, Dr. Louis Pribyl, that there might be unintended side effects to the genetically engineered foods and that, as Pribyl wrote, "there is no data to back up their contention" that the foods are "safe." According to Burros, Maryanski, however, held steady that "as long as developers of these foods 'follow the agency's guidelines and do the testing that is recommended,' though not required, genetically engineered foods were 'as safe as any food on the market.'" To further back up industry, Vice President Dan Quayle stated that the United States "was the world leader in biotechnology" and that the government wanted "to keep it that way." In other words, let her rip.

If regular food-buying Americans were paying attention to this circus going on in Washington at all—which most, frankly, were not—they understood, perhaps in some vague terms, that in Europe activists and consumers were rejecting GMOs just as the U.S. regulating agencies were effectively dodging any notion to proceed with caution. Burros writes, "Now many British supermarkets require labeling of genetically modified products." That was 1999—five years after the first GMO, the Flavr Savr tomato, appeared on supermarket shelves in America, and probably fifteen or so years since GMOs had started being grown outside in the open air, potentially contaminating other crops nearby through pollination, animals, or just human error.

Although, from the distance of time, it seems, by reading news reports, that back in 1999 the case against GMOs was about to blow open and Americans were poised to begin their own battle for their food, no such revolution came to pass. Despite the increasing concern, and the resultant media coverage, the government, and therefore the industry, was able to sit back and rest on the Bush administration's 1992 assertion that "the new foods were 'substantially equivalent' to the old ones; and that they were 'substantially safe,'" according to Pringle. Although the Canadians, too, were well on their way to an open-armed adoption of the new technology, a report from the Royal Canadian Society, Pringle reports, mocked the idea of "substantial equivalence" by writing, "To say that the new food is 'substantially equivalent' is to say that 'on its face' it is equivalent (i.e., it looks like a duck and it quacks like a duck; therefore we assume that it must be a duck—or at least we will treat it as a duck). Because 'on its face' the new food appears equivalent, there is no need to subject it to a full risk assessment to confirm [the] assumption." In other words, GMO foods are innocent until proven guilty. Furthermore, Pringle writes, in Britain, at the University of Sussex, "researchers argued that there was 'intentional fuzziness' here. . . . 'It is exactly this vagueness which makes the concept useful to industry but unacceptable to the consumer.'"

In Europe, health officials were claiming that "substantial equivalence" did not mean "safe," and they were busy instituting a comprehensive GMO-labeling law, which allows no more than 0.9 percent of detectible GMO into a supermarket food product (not including meat, dairy, alcohol, and, it turns out, honey). Meanwhile, in the United States, a fog of confusion was generated around the words "substantial equivalence," confusion that would persist into perpetuity, making it almost impossible for the regular consumer to engage with "substantial" knowledge on the subject. As Michael Pollan wryly pointed out in the PBS documentary *The Botany of Desire,* based on his book of the same name, there's "a suspension of disbelief" one must engage in to accept the "substantial equivalence" idea.

The problem with honey began, I told Dan, when beekeepers started to become concerned that honey had been overlooked in the labeling laws—it had been thrown into the "animal products" category—wherein it's inferred that foods of animal origin may be considered to be produced from a GMO only if the animal itself has been genetically modified—with very little consideration for the fact that if there was any one food product that would come into direct contact with GMOs, it would be honey. As beekeepers and honey distributors saw it, both honey sourced in Europe near GMO fields and imported honey from other countries could be contaminated with GMO pollen and nectar. How would it be labeled? beekeepers wanted to know. How would their consumers react? What began as a question mark on the part of a few German beekeepers developed into an enormous Europe-wide debate, which went all the way to the Court of Justice, Walter had told me.

Dan was listening to all this while he made us some tea from fresh mint I'd grown in our garden and then dried. And then, ever my cheerleader, Dan said, "Go for it! Sounds really interesting. In fact, aren't Uncle Tom and Aunt Sally still at their house in Italy? How about we all go?"

So, on a cold November evening, Marsden, Dan, and I said goodbye to Hopper and our cat, Hemingway, piled our duffel bags into the back of the car, and drove from Portland down to Boston to catch a plane to Rome. This was Marsden's first time on an airplane, which thrilled him.

Our flight left Boston in the middle of the night, after numerous delays. It was full of older Italians. I couldn't help but remember the story my mother had told us of a similar trip she and her family took when she was fifteen and they decamped from New York City to go live in Mallorca, Spain, where her father set about trying to write the great American novel (that is yet another tale for another time). They took the *Vulcania*, a big, lumbering ship, and traveled steerage because her father thought that was how all the interesting artists traveled. Well, my mother tells us, steerage, it turns out, "was full of Spaniards on their way home to the motherland to die."

On our trip, the minute we boarded the plane, we were already in another country. No one spoke English as their native language. So I found myself dusting off and stumbling through some twenty-year-old ItaloFranSpanglish to order our dinner. After eating at the stylish hour of 1:00 a.m., all the lights went out. And then, across from us, a sleeping Italian man began crying out in his sleep in garbled yet religious-sounding Italian, waking himself up, mumbling some Ave Marias, then falling back asleep. He sounded in pain. Every time he yelled, I'd jump and my eyes would shoot open. The woman next to Dan was snoring, mouth open, a little stream of drool coming down her cheek.

During the night, everyone on the plane used the toilet, which was right next to our little banquette of seats. Each time someone new went in there, slamming the door shut and then making themselves comfortable while wafts of shit-smell emanated from under the door, I'd turn to Dan and say, "How is it possible that everyone on this entire plane needs to poop?" By the time the pooping started—now well after 2:00 a.m.—and even though I'd made many preachy pronouncements about how I was not planning on sitting my four-year-old down in front of a bunch of movies the whole flight (I'd prepared with games and books and crayons and, somehow, insanely, I'd imagined he'd actually sleep), I quickly threw this notion out the window and allowed a Charlie Brown episode about a pumpkin (over and over), even though I find Charlie Brown rude and annoying.

After seven hours that felt more like one hundred, we descended to a steaming-hot tarmac and balmy Roman fall weather. We immediately made a beeline for the airport espresso bar and then began trying to earn a quick engineering degree from MIT in order to put the Italian car seat into the back seat of our rental. Finally, we piled in and headed north to Tuscany. As we drove, we passed fields of winter wheat growing fresh and green in soft, brown, fertile soil, interwoven with farms that grew kale, broccoli, fennel, potatoes, olives, lettuces, and chard. Although Italy is trending in the direction of America, with big agri-farms starting to patch up the landscape as younger Italians jettison the provincial ambitions of their forebearers and go off to college and beyond because they are hoping for bigger-paying jobs, the country still maintains a kind of holistic farming rubric that has not been seen in many parts of America for decades. *What a contrast*, I found myself thinking as we passed a rainbow of crops, *between this and the walls of corn in Iowa.* Finally, we took some curvy streets through sepia-stone buildings and found my aunt and uncle's red-roofed *villino* near a lake.

The next morning, Dan and Marsy went to work with Uncle Tom, harvesting olives to make olive oil. As they worked outside, I worked inside, getting myself ready for my trip to meet Walter at Beecome, the beekeeping convention being held outside Brussels. Walter had laid out the itinerary for me: After three days at Beecome, he and I were going to take the train north to Cologne to meet Wolfgang Koehler (the lawyer who had worked in the German government in the Ministry of Food Safety, Agriculture and Consumer Protection overseeing the labeling of GMOs in the early 2000s). From Cologne, we'd take an overnight train to Walter's home city of Munich, where he was going to introduce me to Karl Heinz Bablok, the guy with the contaminated honey. Although I was a little daunted by the logistics of how I'd catch as many planes and trains as seemed necessary to make this all come together, I put on my game face and started mapping it all out.

That night, I went for a run, the sun setting quickly. In the dark I took a narrow road that wound through olive groves and vineyards, past farms with chocolate-earthed and fragrantly fecund fields. As I ran, the moon came out—a tiny white fingernail, hanging like a delicate, shiny charm on a necklace in a pitch-black sky. As I passed a large chestnut tree, an owl startled and flew away; on my way back, it startled once again (having figured, I suppose, I was gone for good the first time). I remember thinking as I ran in the dark, the olive trees almost audibly breathing on the sides of the road, that I didn't know if I'd ever felt quite so peaceful.

The next day, after managing in our jet-lagged state to sleep through the alarm, we got up quickly and ate some fruit and hard-boiled eggs for breakfast. Then we began an epic car ride with Dan speeding through the curvy roads of the Italian countryside until Marsy puked eggs all over himself and the car seat. When we finally got to Orvieto, where I needed to catch my train, not one person in the whole town could tell us how to get to the train station. Everyone knew where the tracks were. But the station itself was mysterious. Finally, somehow, after driving in circles, we found it, ran in, and bought my ticket from a woman who seemed to think we were very amusing, rushing around like the overcaffeinated Americans we are. After saying good-bye to my family on the platform, I took a train by myself back to Rome, through the lush river valleys along the Tiber River. In Rome, I caught a train to the airport where I flew to Brussels, through the most incredible turbulence and wind I think I've ever experienced. While bouncing along on the airplane, I was able to catch up on the news back home from a *New York Times* I'd picked up in the airport. I found that the labeling initiative in Washington State that Dave and Lisa had been working on had been defeated. Again Biotech had far outspent the opposition and GMO labeling was not going to be a thing of the immediate future for yet another state. Then, after a long train ride out of Brussels and finally getting off in the dark and pouring rain at the wrong, deserted stop in a small Belgian town, I finally made it, via taxi, to my hotel, which, by then, looked like the promised land. I ordered steak frites for dinner and a big glass of red wine, and called Dan. We talked while I ate, both of us relieved I was there after what seemed like a crazy trip to travel just a few hundred miles. After my dinner, I went up to my hotel room, where I took a bath and agreed, via text, to meet Walter in the lobby the following morning.

chapter 13

Morning came quickly, cold and rainy. Walter was waiting for me in the lobby and was dressed in faded designer jeans, a collared shirt, and an army-green Bavarian jacket (a traditional and handsome style of jacket made of boiled wool, with no collar and shiny buttons that march in a line up the front). His friend Karl Reiner, also a beekeeper, was pulled up outside in his minivan. Walter and I hustled through the rain and piled in. Soon we were on our way to the convention, which was held at the low, gray campus of a Catholic university called Université Catholique de Louvain. The three of us unfolded out of the minivan into the pouring rain and made our way inside.

Over three floors, vendors from all over Europe had fanned out and were setting up long tables of honey jars that varied by region, flower pollination, and time of year they were collected. They ranged in color from the lightest amber to the darkest molasses. As I went from table to table sampling the different honeys on little spoons, I was amazed by the range of flavors and different levels of viscosity.

The most sublime honey I tasted that day was a coriander honey from Hungary—it was almost peppery on the tongue, with a lemony cilantro aftertaste followed by an intense hit of sweetness. (I am still, to this day, kicking myself for not purchasing it immediately. Thinking it was still early, I told myself I'd go back. By the time I did, it was all sold out. So I settled, instead, for an herbaceous chamomile honey.)

Tables were filled with everything from bee hobbyist paraphernalia—bee-covered mugs and dishes (I bought a sweet white bumblebee-covered mug and a matching eggcup for Marsy), bee stuffed animals, bee-emblazoned flags, signs, buttons, books, and curiosities—to more serious beekeeping necessities such as bee boxes, big stainless-steel honey extractors, clothes, hats, gloves, smokers, queen-rearing kits, and jars. I felt a little like Alice; I'd fallen into an alternate universe.

Overwhelmed by the sheer volume of bee products (many of which I had no reference point for), and a tiny bit of convention fatigue that started to waft over me like a fog, I tagged along, following Walter here and there, standing back and listening as he said hello to people he knew from past conventions. As he made conversation about his thoughts on, for instance, "flower power," a concept he's developing to replace corn biodiesel with diesel made from "bee-friendly" flowers grown in rotation as cover crops by farmers, I found myself chatting on the periphery of his conversations; for a time I sat with a silver-haired Irish man sporting a gray suit.

As Walter and I traveled through his day, a picture started to come together for me: Walter was a kind of "green knight"; in every interaction, whether his subject was bees, biodiesel, what he called the "maizification" (or cornification) of our planet, or food, he was consistently interested in moving his environmental agenda ahead, and he was always looking for solutions to the questions that loom like thunderclouds on most environmental agendas. Unlike much of the fear-based messaging from many environmentalists, Walter always seemed perky, game, upbeat, and never fatalistic about any of it.[1] Later, in the evening, I joined him in an enormous amphitheater full of beekeepers, politicians, and European dignitaries to listen to speeches on the subject of bees. It was here that the convention took a hard right turn into the GMO topic, any fluff and puffery surrounding beekeeping left behind for good.

The beekeepers' speeches, in particular, were fiery, with beekeepers from around the world (including Walter) taking the EU to task for pretending to be friendly to bees while still leaving the door open for the biotech industry. A Spanish beekeeper named Manuel Izquierdo García, from COAG, the largest farmers union in Spain, gave an impassioned speech condemning the widespread cultivation of GMOs in Spain and how it's affecting bees. (Colony collapse disorder—or CCD, a condition affecting massive bee losses—rates in Spain are some of the highest for all of Europe, and the Spanish and Portuguese governments, unlike much of the rest of Europe, have embraced biotechnology and continue to cultivate GMO crops.)

When the EU director of the Safety of the Food Chain at the European Commission, Eric Poudelet,[2] a small, thick-lipped Frenchman, took to the podium, the theater full of five hundred or more people booed vociferously. Over their booing, he tried to convince them, essentially, that he is "acting in the best interests of the beekeepers." Bees, he told the audience, were a priority for him when he considered any industry proposals. Thunderous booing in response. He persisted and got through his speech, though, truth be told, I'm not sure anyone heard much of it.

Next, a parliamentary member named Mariya Gabriel from the European People's Party took the beekeepers to task for standing in the way of GMOs, saying that GMOs were entirely safe and had been

---

[1] He wrote me an email as I was finishing this book to tell me about a concept he's developing for "digital plant protection" to replace "chemical plant protection." He wrote, "this is not just a fight against something but also a quest to create alternatives."

[2] Poudelet has now retired from this position and some say he's engaged in beekeeping somewhere in rural France.

proven so, so why such difficulty from the beekeeping sector? More booing.

Finally, Walter, scheduled to give the closing remarks for the evening, took a cue from Marc Antony's famous speech "I come to bury Caesar, not to praise him" and began with an uncharacteristic, though smirky, apology to Mr. Poudelet, saying, "I would like to apologize to Mr. Poudelet. He was unjustly accused of taking the side of industry. This is entirely our fault. We are not often enough in his office. [We leave] him so much time to listen to the stories of industry, that he now honestly believes them to be true." Uproarious laughter. He went on to eviscerate Poudelet for understanding absolutely nothing about the gravity of the situation, and he listed the planetary challenges of a world without bees (no crop diversity, food scarcity, etc.). Oddly, I expected Poudelet, sitting in the front row, to look uncomfortable, or at least perturbed. But he smiled gamely and then, at the end of the speeches, stood around yakking with colleagues and even a few beekeepers in what seemed to me to be an unusual camaraderie. The presentations now over, Walter told me that the speakers and audience had been invited "for drinks and snacks" and that he "need[ed] to do some lobbying."

I followed Walter into a large, packed reception area where canapés—all made with some kind of honey ingredient, either drizzled into a sauce or baked into a crust—were being passed and honey-brewed beers were poured. People stood in small, hungry groups, speaking intently about bees and honey. I remarked to Walter on how the atmosphere was distinctly collegial and he told me that many of the European beekeepers know each other by now; they see one another at yearly conferences like this one. Because he seemed to be feeling more open with me than he had been earlier in the day, Walter introduced me to colleagues as we made our way around the room.

Almost immediately, he deposited me at the side of a dark red-haired female scientist, whom I guessed to be in her late forties or early fifties. She was from Greece, she told me, and her name was Dr. Fani

Hatjina. Fani, whose smile seemed to create an orb of light around her, was schooled in Greece and the UK, where she clearly chose early on that her specialty would be bees—and she never looked back. Her résumé is singularly impressive—she has been published in numerous books and journals, has lectured at universities and scientific conferences around the world, and is on board as a referee at numerous apicultural journals and awards. She is known for her work analyzing bee pathology, looking at bee risk assessment, and studying how biodiversity (or, for that matter, monocultures) affects bees. More recently, she has turned her focus to the effects of pesticides and pollution on bees.

She told me that she has been trying, for a long time now, to get her hands on some Cryproteins—she has requested 10 micrograms—from Monsanto's European headquarters in Brussels[3] so that she can conduct some risk assessment on bees. But she has been denied. She did say that some reps from Bayer CropScience (the biotech wing of the pharmaceutical company Bayer, makers of aspirin, among other things) came to Fani's office and offered her their results from studies they had done. They suggested that she work with them, but that she would need to do the research on their terms, and only publish the results if they agreed. She apologized for being unable to join them.

As Fani and I huddled together in the overwhelmingly disproportionate sea of men, she told me that she felt that she and other scientists have "so much evidence [about the dangers of GMOs and pesticides to bees, given the number of studies that are coming out from all over the world about pesticides used in areas of intense industrial agriculture where GMOs are grown and their effects on bees]. But we need to find more." Where it stands now, she said, is that she believes GMOs and pesticides work together to compromise the immunity of bees, though they might not outright "kill all the honey-

---

[3] Though headquartered in St. Louis, Missouri, Monsanto has offices in sixty-six countries throughout the globe, which their website describes this way: "variously administrative and sales offices, manufacturing plants, seed production facilities, research centers, and learning centers—all part of the corporate focus on agriculture and supporting farmers."

bees on the planet," but "GMOs are often engineered to produce pesticides themselves. The proteins they produce are toxic to insects. Therefore they belong to the same 'large' category of 'insects killers.'" She said that scientists like her are always searching to find an ace in the hole, and that one study never feels like it will be enough to tip the scales against the incredibly powerful reach of Biotech. She said, "There are quite a lot of studies from the industry. They invest a lot of money in this." But the problem remains: if Biotech is doing their own studies, are they accurate? As we know by now, they certainly aren't independent.

In Fani's statements, I was hearing echoes of something Lisa Stokke had said to me during a phone call after I'd been in Iowa: "Our side—the activists—don't get this right because they've [the biotech industry] got science—or so much more science. And the second our side has a little bit of science, they rip it to shreds." David Michaels, the assistant secretary of labor for Occupational Safety and Health, wrote in his 2008 book, *Doubt Is Their Product,* that the corporations, taking a cue from the tobacco industry, now double down on what they call "the science": "Industry," he wrote, "has learned that debating the *science* is much easier and more effective than debating the *policy*." "In field after field," he wrote, "year after year, conclusions that might support regulation are always disputed. Animal data are deemed not relevant, human data not representative, and exposure data not reliable."

When I brought up this problem to Simon Hogan, he nodded vigorously. He said that the pro-GMO side "has an abundance of science to point to. They are world leaders in that. But when it comes to the consequences of the plants themselves, instead they have an enormous amount of circumstantial data, which, ultimately, they will try to drown you with. That's where the strength of their argument is—you're going to struggle to beat [them at this]." Furthermore, Simon said, "It's going to be extremely difficult to have a positive outcome in moderating the conversation without some more substantial evidence to indicate that GMOs are having a negative impact on human health. . . . [I believe] that evidence is probably there, but it's just being able to find it." In other words, tighten your chin straps, scientists, because this is not going to be easy! (And, I guess, should it be? Despite the obvious hurdles—funding, and the powerful reach of Biotech being the most instrumental—we will need good, sound scientists asking tough questions and trying to prove or disprove their own questions so that this GMO question can be unraveled effectively—and clearly—before it's completely too late.)

Call me an emotional sponge, but I noticed as we meandered around the room that Walter was becoming increasingly tense; Eric Poudelet had arrived and was milling around and Walter was waiting for the moment when he could corner him. I stood to the side, smiling benignly at whoever looked my way. Suddenly, a French beekeeper named Étienne, who has furtive eyes and long, shaggy hair cut in a grown-out punk rock do and who was wearing skinny jeans and a slim gray jacket, approached me and said, "Aren't you the American journalist whom I gave a press pass to?" I told him that I wasn't sure since my pass had been left for me in an envelope at the reception desk, but nonetheless I introduced myself and thanked him for procuring my pass. "Stay here," he said. "Mr. Poudelet will want to meet you."

When Mr. Poudelet arrived at my side, an ironic smile stuck on his face, as if the whole shindig was enormously amusing, I asked him what he thought of being booed by the beekeepers. He laughed and, while exchanging a look with Étienne, told me that he believes he is a friend to the beekeepers. He told me that he, himself, has bee boxes on the balcony outside his office at the European Commission. (When I asked Walter about this, he said this gained little credibility with him. "He is trying to make hay with us," he said dismissively.) Poudelet went on to tell me that he is doubtful that GMOs are harmful. He said "there is no evidence" to convince him. He insisted, instead, that I should pay attention to his efforts on the two-year ban of neonicotinoids, the systemic pesticide, which was set to go into effect a few months after I met him, in the spring of 2014. (This ban was the result of numerous European studies on neonicotinoids, including one from Italy, which indicated that they disrupt the immune systems in bees.)

Neonicotinoids, or neonics, as some farmers call them, are, as the word "systemic" infers, a kind of pesticide that is taken up by the plant into every cell of its leaves, pollen, flowers, fruit, guttation drops,[4] and seeds. They are made from nicotine and used on both GMO and non-GMO crops (not to mention that neonics are used as tick- and mosquito-prevention sprays on lawns, to treat shrubs and flowers we buy at the garden store, in termite and ant treatments, as top-spot treatments on our dogs and cats for fleas and ticks, and in wasp sprays). It takes less neonicotinoid to kill a rat than a fly, interestingly (and terrifyingly), which may speak to how they affect mammals. At any rate, neonics have been fingered—most decisively in Europe to date—as the cause for the worldwide and devastating losses to honey-bee populations due to the condition called colony collapse disorder, or CCD.

The term "colony collapse disorder" was coined by Americans in 2006,[5] after a significant rise in bee colony disappearances in North America (coinciding with both an explosive growth in the use of neonics in 2005 and the enormous expansion of GMO crops, which carry their own insecticide, taking over more than 90 million acres of farmland for just corn alone, as stated earlier). CCD is characterized by a hive in which an entire colony of bees has just vanished. Only the empty hive is left, sometimes full of honey, often with a brood of unhatched larvae, and always with a forgotten queen languishing at its heart. Most peculiarly, the honey in these abandoned hives—which researchers have found to contain no presence of pathogens or

---

[4] Little drops of sap on the tips or edges of the leaves that the bees drink. (In a study published in *Ecotoxicology Journal* in 2009, bees fed a water solution that mimicked the amount of neonics in guttation drops found that the bees became intoxicated and then died.)

[5] The English initially called it Mary Celeste Syndrome, after an 1872 merchant ship that left port in New York and was found four hundred miles east of the Azores by another ship. When the sailors from the second ship boarded the *Mary Celeste*, they found it empty—no captain, his wife or daughter, and no crew. Oddly, the ship was well stocked with food and water and the cargo was still there.

mites—isn't robbed by other bees or hive pests, like the wax moth, the small hive beetle, or ants. Why would the robbers stay away? researchers wonder. What's happened? One theory rests on the idea that the bees get sick and either disoriented about where home is or, in an act of selfless honor, fly away from the hive so that the larger hive does not get sick. The problem seems to lie in the fact that if all the bees are sick, they all disappear (except for the queen). Researchers are still trying to understand this phenomenon, and with no dead bees to dissect and test (since the hive is empty and the dead bees have effectively vanished into thin air), it's been challenging. The most solid conclusion seems to boil down to some combination of the "three p's"—pesticides, pathogens, and parasites. Of these three, many researchers are focused primarily on the increased use of pesticides worldwide, because pathogens and parasites have, for the most part, always existed. Researchers have found more than 150 chemical residues in the honey, pollen, and wax gathered from CCD hives, and many wonder about the synergistic effect of a toxic soup of insecticides, herbicides, and fungicides. Researchers in Massachusetts have found that in every hive affected by CCD, there is neonicotinoid residue, a fact that just blows my mind when I think of honey as a medicinal, healing substance, which may have been turned, by our modern world, into a kind of poison. And yet, to date, in the United States, with our usual reluctance to get on the bad side of any multinational chemical companies, we have been slow to ban or restrict neonics, as has been done in Europe. The EPA states that we need more evidence.[6]

While we wait for more evidence, the most devastatingly enormous losses due to CCD are being suffered by American migratory

---

[6] In November 2015, the EPA issued a cancellation order for Dow Chemical's sulfoxaflor, a subclass of neonicotinoids, after six years of petitioning from the Pesticide Action Network, the Center for Food Safety, and Beyond Pesticides, and a court case from the American Honey Producers Association and the American Beekeeping Association. In the original petition to the California Department of Pesticide Regulations, it's written, "All neonicotinoids kill insects by interfering with their central nervous systems, causing tremors, paralysis and death."

bee colonies—in other words, those bees that are physically transported around the country to pollinate crops (they are the migrant
workers we may never even think about, who have no rights or voice,
and yet, like other migrant workers, are imperative to our food economy).[7] Every year, huge truckloads of migratory hives will arrive in
California to pollinate almonds and then go north and east to the
Dakotas and the Great Plains, then to the Midwest, then up to my
home state of Maine for the blueberries, then south and then back out
to the Midwest again before going back to California—following the
growing cycles of crops that need pollinating. Some services even
ship bees by 747 from other countries like Australia to come pollinate
in the United States. This is a big business. Not only do farmers desperately need bees because over one-third of the world's agricultural
crops need pollinators to produce, but 90 percent of our wildflowers
need them to survive and thrive. One of the biggest businesses in
America that depends entirely on bees is the California almond business, which comprises 80 percent of the nation's almond groves (and
supplies close to 90 percent of the world's almonds in trade) and is a
multibillion-dollar business.[8]

Some contend, probably correctly, that a world without bees is
one that will become inhospitable to people. At the very least, it will
be enormously expensive for humans to figure out how to pollinate
their crops without bees—though it's worth noting that in some
parts of China, where bees have all but vanished, crews of people are
being deployed into the fields with small Q-tips and paintbrushes to,

---

[7] Watching Internet videos of beehives being loaded on trucks for a long trip down the interstate made me wince; there's something inherently emotional about watching the bees flying
around their hives, desperate and confused as their home base begins to move down the road.
Sometimes huge nets are used to contain the bees; sometimes bees are just left behind. It's
best, I'm told by my beekeeper friend Jodi, to move the bees at night, when they are sleeping.
This is not always possible, she said—deadlines need to be met, crops are in flower, money
needs to be made, and people's schedules can't afford the extra time.

[8] As a tangential thought, while researching this subject I vowed never again to feed my children or myself another inorganic almond; almond groves are coated with neonicotinoids. I
can't imagine that if they cause immune problems in bees, they wouldn't, even in small
amounts, begin to disrupt our own immune systems.

essentially, do the job of the bees. And though these workers are not nearly as good at it as the bees, do not lose all hope: researchers at Harvard have come up with a mechanical robot, the RoboBee, which will take on the bees' job, and scientists at a university in Germany are working on a genetically modified bee.

In the middle of my conversation with Poudelet regarding his work on banning neonics, an earnest-faced beekeeper, whose accent sounded to me to be from the South of France, approached and implored Poudelet to do more on behalf of the bees. Poudelet seemed to barely listen; the man's entreaty became a source of fun for him and Étienne; they giggled and exchanged looks. For me, it was painful to watch Poudelet laugh so openly—and with such an unabashed lack of respect—as the man described the plight of his bees and his concerns about GMOs and agricultural chemicals. I'm not sure Poudelet meant to be rude, actually—it might have been nervous laughter of some kind, since I was standing there; and I'm not sure I understood the relationship between Poudelet and Étienne, the latter of whom I just assumed would be working on the side of the bees. But it was awkward, to say the least. Poudelet laughingly told the beekeeper that "the problem with you all is that you're not organized. Get organized!" His point seemed to be that if the beekeepers could mobilize specifically against GMOs, they would move mountains. He ended the conversation claiming that beekeepers had "all of the sympathy of the Commission—more than any other farmer in Europe!" "Remember you presented us with two million signatures!" he said. "*Deux million!*" he exclaimed again, putting up two fingers for emphasis, reminding the beekeeper of the referendum on neonicotinoids that was presented to the Commission. (Walter told me that actually there was a second petition that was circulated and that, in total, the Commission received more like six million signatures on the subject of neonics.[9])

---

[9] To compare: the USDA's public online forum on the new 2,4-D–resistant crops and their accompanying pesticide, Enlist Duo, made by Dow Chemical, received five hundred thousand signatures against their approval. And yet they were still approved.

Poudelet, all smiles, turned back to me, effectively done with the French beekeeper.

Over the heads of the people milling around us, I could see Walter's eyes flashing. He wanted to get to Poudelet and here Poudelet was waylaid by that damn writer he'd brought along! Soon, Poudelet was pulled off in another direction and I stood talking to a beekeeper standing nearby. For the rest of the evening, Walter hovered just outside of wherever Poudelet stood, trying to get his attention. Finally, as the reception drew to a close, Walter was able to make his move. In a hushed conversation, he and Poudelet went into a huddle—heads down, iPhones out, affirmations made—and a meeting was set for the next morning in Brussels. After that, Walter relaxed a little bit and said it was time to go.

As Karl, Walter, and I made our way to Karl's van, Walter erupted at me, furious that I'd gotten some one-on-one time with Poudelet. He claimed that Poudelet was pandering and sucking up to me and that it made his job harder. We drove back to the hotel in a stony silence after that outburst. I was unsure of how to go forward.

Later, over dinner back at our hotel, I pasted a smile across my face and ordered a delicious seafood stew, full of fish and mussels and clams in a simple broth of tomatoes, onions, garlic, and wine, made by a chef who proudly extolled the simplicity of his ingredients to me, while Walter tucked into a burger with fries and a beer. As the blood sugar numbers went up, everyone seemed to cool out a bit. As we ate, Walter wanted to talk about our plans for the morning, when he would meet Poudelet, then a Green Party contact, and then some members of the Parliament. However, Walter told me that after seeing how my presence had affected Poudelet at the conference reception, he was wary of my influence as an American, as a journalist. He reiterated to me, "It's not a question of intention. . . . [But] whether you want it or not, it alters the course of events."

Finally, after some deliberation, while his friend Karl looked increasingly nervous and tired, he decided that the Green Party meeting would be fine for me to be a part of, conceding, "Their stance with us is their public stance." But in the other meetings—with Poudelet and some parliamentary members—Walter said he'd fly solo. I nodded, and shortly thereafter I begged off dessert and made my way back to my hotel room.

When I finally got back to the small, clean room I called my own, I phoned Dan to vent. "It's so irritating!" I moaned. "He's so arrogant and controlling and privileged and *rich*." I inexplicably threw that last word in as a final mark against Walter. "I came all this way and now I'm cut out. And even more, I want to like him because he's doing important work, but I can't like him because he's a *jerk*." I started to cry a bit. Suddenly I wished I was back in Nebraska on Zach's tractor, or driving through Iowa listening to Ryan Adams.

"Cait," Dan said, "you don't have to like anyone you're writing about. You just have to listen to them and write about what they do and say and what they are working for or against."

"I guess," I sniffled, only slightly mollified. After we hung up, I pulled out the little glass jar of honey I had purchased that afternoon from the Hungarian couple at the conference. I held it up to the light. It was so clear and yellow, like the golden tip of a chamomile flower. With the hot pot provided by the hotel, I made myself a cup of chamomile-lavender tea (my nightly ritual—last summer Marsden and I grew both chamomile and lavender and dried it to make our own) and tipped in a generous pour of the sweet honey. Before tasting the tea, I stuck my spoon back into the jar, filled it, and guided it to my mouth. Conscious, as I stood there, of the floral and fragrant substance in my mouth, I realized that I had come this far—across the Atlantic—with only shreds of knowledge about GMOs, bees, honey, labeling, pesticides, and the politics that surrounded all of the above. As I traveled further into the topic, I was slowly starting to put the pieces together, but there was still so much I didn't know and didn't understand. Each day was proving to be both revelatory and arduous.

chapter 14

The next morning, I was up and ready to travel to Brussels and on to Germany with Walter. Something about the early start, the darkness surrounding us, and the slightly bleary yet excited beginning of a trip together seemed to shorten the space between us ever so slightly. In the dark, with a marauding sky spitting rain, we sped through the Belgian streets to the train station in a taxicab, talking easily. Inside the busy, shiny station we bought our tickets and boarded a train full of early-morning commuters to Brussels. Women dressed in stylish jeans and high heels stood reading books as the train bumped along; college-aged kids with full backpacks and Timberlands closed their eyes, catching a few extra z's; almost everyone had their earbuds plugged into their ears, affording them each their own private universe.

Walter and I sat separately, alone with our thoughts. Soon the train came to a halt at Bruxelles-Midi station and we filed off. Walter knew his way and effortlessly negotiated us through the dreary station, rolling his suitcase toward some lockers. I followed with my own rolly bag and, witnessing now how streamlined his travel gear was, I realized how bulky and impractical my own was. A few moments later, we boarded the subway and traveled to the European Commission, the executive body of the EU government.

On the subway, Walter told me that at that moment the Parliament was considering a labeling vote that had been proposed by the Commission (and Mr. Poudelet) and which would directly affect beekeepers, because it would reverse a decision made in the European Court of Justice in 2011 that required honey to be tested and labeled if it contained GMOs (hence the California scientist Ignacio Chapela's efforts to come up with a good, affordable testing device). The Commission was essentially saying that honey was its own entity and was neither a lableable ingredient nor an animal product, so therefore it was no longer necessary to label. If allowed to go through, this decision would undermine years of Walter's work.

Walter said the whole ordeal had a déjà vu quality to it. He told me that when he first addressed the labeling issue, back in 2003, he had met with Wolfgang Koehler at his office in Germany's Federal Ministry of Food Safety, Agriculture and Consumer Protection. Through Walter, I had talked some to Wolfgang on the phone from Brussels in anticipation of our meeting. Wolfgang told me that Walter had approached him about the EU's oversight of honey back when the EU had started making laws that required the labeling of foods containing GMOs. Honey, Wolfgang said, didn't fit into the legislation for animal products (which allows animals to be fed GMOs, a result of the trade alliances and the deals that were brokered between the EU and the United States) or into the products *made* with GMO ingredients. Honey wasn't thought to be connected to the cultivation of GMOs, where the bees would surely forage and bring back not only GMO pollen but also GMO nectar. And, he said, the "beekeeper had been forgotten" in the legislation. But when Walter came to visit him and started asking questions about how the government could protect bees and beekeepers from GMOs and the labeling laws, Wolfgang realized there might be a problem. At first, Wolfgang said he told Walter to "just be quiet; you have nothing to do with GMOs, so don't wake up sleeping dogs." But Walter would not keep quiet on this, Wolfgang told me. "That's Walter's problem, he is never quiet."

So, on this bleak, gray day in Brussels, with icy rain coming down in fits and starts, Walter was extremely concerned that the Parliament could, essentially, override the European Court of Justice—a battle that he had fought for a long eight years—and decide to group honey with all other animal products. For this reason, he had set up meetings in the Parliament with anyone who would listen to his reasoning.

But first up this morning was Poudelet, with whom Walter's job was twofold: First, to warn him against the cultivation of Pioneer's TC1507—a GMO corn variety the EU was currently considering approving for widespread cultivation, restarting the early EU battles that eventually led to a GMO cultivation ban in many EU member states. And second, to entreat him to work with the beekeepers to help protect honey from GMOs in the first place. According to Walter, Poudelet was at the helm of a team at the Commission who were trying to undo the now famous Court of Justice decision "with some legal trickery." He told me that the "bottom line of the Commission's trickery is the claim that as soon as GMO pollen enters honey, it somehow, magically, becomes a natural product." Walter's hope for his meeting with Poudelet was to dissolve the stereotype of unworldly, frumpy farmer-type beekeepers and have a sophisticated, beekeeper-to-beekeeper talk with Poudelet.

Walter left me in a coffee shop next to Poudelet's Commission office, where he found me a little over an hour later people-watching, sipping a jasmine green tea, and eating a darling little French yogurt that came in an old-fashioned glass yogurt jar. I had been imagining the lives of the polyglot crowd that came in and out of this place to have coffee and eat lunch. Walter sat down heavily. He looked weary, and, for the first time since I'd met him, the tiniest bit vulnerable. I asked him how it had gone. He told me that, at the very least, he felt he had achieved his goal of helping Poudelet understand the predicament beekeepers now faced—with no labeling, they could not convince their consumers their product was safe.

From the teashop, I followed Walter to the subway. A few stops later, we ascended and wound our way through streets flanked with important governmental-looking buildings until we came to a small restaurant for our scheduled lunch with his contact from the Green Party. The restaurant was half dining establishment and half curiosity shop, with anything from funky handbags and unusual toys to some clothes for sale. The proprietress was dressed in a skirt and sweater, had a long dark braid down her back and a friendly, pretty face. We found a table without any trouble and Walter ordered tea with lemon while we hung our wet coats on a rack along the wall.

After a few sips of the warming tea, Walter was ready to give me more information. It was in these down moments with Walter that his incredibly accurate and scientific mind began to shine; in short, his ability to break down the GMO issues in regular parlance was exceptional. Walter turned our conversation to his understanding of some scientific research done at the University of Jena between 2001 and 2004 by a German scientist named Hanz Hinrich Kaatz. The way Walter explained it, Kaatz had been evaluating the effects of Bt (the pesticide bred into GMO corn, soy, beets, potatoes, alfalfa, and cotton) on honeybees. When fed Bt insecticide (which Kaatz provided at a concentration ten times higher than what some scientists believe would be the normal amount of Bt a bee would come in contact with), he speculated, the honeybees were more susceptible to nosema, a common bee disease caused by a microscopic fungus called *Nosema apis*, and were more likely to die from the condition. However, when the bees were treated prophylactically with an antibiotic, they seemed to weather nosema and survive. Kaatz speculated that the Bt toxin may have "altered the surface of the bees' intestines, sufficiently weakening the bees to allow the parasites to gain entry—or perhaps it was the other way around, we don't know."[1] Kaatz said that he wanted to continue studying his findings but that he was not able to secure any more funding for the pursuit. In the end, the conclusion drawn by Kaatz was that Bt in small doses was probably okay for healthy honeybees. However, Walter explained to me that nosema spores are present in almost every beehive—even healthy ones. He went on to say that healthy bees that are affected by nosema suffer no clinical effects. But when Bt is added to the mix, he believes, it may create a situation in which nosema is much more toxic to an already compromised bee.

To understand this, he told me that the way Bt works when it's inside a GMO is that it punctures the walls of, for example, the corn borer's gut and allows bacteria to then enter the gut. If treated ahead of time with antibiotics, Bt will still puncture the intestinal wall, but septicemia—blood poisoning from bacteria—will not take place. What does this tell us? I wondered.

According to Walter, Kaatz's study proves, then, perhaps inadvertently, that Bt will damage a bee's gut and therefore lead to increased immune problems and susceptibility to disease that the bee would have weathered as just a normal course of life before the introduction of GMOs. Walter's question was, What does this tell us about Bt and insects and the way the toxin works? He pointed out that in the United States, where antibiotic use is still legal for beekeepers (it's illegal in the EU because antibiotic residue is left in the honey), the bees are often being prophylactically treated with antibiotics. Perhaps coincidentally, he thought, this may help some cope—to some degree— with the Bt crops for longer than they might otherwise. (In large-scale honey operations, especially those that migrate, antibiotics are de rigueur; antibiotic residue is found in most honey if it's not organic.)

---

[1] This conclusion is similar to a more recent one two USDA scientists, Jonathan Lundgren and Jeffrey Pettis, came to as well. Their research shows that pesticides somehow weaken the immune systems of bees and make them more susceptible to disease. Both Pettis and Lundgren came under heavy fire from the USDA for this conclusion, and Lundgren has filed a whistle-blower suit, claiming the USDA tried to muzzle him for implicating pesticides.

What we don't know, of course, is whether the antibiotic use helps the bees cope with the assault to their systems from pesticides, parasites, and pathogens over the long term or if, after a long period of antibiotics coupled with the assault from a variety of environmental factors, they are actually further weakened, making CCD more likely. All this is still a mystery.

Walter went on to tell me about a study called "Midgut bacteria required for Bacillus Thuringiensis insecticidal activity," a 2006 University of Wisconsin study. In this study, evaluators essentially were able to prove that for Bt to work on gypsy moth larvae, indigenous midgut bacteria need to be present. Similar to Kaatz's study, if the insects were prophylactically treated with antibiotics, the Bt will not work the same way, because the bacteria will have been destroyed. Walter explained it this way: "If you lay siege on a medieval city and manage to puncture the city walls, but have no soldiers to enter, then the hole is of no consequence."

This interested me because I, like many people, have been following some of the research into antibiotic overuse and the lack of important microbes in our bodies, which may, some research seems to indicate, be affecting our gastrointestinal health and leaving us more susceptible to inflammatory disease. So, like many people, I pop a lot of probiotics with the hope that I might be able to reverse damage from the many years of taking antibiotics when I had simple colds. As Walter was talking, I started to wonder if, perhaps, a possible problem for humans eating foods that are genetically engineered to carry their own pesticide, or Bt, might somehow be connected to our microbes, the amount of antibiotics we've taken, antibiotic resistance in people, and that "gut leakiness" everyone seems to be talking about lately (which is, simply, small holes or perforations in the gut, which allow toxins and proteins to escape into the bloodstream, causing allergies and inflammatory disease). And if I add to that the possibility that our gut pH may have been changed by the overuse of antacids and PPIs, like Maalox and Nexium, it made me wonder if Bt, or other proteins tested by Monsanto in tubes but not in animals (since Monsanto has deemed those studies to be "not valid"), could, indeed, pass through our intestines and make us sick simply because we do not have the right amount or right kind of microbes, and/or our pH is too alkaline. This was nonscientific thinking, to be sure, and I didn't know where to go with it because the issue at hand was bees and their guts, not humans. But it did get me lost in thinking.

Several months after I got back to the United States, I was still thinking about these questions. Since I'm neither a doctor nor a scientist, I still wasn't sure how to put all those pieces about gut microflora and Bt proteins together into any kind of cohesive statement, if indeed one were warranted. So, when I was working on this section of the book, I called up Dr. Martin J. Blaser, the director of the Human Microbiome Program and professor of microbiology at the NYU School of Medicine. Dr. Blaser authored a book called *Missing Microbes*, about how our overuse of antibiotics is fueling our modern plagues and, more specifically, how early-life perturbations of our microbiome—the beneficial cadre of good bacteria we need in our guts to fight off disease and be healthy—may cause "inflammatory disorders such as type 1 diabetes, asthma, psoriasis, and skin infections."

Dr. Blaser told me that he did not have any answers specifically about Bt. But he did say that if what's inside a GMO is an insecticide or a pesticide, then "insecticides and pesticides often have an antibacterial function, so that's an important question." He said, "I think it's possible." Because of this, he is now turning his own research to try to understand what happens when we ingest these pesticides. What are they doing to our microbiome? he wonders. Could they be part of the problem? Just to play devil's advocate for a second, I asked him if he believed animal models would be the way to start to get some answers. "Absolutely," he said emphatically. "We mammals are enough alike that if we find such a relationship in one, it would very likely be found in another." Would bees predict anything in humans? did he think. He was cautious in answering this question. "The farther the animals are from humans," he said, "the less likely that the information is transferrable. That being said, we have learned a lot from fruit flies and worms about human genetics and physiology. In the interface between microbes and their animal hosts, there is deep conservation, which implies the utility of studying what happens in other life-forms when microbial populations are perturbed."[2]

Back in Brussels later that day, my tangential microbe reverie was interrupted by Corinna Zerger, from the Green Party (in Europe this is called the Greens/European Free Alliance Group), who had arrived for our lunch. Corinna is a wan, blonde-haired woman who works as an adviser on food quality and food safety for the Green Party. As soon as she sat down, we all set about to order: a green salad for me, savory tarts for both Walter and Corinna. While we ate, the two talked strategy (despite the fact that they are both German, they conducted their conversation in English so I could listen in).

Walter's role throughout all this appeared to be mostly as the interpreter for Corinna of what the issues are for European beekeepers vis-à-vis GMOs. He briefed and prepared her with all the possible arguments the Greens could go up against as the labeling vote disseminated through the Parliament. He told her who in Parliament thought what, what their weak points were, why they were strongly for or against labeling, and why and how the Greens could help inform those members and with what information. Again and again he brought the conversation back to his salient point: "All we're asking is that honey be treated like other foods [and continue to get GMO testing and labeling]." (As a side note, Walter has also made it a habit of leading his audiences when he gives speeches and talks on the fate of bees in a sing-along that goes like this: "All we are saying, is give bees a chance.")

---

[2] While I had Dr. Blaser's attention, I decided to ask him via email about chronic Lyme disease, which I was treated for with copious amounts of antibiotics that made me worse, and likely damaged my microbiome. He wrote, "This is a long and more complex subject, but in brief, I think you understand it well—many patients have been victimized and brainwashed by unscrupulous caregivers who have fed them a line which is dangerous to them."

. . .

SOON OUR LUNCH was over and we made our way to the capacious
parliamentary building. Passing through metal detectors, we followed
Corinna up carpeted hallways, under gleaming chandeliers, and by
groups of men and women conducting hushed conversations with
heads leaned in toward one another, nodding intently. I was deposited
in a large cafeteria outfitted with plush chairs and small tables, where
throngs of aides and various politicians gathered for afternoon coffee
and tea. I found a spot near a leaky window and prepared to wait for
Walter, who had fortified himself enough at lunch with tea and food
to begin lobbying in the bigger leagues. He was excited, it seemed,
to be in a building where he could optimize his influence in a few
key areas.

I settled down, feeling dejected that I wasn't going to any of these
meetings, and spread my coat over myself to keep out the draft from
the window. I watched a lonely red-billed chough sitting in the rain,
its shiny black feathers soaked. Corinna came back out to check on
me and to hang out a little bit. While I sipped a warm coffee, I asked
her what her party's position on GMOs was. She said point-blank that
it has always been to get GMOs out of Europe. But she said it's been
complicated. Take animal feed, for instance. Because Europe has
been in a position of importing animal feed from the United States,
Canada, Brazil, and Argentina, animal feed is allowed to be GMO in
Europe, because Europe hasn't been growing its own "protein plants."
This, along with a dietary shift ("Europeans [like Americans] are eating more and more meat and the production is more and more prof-
itable. . . . "), has increased the demand for animal feed, because, like
in the United States, "you can have thousands of pigs and poultry
without having enough soil to feed them." Grain, she said, is cheaply
procured from the United States, Canada, and South America—
thanks to trade agreements made by the World Trade Organization.

When she mentioned the WTO, I remembered that Walter had
told me that the WTO essentially bullied the EU into taking GMO

animal feed by threatening "punitive tariffs" against the importation of German cars, French cheese, Italian prosciutto, etc.

Later, back in the United States, sitting in her ample yet modestly decorated office housed in an old fish-processing warehouse overlooking Portland Harbor on a clear-as-a-bell fall day, Maine's congresswoman Chellie Pingree would ratify this when she told me, "I'm opposed to our current trade agreements. [I] don't like the behind-the-scenes wheeling and dealing and [I] don't like the fact that we say, 'You're going to have to take our GMO feed or we won't sign the agreement.' . . . The trouble with trade agreements is you get pressured by the people who stand to benefit, and nobody tells you all the deep dark secrets that are in the agreements."

The WTO pressure is the result, Walter went a step further, of deals brokered when the large multinational chemical companies—whose influence in D.C. had been described to me by Chellie Pingree as "massive"[3]—began to get nervous about the fact that Europe was leaning toward going totally anti-GMO—animal feed and the whole nine yards. "The EU regulation of GMOs—the rules we have here—are not the result of a democratic process in Europe," he told me. "It's a big compromise between what was desired by the people [and what was] forced down the EU's throat by the WTO."

Now, sitting in the doldrums of the Parliament with no access to the offices where Walter was leaning on various parliamentary figures about bees and honey labeling, I asked Corinna the question I had been wondering since I arrived in Europe: Did she believe that this fact—that the animals in Europe are fed GMO animal feed—somehow undermines (or even undoes) the European position of labeling foods? I asked this because in the few days I was in Italy, I saw some chicken in the local grocery store with what's called a positive label: it said "No OGM." (In Europe they call GMOs "Organisms Genetically Modified.") This is the kind of label we're seeing with more and more

---

[3] Severin Beliveau put it this way: "Money is the mother's milk of politics." And, he said, "They [Monsanto] have tremendous influence in Washington, both sides of the aisle."

prevalence in the United States (think of the Non-GMO Project[4]). A positive label campaign basically circumvents the significant problem the various ballot initiatives have encountered, which is that industry—Monsanto, Dow, Pioneer, Pepsi, Coke, Morton Salt, etc.—have all outspent each initiative to such a huge degree that it's been almost impossible for any state (except Vermont) to get an effective legal labeling effort through. So, the only other alternative has been this "positive labeling," which is paid for and done by the companies that want to advertise their food as "GMO-free" themselves and requires nothing of the government agencies.

I told Corinna that when I asked some local Italians how they felt about GMOs, they adamantly told me that there were no GMOs in Europe. I pushed the matter and asked, "Anywhere? Even animal feed?" The resounding answer seemed to be that their country—Italy—was, to the large part, an anti-GMO zone, and that, for the most part, all of Europe followed suit.

Corinna paused for a second and looked at me quizzically. Slowly she said, "I suppose many Europeans, yeah, simply do not know that the meat they eat might, if it's not from organic animals, have been fed with GMOs. . . . That's more reason to label. If it was put on the label that this milk comes from cows who have eaten GMOs, then I'm sure people would buy other milk. . . . Of course there are more and more of these 'GMO-Free' labels appearing in the member states, which is, of course, the second-best choice."

What Corinna was saying intrigued me because I realized—in a clouds-parting kind of moment—that although many of us in the

---

[4] When I asked Dave Murphy to explain the Non-GMO Project to me—as in, *what is it exactly?*— he said this: "The Non-GMO Project was set up by the organic companies because they were concerned about contamination. In a lot of ways, it's a good transition label. But the real problem is that it undermines organic. You have to remember that there are pesticides, and herbicides and systemic chemicals still being used [on non-GMO food]. Just because you bought a non-GMO doesn't mean you avoided the gambit of pesticides used on most nonorganic crops." In other words, the only way to avoid GMOs—because anyone can slap a "GMO-free" label on their products—is to buy organic (this will be even more the case if the FDA is able to require that positive labeling like "GMO-free" now has to be supplanted with longer, more complicated language, as their draft guidelines issued in November 2015 suggest).

United States seem to think that they have it all figured out in Europe, they don't, exactly. It's complicated there, too. (Or, as Greg Brown sings in his song "In the Dark with You": "It's weird here, but it's weird there, too!")

What I started to wonder that afternoon in Brussels was, were Europeans duped when they got the victory over labeling *most* of their foods? Did anyone take the time to point out the fine print? Is this kind of like the trade agreements Chellie told me about when she said, "So a lot of times [the voting on trade agreements] is so fast and members get so much pressure unrelated to that issue, it'll be about shoes or steel or something else that's important to your district, and suddenly you get to the vote, you make the decision, and you're like, 'Oh my God, I didn't know that they were going to dump toxic chemicals on my backyard. Jeez, no one told me that part.'"

Soon Corinna needed to go. She was working, she told me, on the labeling proposal Walter was behind closed doors discussing. But I had one more question for her before she left. I had been hearing—all over the place, it seemed—that the Europeans tested their food more rigorously for GMOs and also had done more testing than the FDA requires in the United States. This was always intriguing to me, because I wondered why those tests—if they had indeed been done—hadn't been decisive one way or the other. In other words, why didn't the tests either (a) make GMOs downright illegal or (b) persuade the activists in the United States to accept GMOs if the Europeans found them to be safe?

"Do you do rigorous testing in Europe before a product is put on the market?" I asked.

Corinna looked a little shocked by my question. "Not rigorous," she said. "I mean, at EFSA—at the European Food Safety Authority—they just rely on what the companies present them."[5]

With that, Corinna picked up her bag and went off to work. But, geez, that sounded awfully familiar. . . .

---

[5] EFSA says that they are more involved than in the United States and will conduct their own research if they feel that there are holes in the data provided by industry.

chapter 15

By the time Walter texted me, saying he was done with his meetings and wanted to meet me outside, it was dark out. I had fallen asleep for a little while in the cafeteria, huddled under my coat like that wet chough outside, ignorant to the comings and goings of Europe's political leaders.

Rejuvenated by the quiet time I'd spent just sitting and dozing, as I'd had nowhere to be for a few hours, I hastily picked up my things and descended through the brightly lit building, still full of people networking, even though it was well after six at that point. Walter and I found each other under a street lamp on a corner and began our walk to the subway, which would take us back to the train station and, finally, north to Cologne.

Walter was, for the first time since I'd met him, moving slowly, like the marathon was over. Though he told me that his meetings had all been positive and that he'd been given ample audience, his limbs looked limp under his tweed jacket and raincoat, as if he'd been to battle using only a slingshot and his wits. "On a day like this," he told me, "you can see how much could be accomplished if I were in Brussels more often—if I were willing to endure the pain and suffering." He went on, "One of the things that gives [me] credibility is, I'm not getting paid. I'm not a paid campaigner on an issue. If someone can convince me that it's a nonissue, I'm more than happy to go sailing." I found myself wondering aloud if an American beekeeper would have the same traction. "Well, you have to understand," he said, "ten years ago this would have never happened, okay? This level of attention you have to earn. You have to essentially be enough of a problem. . . . I mean, we won a GMO court case against the European Commission and Monsanto, okay?" Still, it was undeniable to me that evening, after seeing Walter in action, that his demeanor, CEO experience, and the incredible power he's leveraged since taking up the cause of bees have made him, essentially, a lobbying power broker. And his currency is honey.

In the train station we stocked up on Belgian chocolate (my favorite!) and bottled water and found a drab waiting room with hard plastic chairs where we could sit and wait for the train. Sitting together and drinking our personal waters and munching our personal dark chocolates, we began to laugh and talk. The biggest part of our journey now over, Walter and I could just interact as people. I felt he had finally started to like me, for the first time since we'd been traveling together. And, somehow, just thinking he liked me made me like him. Also, watching him from the sidelines during this long day had made me respect him. I knew he would stop at nothing to get his job accomplished; he had gotten up early and navigated numerous personalities and environments with aplomb, even when I could see that he was getting tired.

On the train, Walter sat just ahead of me. I sat next to a German cellist on his way home from having his cello fixed in Paris. The train was full of people, quietly working, talking, or reading. I had a bag of the most sublime Sicilian clementines, which I'd carried all the way from Italy and had been eating since I left. As the train swayed and clanged, I peeled them, their tangy perfume making the night feel like a holiday in a storybook far away from home on a European train.

Across the aisle from me sat two American men from Wisconsin—one a big, heavyset blond wearing khakis and a collared shirt, and the other a smaller, dark-haired man wearing glasses—who sold agricultural parts for combines to companies like John Deere. What a funny synchronicity, I thought, that I've crossed Nebraska and Iowa, then come as far as Europe, only to meet up again with American Big Ag. With wireless that somewhat worked on the train, I was happily writing emails and logging on to Facebook when the train came to a screeching halt and an announcement sounded over the loudspeaker in German only.

I turned to my friend, the cellist—with whom I'd become quite chummy because the little trash container between us would fall out of its holder every time I tried to deposit my Clementine peels and he'd taken to gingerly holding it for me each time I finished a tiny fruit. I asked him to translate what had been said over the loudspeaker.

He said, "There has been a bump alert."

Oh, a bump, I said to myself as if this made perfect sense, and tried to imagine the height and girth of a bump that would bring a fast-moving train to a full stop. I thought of the children's story "Strange Bumps" in our bedtime standard, *Owl at Home*. In this story, Owl gets into bed and sees two strange bumps at the bottom of the bed. He jumps out of bed and the bumps disappear. He gets back into bed and they reappear. Poor Owl gets hysterical trying to find the bumps—they keep reappearing and then they seem to grow, getting more and more terrifying. Finally, exhausted, Owl gives up and goes down to his living room and sleeps in his favorite chair.

On the train, next to the cellist, as I tapped away at emails and "liked" things my "friends" were doing on Facebook, I thought of Owl's feet at the end of his bed making those nefarious bumps, and just as Owl's bumps grew, the longer we sat on the train, the bump on the track began, also, to turn into Kilimanjaro for me. Finally, though still in very good humor due to clementine nectar and little sips of Internet surfing, I got up and walked to Walter's seat, where I laughingly proclaimed that I worried I might never meet Wolfgang if we sat there any longer.

Walter said drily, "Yes, it's a bomb scare. I have no idea how long we'll sit here."

"A bomb scare," I squawked, turning to my cellist friend and accusing, "I thought you said it was a bump alert! I was picturing a really, really big bump on the train tracks!"

Everyone around us broke out laughing. Despite my preternatural proclivity for disaster-prone thinking, the joke of the bump became much bigger than the fear of the bomb. (My dear friend Craig wrote to me that perhaps I was really sitting next to Inspector Clouseau in disguise: "*Excuze-moi*, but zer is a bump alert!") Soon, "the bump" was dealt with and the train moved along.

Not long after, Walter and I ascended the escalator out of the station, toting our bags behind us, and arrived at the central square of Cologne, the magisterial Gothic cathedral called Kölner Dom rising imperiously in front of us. Because Walter was hungry, and Wolfgang was waiting, we quickly made our pilgrimage to the Gaffel Am Dom pub, a large, open, and brightly lit space, filled with long wooden tables. As beer was swilled, I did as the Germans did and ordered those aforementioned blood sausages served with applesauce and mashed potatoes, which Walter told me he gets every time he stops in this pub. (The blood sausage, though I worried it might be disgusting, was oddly creamy inside and actually delicious along with the sweet applesauce and soft mashed potatoes. This was, indeed, a comforting meal, just as Walter had advertised.)

With not a moment to spare, we tucked into our meals, and it was time for me to hear Wolfgang's story of how he came to be involved with Walter and the beekeepers and what his role was in the German legislation around GMOs.

Wolfgang began by telling me that he was trained as a lawyer and eventually ended up working in what he called "political management" in the chancellery of the German government. Then, in the late nineties, he was given the job in the Federal Ministry of Food, Agriculture and Consumer Protection, despite the fact that "nothing in my life had ever had anything to do with agriculture," he said. (Except that "I like eating," he quipped.) In the first two years of his tenure, he was responsible for the legal language that was used in food labeling—allergens, ingredients, preservatives, etc. Then he was asked to take over the "GMO Unit" (not to be confused with the Bloodhound Gang . . . er, did I just date myself?), called the Division on Biotechnology and Genetic Engineering. This was around 2003, he said. He said he wasn't sure he wanted to do it because the only thing he knew at that time about GMOs was that "it was a big struggle, big discussions everywhere." He also knew that Germany was very influential in the greater EU and whatever he did would have larger ramifications—both political and, perhaps, healthwise. He said, "The German vote is quite important for this. So if the Germans say yes, it's much easier to have authorization, and if the Germans say no, sometimes it doesn't work." He told the committee that he would think about it; it seemed like a big, and perhaps complicated, job, one he really wasn't sure he wanted. "Then, a half hour later, I had the Minister [of Agriculture] on the phone telling me congratulations, you can have it." At this, Wolfgang laughed into his beer.

After his appointment, Wolfgang set out to learn everything he could about the GMO debate and about GMOs themselves. What he realized immediately was that it was a tangled issue and that there wasn't yet a coherent framework with which to address all GMOs—in animal feed and therefore meat and dairy, prepared foods, alcohol, and honey.

Initially, he said, he thought he'd deal with labeling grocery store items. Animal products were complicated because of the feed, and honey was just not on his radar much at all at that point. That is, until Walter and his cohorts started visiting him. Wolfgang told them that in his legal opinion he felt there was no place for a discussion of honey in the GMO debate. He said that his first take on Walter was that he felt that Walter was using honey "as a trigger to just defeat the GMO issue in Europe." And he didn't want to be involved in that. Furthermore, he told them, "you don't need to label it, you are out of the GMO case because it's not an animal product—honey is . . . something special." He argued that since honey is not metabolized by the bees, it would never be labeled as an animal product and, also, honey didn't technically contain GMOs as an "ingredient," like in a prepared food. According to Wolfgang, the regulations were done and no one in the dairy or meat sectors were protesting, so his legal opinion was that Walter should go home and stay quiet. But in his personal opinion he, like Walter, started to wonder if honey might become an important issue. "There was a big curtain, a big black cover-up on this whole issue," he said. He knew already that when the labeling discussion was initiated, the food industry had pushed back when some lawmakers suggested that dairy and meat needed labeling. This was complicated, and he said, because even though he told me that he thinks it's widely understood that, for instance, you can find fragments of the Bt DNA and Roundup residues in the milk and meat from animals fed GMOs, the consensus has been that they don't do anything to the consumer. "If you eat pork, you don't get pork ears," he said. So the thinking went that "even if you feed your pork with GM soy, the meat will be the same. . . . I'm not sure if that's true. But that was the excuse to exclude [meat, eggs, and dairy]." It was a loophole—one that many, like Wolfgang, thought would just be ignored.[1]

I wondered out loud to Wolfgang whether he felt that the European people had effectively been duped—by people in government like him—into thinking that there were "no GMOs in Europe." I looked around the busy pub where we were eating and asked him if the people at the pub didn't really know that, indeed, most of their

---

[1] Obviously if Bt can show up in human pregnant mothers' cord blood, it's going to show up in cow meat and milk. Swedish researchers proved the "Bt in milk" point, and in 2014 German researchers found glyphosate—Roundup—in milk.

animal products were produced with GMO feed (including, perhaps, those blood sausages I was eating at that moment).

Wolfgang told me he thought it was unlikely that most people sitting in the pub had any idea—that they likely assumed most everything they ate had nothing to do with GMOs. He said he thought it was a political mistake to write the laws this way, and that he felt this might eventually come back to haunt the EU lawmakers. As far as the consumers go, he said, "They wouldn't be very happy with this" if they understood it clearly. Wolfgang went on to say that "if we change the GMO-labeling system on the European level, if we could succeed in the labeling of animal food, you can be sure that the question is resolved in Europe because nobody will buy a steak that is labeled 'produced from GMOs.'" Later, he said, "That would be the death, the real death, of GM products."

To me, there were two incredible revelations here: First, that the GMO industry could be effectively killed (at least in Europe) if animal feed and animal products were labeled. And second, that the majority of the European people think that the government has taken care of the GMO situation for them and are blithely buying their meat and dairy at the supermarket, just assuming it is likely non-GMO. From my American vantage point, where we seem to be engaged in a big brawl about labeling, this was eye-opening: America, it turns out, no matter how rhapsodic we get about Europe, isn't the only place that doesn't give full transparency to the consumer.

With a final pull on his beer stein, Walter told me that we needed to go—our night train to Munich would be leaving shortly. We gathered our things and said good-bye to Wolfgang, who went off into the night. Like everyone I was meeting to write this book, there went another stranger who had become familiar for a few short hours, and then he was gone.

chapter 16

Morning in Munich was resplendent. Walter and I disembarked from Vronsky's dark horse, came through the slick metal corridor of the station, and cascaded into the sunlight-filled atrium before heading straight for the Coca-Cola logo, scrawled in red letters over a huge glass façade. Blinking in the morning light, I followed Walter, who walked with officious confidence toward an old Munich hotel called the InterCityHotel where he likes to have his breakfast after taking the overnight train. On our way, he stopped in front of a homeless man loitering in front of the station to hand over the bag breakfast that Vronsky had given him as we got off the train. Hardly aware that I, too, was carrying this breakfast, the morning still so bleary for me, I opened it and peeked inside: a small pouch of honey, a roll, and a piece of cheese. Following his lead, I, too, handed mine over.

Together, we found a cozy seat near a tall window looking out at the city, then stood up to take in the sumptuous breakfast buffet: every kind of egg you could wish for, yogurt, muesli, meats, fruits, cheeses, honey, red berry jams, and thick brown breads. I filled my plate with fruit, two hard-boiled eggs, and a small bowl of yogurt with honey and sat down, gratefully, at the table. Walter and I ate quietly and congenially, like two old friends. We talked about books and movies and music. He told me his favorite essay is "The Whole Horse" by Wendell Berry and promised to send me a scan when he got home.

In the easy and expansive energy between us, I brought up that Wolfgang had mentioned the night before his belief that when Walter first came to him, supposedly on behalf of the bees, it was really just looking for a way to defeat all GMOs with honey. I asked him if that indeed was his intention—and if bees and honey were really just a red herring. He snorted. "Our original intention," he said, "was just not to be roadkill." He told me that his first suggestion to Wolfgang was that they figure out a way for the biotech companies to pay for analysis costs, so that beekeepers could at least have a handle on their contamination and then decide, on their own, beekeeper by beekeeper, what to do about it. It would have cost Biotech "peanuts," he said. But Biotech, he told me, said no. So, he said, "By not addressing the concerns of the beekeepers, they ended up with a situation where we were part of a movement [against GMOs]." And it was only when Biotech rejected them, he said, that he began to organize his search for a beekeeper who could become his poster child. He found that in Karl Heinz Bablok, the beekeeper whose honey was contaminated (and wasn't happy about it), and whom we were scheduled to meet later that afternoon. With Karl as their cause célèbre, beekeepers quickly went from being a small thorn in the side of Biotech to a legitimate roadblock.

When Walter and I disbanded from breakfast, we agreed to meet at Marienplatz, or Mary's Square, the central square in Munich, in the late afternoon, where Karl said he would be waiting for me. Walter would come along to play the role of interpreter.

Since it was a lovely, crisp fall day and I'd been sitting for what seemed like forever, I decided to walk to my hotel. I had never been to Germany, and since my gap year in Paris between high school and college, I'd been trying to find a way back to the feeling of discovering Europe for the first time. All those years ago the world had felt so innocent, so full of possibility.

With a map in hand, I took my rolly suitcase and walked down Bayerstraße toward Bahnhofplatz, and then turned to meander down small side streets with gray stone buildings on either side that housed bakeries boasting thick loaves of rye bread and fragrant pretzels, cakes, and cookies until I finally came to the tiny pension where I had booked a room. Inside my small but immaculate space, I showered and then lay down on the futon frame bed to write my notes. Under the warm weight of another clean, white cotton duvet cover filled with another thick wool blanket, I dozed off.

When I awoke, it was late afternoon. I was due to meet Walter and Karl in a short half hour. I hurriedly dressed and made my way out to the street. The air was pleasingly cool as I walked down the Munich streets toward the Marienplatz. In vain I searched for a local coffee shop and found only a Starbucks, where I ordered a dark roast, tall. Then I continued on my way down the street. Karl had told me he would find me under the square's tall, central column, which was adorned on top with a golden statue of the Virgin Mary standing on a crescent moon. (He told me that the statue was installed by the Germans in 1638 to celebrate the end of the Swedish occupation.)

My Starbucks in hand, I found Karl Heinz Bablok faithfully waiting. He is of medium height, with gray hair and glasses. He wore a leather jacket and a pair of jeans. He was shy, with a gentle handshake, and a diminutive aspect; he hardly seemed like the kind of person who, with his bees and contaminated honey, would want to become a fundamental lynchpin in the European discussion of GMOs.

Once Walter had joined us, he and I followed Karl into a cavernous, basement-level Bavarian wine and beer cellar, called Ratskellar, located underneath Munich city hall. The ceilings and walls of Ratskellar were adorned with beautifully painted frescoes and oil paintings and crisscrossed with shiny wooden beams that looked almost church-like in their buttressy patterns.

We sat down and the men ordered beer and I ordered a Bavarian red wine, which came decanted in a small glass bottle. We ordered some cheese and bread and I got a salad, which had fried buckwheat on top of tender greens; it was divinely crunchy and fresh.[1] I ate it with gusto—second to that bowl of seafood stew I'd had in the hotel outside of Brussels, this was the best meal I'd had since leaving Italy. And then we began to talk. I asked Karl to tell me, from the beginning, what had happened with him and his honey, how he had become the face of beekeeper resistance to GMOs, and how he felt about that role.

Karl told me that he lives in a small town an hour outside of Munich, ten kilometers from where he was born. A self-described "blue-collar worker," or "arbeiter," he has worked for the past forty years at the BMW factory in Munich. He said that he was always under "neon lights, with artificial lighting all the time." One summer, before his children were grown, twenty-five years ago, he was driving home from Munich and he saw farmers harvesting wheat on the side of the road. This vision was followed by a kind of Levin-like epiphany:[2] "I figured I have to do something so I can actually experience nature," he said. Because he had always been a person who was interested in small things—the plants in his garden, insects, things you might have to investigate under a microscope, he decided to turn his attention to bees. The reason for bees was that he had been moved, he said, by a

---

[1] This has become one of our favorite salads at home: Dan fries buckwheat groats, which he's cooked the night before in just water and salt, and we mix them into a lovely green salad, sometimes adding a little goat cheese and caramelized onions. I like to toss the salad with an apple cider vinegar, olive oil, and honey dressing.

[2] I refer to Konstantin Levin, the agrarian idealist in *Anna Karenina* who falls in love with the beauty and grit of farming in the springtime, and, in one passage of the book, visits his "bee house." Tolstoy writes: "It made his eyes giddy to watch the bees and drones whirling round and round about the same spot, while among them the working bees flew in and out with spoils or in search of them, always in the same direction into the wood to the flowering lime-trees and back to the hives."

beautiful traditional bee house—a small shed that is fashioned to hold many hives—which his mother's second husband had constructed on his property not far away. One day, upon hearing about his stepson's desire, the stepfather offered to give Karl two of his bee boxes, which was no small gesture because, according to Karl, it was like "ripping [out] part of his heart." Karl accepted, took them home to his house, and set them up in the garden.

He said he felt an immediate tranquillity come over him when he was with the bees, a calm he had never felt before.[3] But what moved him, he said, was that bees were "holistic." It was never about a single bee, he said. Instead, the beehive is cooperative, comprising worker bees, which forage and clean the hive; the drones, or males, who mate with the queen; and the queen, who lays the eggs. All of them have their separate jobs, but their collective goals are the same: to protect the queen, hatch the pupae, and make enough honey to feed not only themselves and the baby bees but also to leave a store so that the queen and a few worker bees who stay with her can survive the winter and thus ensure that the species continues to exist.

Eventually Karl Heinz began building his own bee boxes and taught himself about different kinds of flowers that bees liked so he could plant them; he learned about possible dangers to his bees. As he went along, he went from two to four to six to thirty to many more bee boxes—eventually managing close to a million bees. He began to make things out of the wax to sell, in addition to honey, at local markets.

After the Chernobyl disaster, which had brought nuclear fallout on the prevailing winds into central Europe, both he and his wife began

---

[3] It was interesting to me that Karl used the word "tranquillity" in terms of working with bees—an insect that can sting you if you aren't careful. But Karl Heinz was not the first person to use this same language. Karl Reiner, Walter's friend who had been chauffeuring us around outside of Brussels, also described his father, who ran a stressful dentist practice, as finding peace and "relaxation" with his bees, which Karl witnessed and eventually wanted to replicate in his own life, becoming a master beekeeper. Walter, for his part, told me that his bees mean more to him than he can quite express, except to say that he is continually mesmerized by "all these bees determined to bring something back to the hive."

worrying about the environment and how it would affect their children. But with their acquisition of bees he said they began healing from that intense period of worry and that innocence had been returned. It was a special time.

In 2000, Karl's innocence came to an abrupt end. He said that Edmund Stoiber, the minister president of Bavaria (who is known for coining the phrase "Laptop and Lederhosen," referring to Bavaria's unique ties to both tradition and technology), announced that Bavaria was going to try out "this great new technology"—GMOs—on a nearby research farm, where Karl had already been hired to help pollinate canola with his bees. Because his relationship with the canola farm had been, until then, going well, Karl had bought a small piece of land next to the canola fields and had built a bee house there. He was growing some vegetables, too.

At first, the research farm started with "one square meter of little plots of MON810, GMO maize," manufactured by Monsanto. "By 2003," said Karl, "it had grown to one thousand square meters." Walter had told me, explaining the climate that surrounded Bablok's discovery of GMO pollen in his honey, that "This is where the state of Bavaria ended up on a collision course with Bablok." Karl became concerned and expressed this to the research farm, but he was rebuffed by an expert affiliated with the farm and told that the corn cultivation would not affect his bees because the bees "were not collecting pollen from maize and therefore there is no risk for contamination." (Poudelet said the same thing to me when I interviewed him back in Belgium: that bees do not gather pollen from corn. In response to this, Walter said, "It's actually the most collected pollen in our agricultural landscape.")

However, Karl could see his bees foraging in the corn. Taking matters into his own hands, he set up two hives close to the field and also installed a pollen trap. (A pollen trap is a mesh grid through which pollen-carrying bees must crawl in order to enter their hive. As they crawl through, bits of pollen pellets are scraped off their legs and fall into a container, which stores the pellets. Some people like to sell this pollen as a nutritional supplement, which can be sprinkled atop yogurt or cereal. It has a distinctive nutty flavor.) He was hoping to verify that what he was seeing with his own eyes was actually true. He said, "I didn't know the larger significance of what I was doing."

When Karl had gathered enough pollen, he sent it to a lab to be analyzed for GMO DNA. It cost him three hundred euros (around $400). Initially Karl says that all he wanted to do was prove the "expert" wrong. But then, it became bigger for him. He had been reading about GMOs and, he said, "I'm a technician, you know—technically trained. I'm trained to look closely and understand. So when I understood the technique [to make GMOs], it became clear to me that they really cannot control what they are doing. The whole plant is toxic, from bottom to everywhere. This is not good for myself, this is not good for my bees." In the midst of this, Karl started to examine the zoning and property lines around the research farm. He realized that some of the farm's land overlapped with the protected habitat of a nature preserve. This was a galvanizing piece of information.

He then started writing letters to the various authorities—anyone he could think of—that essentially said, "Okay, you're planting these crops here in this nature preserve and this doesn't seem to be right." Over and over he got the same response: "No problem . . . there's nothing to worry about, no harm for your bees, you can eat it. . . ." This pissed off Bablok because he didn't believe these crops were harmless. If there was anything Chernobyl had taught him, it was that people could introduce dangerous things into the environment in the name of progress.

He responded by sending the invoice for his DNA analysis to the research farm and attached a copy of the results, which showed very clearly that GMO pollen was being brought back to his hives by his bees. For Karl, who had seen his bees as a kind of refuge in an increasingly hectic world, this whole thing was starting to unravel his dream. He said, "In Germany we have [an expression] called 'the St. Florien' . . .

where you pray to Saint Florien, and you say protect my house, burn another one. . . . If they had gone somewhere else that wasn't interfering with what [I] was doing, that would have been fine with [me]."

Eventually, Karl was contacted by the organizer of a German beekeeping association named Thomas Radetzki, who had gotten wind of his situation. He asked Karl if he would be willing to become the face of the beekeepers' struggle with GMOs. Walter said, "So this is essentially the point where the personal, the individual struggle of Mr. Bablok, met up with the struggle of the beekeeping community as a whole."

The case became a national media sensation and Karl ended up, eventually, in the European Court of Justice, pleading his case of contamination. Initially Karl and his lawyers had aimed their case only at the state of Bavaria and their research plot. But then Monsanto entered the case, sent a cadre of their big-shot attorneys, and also procured scientists to prove their points (in Maine we call rigged science used for political benefit "eyewash"). Karl said he took one look and said, "It was a roomful of high-powered people against [me] and two attorneys." He figured they were dead in the water.

When I asked him what it was like to be in that courtroom, he said, "It didn't feel good." I asked him if he was scared. And he said, "No. I'm fearless." After all, he told me, he was born during "The War," meaning the Second World War, and afterward he and his family were refugees. Sitting there in that courtroom, he assumed that there was no way he could possibly win. The scientists vouching for the other side had essentially said there was no way his honey could be contaminated, despite the fact that he had proven it was. Then, unbelievably, the court decided that the research plots growing MON810 needed to be halted. He was now in the middle of a huge victory—and this became a cause célèbre. In the end, the farm that had allowed the GMO plots turned to researching organic agriculture and cultivating only organic herbs. So, he said, "It's completely changed. It's like an oasis."

I asked Karl if it had all been worth it to him. Even today he still gets media attention and is still involved in legal hearings about contamination in the onward push by beekeepers to eradicate all GMO cultivation across Europe. And the fight is not over; just the day before our meeting, Walter had been at the parliament lobbying against the proposal to overturn his case.

Karl said that without a doubt, his life has been changed enormously. The peace he had been seeking that summer afternoon as he was driving home from his job has all but been lost. But, he said, he is sanguine about even this: "You cannot achieve all goals [in life]." Nonetheless, there is still magic each time he first opens a hive: "The smell from the beehive, especially when they are making the honey, that's special. . . . And when you see the queen, with the brood. . . ." But more important, he said, in the end, he's glad he's made this contribution, albeit "a small one—like a bee sting," toward making the planet a safer and greener place.

It was getting dark by the time we emerged from Ratskellar and back out to the Marienplatz. Walter ran off to meet his wife, whom he hadn't seen for six days, and Bablok and I shook hands under the statue of Mary; then I wound my way back up Sendlinger Straße, looking in the windows of clothing shops. Eventually I found an Afghani restaurant where I was the first early diner. I sat by the window on a cushioned bench and ordered some tea from a young, soft-spoken man who was attentive without being cloying, making me feel comfortable and at peace. The tea arrived and was warm and sweet in a tall glass mug. I ordered a chicken vegetable curry dish with rice and waited. The food came and was hot and spicy—I ate with relish, though I knew that it was extremely unlikely that the chicken or vegetables were organic or GMO-free. The truth was that traveling abroad and trying to eat like I did at home was hard, sometimes next to impossible. By this point in my journey, I hadn't felt 100 percent for a few days. I was run-down, my stomach was a wreck, my skin was slightly rashy again.

But I knew that this was a momentary thing—I could get myself back in balance as soon as I got home.

A calm came over me sitting in the Afghani restaurant. I knew that the next day, I would get on a plane so that I could fly back to Italy, where I'd be reunited with Marsy and Dan. After my meal, in the darkness, I climbed back up the hill, past the shuttered shops to my small pension, made some chamomile tea with a dollop of chamomile honey in a dusty hot pot the hotel had lent me, and went to bed.

In the morning, I was up early. I took the train out of Munich, past fields of mustard blooming yellow against the gray sky, to the airport, where I flew to Paris. On the plane, while sipping a surprisingly good airplane coffee, I read the morning's *Le Monde* and found that already Pioneer's TC1507 corn had been approved by the EU for cultivation. It was that swift. Walter's influence had clearly not been enough to push against the ever-advancing tide of GMOs across the globe.

From Paris, I flew back to Italy where Marsden and Dan met me in Florence. We drove to Siena for a few days on an Italian *tenuta*, or agricultural tenant farm (that looked more like a castle!), called the Tenuta di Spannocchia. Spannocchia dates back to the twelfth century and sits on 1,200 acres of conserved land; and, for the most part, it supplies its own food. There I learned about how that particular farm was managing to avoid any GMOs: they grow all their own black beans and wheat for animal feed (avoiding corn altogether), and almost everything else comes from their own land, which is extremely isolated and nestled in the wooded hills. In the evenings the *tenuta*'s cook, Graciela, a true Italian *nonna*, cooked up extensive meals for us of course after course of fresh meats and cheeses, salads dressed with olive oil from the trees just outside the doors, and chunky fall soups replete with vegetables from the garden, all downed with plenty of the wine made right there, on that same terra firma. One meal in particular ended with a dessert we still talk about in our family: a ricotta chocolate mousse, made from whipped cream, raw eggs, ricotta, grated bittersweet chocolate, and sugar—it was sublime.[4] The last night we were on the *tenuta*, while Marsy slept, Dan and I opened our room's louvered windows (think *A Room with a View*!) and stood gazing at the moon shining over the hills and cypress trees, the air cool and our breath making puffs into the dark night. "This is paradise," I heard myself say out loud.

A few days later, after twenty-four Caravaggio- and Bernini-packed hours in Rome, Dan, Marsy, and I boarded an Alitalia plane and flew west, back to the complicated country we call home. Although I knew that I could perhaps find paradise again sometime, I knew in my bones that the only place that is truly mine is this land of Big Ag, GMOs, and loud fights.

---

[4] Graciela loved Marsden and took him into her kitchen with her, where she made him special cheese omelettes and noodles whenever he was hungry but it was not yet mealtime in Italy or when she thought he might not like the grown-up food on offer for a particular meal. She wrote out her mousse recipe for me so I could make it again for Mars. Ever since our trip, this has become a regular birthday request of Marsy's, right after a big plate of spaghetti and meatballs. Since we always have more than we can possibly eat—her measurements are for feeding a roomful of hungry travelers!—I take the remaining mousse and drop it from a spoon in the form of little Hershey's kisses on cookie trays and freeze them, using them later as garnishes for ice cream.

chapter 17

About seven months later, on a Thursday morning as June shifted from spring into full-blown summer, I called up my friend Jodi, who lives with her husband, Glenn, and daughter, Fuchsia, in a residential neighborhood of Portland. Jodi is a self-proclaimed "novice" beekeeper, even though she's been a city beekeeper for about six years and teaches other people how to keep bees at this point, too. She says there is still so much to learn.

"May I come over and meet your bees?" I asked.

"Sure," she said. She'd been gone for a week in England and wanted to take a peek at the hives herself.

"Cool," I said. "Because I realize I've been writing this section in my book about honey and the European politics that surround honey. And I've been reading about bees and pesticides and CCD. But the other morning I woke up and realized that I don't have any connection to the insects themselves."

With the exception of what Marsden had taught me from visiting Jodi's urban farmlette, as she calls it, I was still pretty fuzzy on life according to a bee. Marsy divulged pithy bits of information, thanks to Jodi, like what a queen bumblebee looked like (big); and he knew that bees died after they stung you, and he'd learned that bees loved certain kinds of flowers like dandelions and clover in the early spring, which helped them start their storage of nectar, pollen, and honey, and that raspberry bushes would later give off a heady, sweet scent, irresistible to bees. More than that was all a bit foggy for me.

I told Jodi as much and she chuckled. "Come over tomorrow. Don't eat any bananas before you come; wear cruddy clothes because the bees might poop on you, and wear long pants, long sleeves, gloves, and cover your feet."

On Friday morning, I got up early and did as I was told: I ate no bananas and even though it was well over eighty degrees by nine, I packed a tote bag with jeans, a long-sleeved linen shirt, sneakers, socks, and gloves (I knew enough about the randomness of severe allergies by then not to tempt fate). I drove over to Jodi's in a light dress, made my way through her big iron-and-wood gate, and meandered through her raised beds and onto her porch. She was waiting for me with a glass of cold water. I took a sip and said, "Let me run in and change!"

When I came back out, Jodi already had her netted bonnet fastened on her head. She helped me get mine on, and then we made our way to the side of her garden, next to the chicken coop, where her hives stood in brightly colored pillars of stacked boxes, painted purples, blues, and pinks.

Jodi told me that we should try to make movements inspired by the kind of mindfulness that is required for tai chi. Well, I've never taken tai chi, but I got her point: I was to move slowly and deliberately, which I did because who wants to be stung by a hundred bees? (I thought of the scene in Little House in the Big Woods when the cousin Charley comes to visit Laura and Mary. He's supposed to be helping Pa and his dad, who are cutting the wheat crop, but instead he's being a pain in the ass. Then, as some kind of divine payback, he gets stung by a swarm of bees—so badly stung, in fact, that they have to wrap him like a mummy.)

In the hot sun, Jodi unstrapped the hive boxes, which were held together with a long belt that looked kind of like those long woven yoga straps used for stretching. In this case, the straps keep the boxes held one on top of the other in the event a bear (unlikely in Portland), some very strong raccoons, or just a kid running for a ball and not looking where she is going happens to knock over the boxes. Then she began lifting the boxes off one another and arranging them in a semicircle around her, where she squatted on her haunches. Slowly and deliberately, Jodi pulled out the traylike frames that sit upright inside each box and have a foundation of wire and wax spread across them. She told me that the bees build wax honeycomb on top of these reinforcements. Their honeycomb, she said, is used not only for storing their glistening amber-colored honey but also for storing nectar and pollen for the bees to eat and for laying eggs and hatching brood (young bees in their larval stage).

With each frame, which she held steadily in her bare hands while the bees buzzed around her, she inspected each individual cell on each side of the frame thoroughly—there were hundreds on each side— all the while pointing out eggs (which look like tiny white petunia seeds); brood, or gestating bees (which looked to me like mushy white rice macaroni); the queen (identified in each hive with a red paint dot on her back); and honey. While she worked, some bees crawled up her hands. She looked unperturbed.

In a quiet and thoughtful voice, Jodi recounted some bee trivia. She told me about the "virgin," or "nuptial," flight of a new queen when she will fly into the air pursued by a fleet of drones (male bees, not the things we've got hovering over Iraq), who will then mate with her literally while she flies, filling her up with enough sperm to fertilize a lifetime of eggs. When a hive gets tired of their queen (either because she's no longer producing enough eggs or because she's injured), she said, the hive will execute her in a ritualized pattern called balling the queen, where they make a huge, tight ball of bodies around her, pressing and pressing until she suffocates and dies.

"Want to see a worker bee?" she asked.

"Yes," I said, taking a step in closer to the orb of smoke from her smoker, in which she was burning pinecones and pine needles. Smoke, it's been understood since ancient times, calms bees. Although the reasons are not yet completely understood by scientists, one part of it is that the smoke masks the alarm pheromones guard bees give off when in danger, and also, it can mask the smell of an intruder. And— this is sort of sad—smoke makes bees think their hive is on fire, which causes a feeding response—they suddenly want to gorge on honey in preparation for escape, and are therefore otherwise engaged in eating rather than stinging the beekeeper. Some people also posit that when the bees start eating, they flex their abdomens in a manner that makes it hard for them to sting.

She pointed to one of the "queen's daughters," who is a "worker," she said. This bee had its butt up in the air while it carefully cleaned an empty cell until it was immaculately polished. She said that worker bees eventually graduate to "forager" bees in the last half of their lives—that foraging pollen is the payoff for becoming a good worker. And, as if on cue, a forager arrived with "saddle bags"—the top part of her thighs—full of light-yellow pollen. Once inside the hive, she did her "waggle dance," where she shook her butt and danced in a circle, telling the other bees in a complicated and incredible bee language exactly where she found some great pollen (bees' communication skills have been widely studied because they are able to describe pollen sources—as far as four miles away—so keenly to their sisters that their sisters can then go out and gather from the same exact plants they've described). More bees appeared, carrying every shade of yellow pollen you could imagine—from dark orange and sepia tones to the palest of creamy yellows.[1]

---

[1] The following spring, Jodi and I were on the phone: "Guess what color pollen the bees are bringing home?" she asked, her enthusiasm infectious. I said I didn't know. "Blue," she said. She said it was from the Siberian wood squill that blooms in early spring. She described the blue as a "cadet blue, like eye makeup" and told me about the "Flower fairie" drawing of Siberian squill, or Scilla, by the famous British artist Cicely Mary Barker. In it, a little blue-clad

. . .

THE SMELLS INSIDE the hive were pungent: the honey that broke open and oozed when Jodi scraped off the "bridge comb"—a bit of waxy comb on the outside edges of the frames—smelled musky and sweet. Along the edges of the frame was some sticky propolis, which the bees make from the resin of pine trees, and is considered by many to be an immune-boosting health food. Propolis, I noticed, has a warm tea tree–mixed-with-cinnamon scent. And then there was the waxy earthiness of the comb itself, and beneath that the mild animal, almost barnyard, smell of the bees mixed in with the campfire smell of the smoker going just behind Jodi's back.

Once, a bee crawled up into my bonnet and stared at me. I asked Jodi, my voice querulous, what to do. In answer, she walked me calmly away from the hives and helped me out of the bonnet.

"Why would she crawl up there?" I asked.

"She's just curious," she said, as if the inner lives of bees were explicable. Luckily I was not stung. (I think it was my Zen posturing!)

As the sun's heat pounded down on us and the morning wore on, Jodi's methodical nature with the bees became a kind of dance; she was in the zone, at one with the bees.

Only once did Jodi squish a couple of bees—she was incredibly careful, despite the buzzing and the legitimate possibility that anyone, even a saint, could become callous about the lives of a couple of insects. Jodi told me she thinks of the bees as both a larger organism—all working together for one goal, which is the survival of the hive through the winter—and also as individuals. She said that it pains her when she mistakenly squishes a bee. (Another beekeeper once told me that there's no sound quite like the "squish and pop" of a bee body.) On one of the last frames, Jodi called me over. "Come watch," she said in a hushed and reverent tone. "This bee is about to be born."

---

sprite stands in between two squill plants, her finger held quizzically to her mouth. I remembered loving my own *Flower Fairies of the Summer* book when I was a child, which I have now bequeathed to Marsden.

Standing next to her, I peered at the honeycomb on the metal-and-wood frame as a tiny bee pushed its furry head out of a thin layer of wax covering the cell where it had matured from egg to larvae to pupae to bee. It looked every bit like a disheveled child waking up from a long afternoon nap, hair standing on end, eyes big and open to the world. The bee struggled to get her whole body out, pushing as hard as she could, flailing her front legs, then falling back into the cell again. None of the worker bees around her pitched in to help; they went about their business, cleaning and readying the hive for the new babies. It must have been maddening, I found myself thinking, to realize that coming into the world is, in the end, such a lonely and private journey. When our heroine finally emerged, she was pale colored and ready to work. She shook herself off and made like the workers around her, barely a minute old.

When Jodi and I were done, and all the frames had been put back inside the hives, which were standing upright again, strapped together, the bees resumed their order and restarted their cycle: some arriving with pollen and others taking off to go gather. We picked up Jodi's tools and gear and made our way to her porch steps where our cool glasses of water awaited us.

As we walked, she handed me the few pieces of waxy "bridge comb" she had scraped off the hives. They were full of gooey, amber honey. Of course, standing there, enjoying the sweetness, I had no idea if the bees that had provided the nectar to make my honey had foraged on any GMO plants or if they had gathered traces of neonicotinoids from gardeners' flowers, or been doused by chemical lawn fertilizers, tick and mosquito sprays, or any other kind of insecticide. But I did know it was sweet.

As I sucked and chewed, she told me how glad she was to see her honeycombs so full. She said, "There will be plenty of honey for not only us this year but also for them."

I said, "What do the bees use the honey for in the winter?"

"All summer the bees are working to lay in enough food in the form of nectar, which they reduce to honey, to keep themselves and their queen alive all winter. They also lay in enough for their first spring brood." As I listened, I spit the wax from the bridge comb off the side of her porch into her hostas. "Their goal is to ensure the survival of the colony, or family. They are always thinking of the future," she said.

As I drove away, it struck me that what I had witnessed that morning was such an amazing constellation of the fecund contradictions in life: sweet nectar and waxy comb; squished worker bees and white grain–like eggs full of possibility; waggly dances of joy at finding good golden pollen and the humdrum of cleaning out cells, over and over; birth and shit; the desire to gather—freely, innocently—to feed our colony and care for our young despite the sobering problem we are presented with that the chemicals in our environment come home with us to our hives, infect our children, change our lives, and sometimes destroy them. All this and yet we still have a very real yen for honey, which reaches back into our DNA, to before Paleolithic times, beckoning us with sweetness and stories of purity.

PART 3

West of Eden

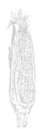

"Once, the whole country faced west."

—IAN FRAZIER, *Great Plains*

"No creature has ever altered life on the planet
in this way before . . ."

—ELIZABETH KOLBERT, *The Sixth Extinction*

chapter 18

It was early 2002 and Ignacio Chapela was digging up his backyard in Berkeley, California. He was "moving earth," he told me, "at four in the morning," while his daughter, Inés slept, oblivious. It was a small house and he'd decided, "The whole water thing was wrong. There was accumulation in the crawlspace underneath—so I decided [the yard] needed new grading. I just moved huge amounts of soil from one place to the other and made it fine, made it good."

At the time he was moving earth, Ignacio was going through a cavalcade of hard things: most recently, he'd published a study in *Nature*, a preeminent science journal, that indicated that GMO corn from the United States was contaminating the landraces, or criollo corn, bred for ten thousand years in the Oaxacan highlands of Mexico. This was in and of itself a startling conclusion because Mexico was officially a GMO-free zone, at least as far as cultivation was concerned. And as a result of his study, he'd gotten into a whole lot of hot water: it was decried by the biotech industry and he was personally and vituperatively attacked. (For the anti-GMO legions, however, his study and the biotech attacks turned him, overnight, into a cause célèbre.) Tyrone Hayes, the herpetologist at Berkeley studying atrazine (who had introduced me to Ignacio), told me, "[Ignacio] was attacked and his career was severely impacted—his research, his tenure, and job were at risk. Lawsuits were involved. There was a powerful lobby against him."[1] Why such a reaction? I asked. "There's a lot of money behind GM and pesticides; ninety percent of the seed business is backed by the chemical companies. So if you're a threat to one, you're a threat to the other," he said.

In the midst of all this, Ignacio had been battling UC Berkeley over a five-year deal it had signed with Novartis, a Swiss biotech company based in Basel that later became Syngenta (one of the "Big Six"— the moniker given to the six most powerful biotech companies—and Tyrone Hayes's nemesis). The company, in an effort to discover the next big thing in the field of GMOs, was offering to give the university a large lump sum (in the 25 to 50 million dollar range, though the actual number is disputed depending on whom you speak to) in exchange for access to research in the plant biology department. Ignacio was an outspoken opponent of the idea, as he felt it compromised the integrity of the university. Also, contemporaneously with his Novartis battle—and to make matters personally more fraught—the university was in the process of denying Ignacio tenure. He hired a lawyer to fight this decision.

As if there wasn't enough stress already, at the same time all this was happening, his complicated marriage to his high school sweetheart, Laura, with whom he'd emigrated from Mexico to America, was falling apart, and he was trying to be the best father he could to eight-year-old Inés. While everything was going on, he said, he would find himself out in the yard moving all that dirt around and "doing physical work to really extreme levels, without being able to fall asleep." But oddly, he said, despite the hardship, he felt there was a light at the end of the tunnel. "It was a very long and difficult, exhausting

---

[1] There was actually only one lawsuit, though it went on for so long it may have seemed like many to some.

but important process of liberation from something that was really bad before that," he said.

How he got to this place of digging holes in the dark while shit hit every fan around him was the reason I was on the phone with him in the first place, back in the summer of 2012, when I was researching my piece for *Elle*. But it was when he mentioned that he'd taken a ride in the back of a black Suburban and he'd felt his life was threatened that I decided I needed to meet him. A little more than a year later, when I was at work on what was becoming this book, I got on an airplane one cold, dark March morning and flew out of the snowy and icebound East Coast across the country to sunny, warm, and hip Berkeley.

chapter 19

I got up at four in the morning in the small rental house we were living in at the time. It was a cozy beige Cape on the banks of the Presumpscot River, just across the Portland line, in the mill town of Westbrook, where Dan grew up. Marsden, then five, had been battling a bad cold and was still asleep. I hadn't slept well—and as I'm wont to do right before a trip, I had left much of my packing unfinished, so I was rushing around in the last hours.

Dan called me a cab, but just when it arrived, Marsden awoke. He was in tears at the prospect of my leaving without his being able to take me to the airport—which, in all fairness, we'd promised he'd be able to do before we realized how bad his cold was. Dan told the cabdriver there was a change of plans, and as the cab turned around to make its way back into the dark without me, we all piled into our car. We drove to the airport on slick, icy streets piled high with dirty, gray snow.

When we got there, we were greeted by a huge line at security. We all waited together until we had to part ways; each time I wave to my child from just beyond security and am about to board a plane, there's a part of me that wonders if this is the last time I will see him.

I suppose this is just leftover anxiety from living in Manhattan during 9/11; or maybe everyone feels this way in the brave new world we inhabit of globalized suffering and rage. Or maybe this is just being a parent with the knowledge that anything could happen; life-altering disaster can sometimes only be a pinprick away.

In San Francisco, I took the BART to Berkeley and rolled my bag up a hill in the startlingly hot California sunlight until I arrived at the Berkeley City Club. As soon as I entered the cool, soothing oasis, I felt a sigh go through my whole body. The hotel was designed in 1929 by the architect Julia Morgan (the first woman to be admitted to the architecture program at l'École de Beaux-Arts in Paris) and it combines Moorish and Gothic styles into a space that is both muscular and incredibly feminine.

A bowl of shiny, waxed apples, free to the guests, sat on a low table. Next to the apples was a small marble Canova sculpture—a study the artist had done for his larger-than-life sculpture of Paolina Bonaparte. I'd just seen the life-size sculpture only a few months before in Rome. Underneath buttresses made of concrete and medieval lighting fixtures, the walls of the hotel were covered with more Italianate art.

The concierge gave me a key to the pool and a bathing cap, and directed me to my room on the fifth floor. Once there, I opened the door into a small, old-fashioned E. M. Forster–like room, with light blue walls and thick yellow, flowered drapes flanking huge windows with views all the way to the San Francisco Bay. Light poured across the bed, and real art hung on the walls. Books—and one of my favorites, *Tender Is the Night*—sat in a wooden bookshelf. The small bathroom had pale beige tiles and creamy white walls. It was the perfect hotel room.

I called Ignacio to tell him I had arrived and we made plans to meet that evening. Then I pulled on my bathing suit and went back downstairs to the pool, which was canopied by a gracefully arced ceiling made of painted concrete. The edge of the pool looked out a full wall of windows that cast lily pads of light onto the blue water.

Blue and yellow tiles accented where the walls met the floor. It was simply the most elegant pool I'd ever seen, which perhaps wasn't surprising since pools were Julia Morgan's specialty. (The "Neptune Pool," which she fashioned for the Hearst Castle—home of the famous newspaper magnate, William Randolph Hearst—in central California, is worth a Google. It is an absolutely stunning study in blue and beauty.) I dove in to swim off the trip and get myself ready for the work I was about to do. Once upstairs, I lay in my towel in an orb of late-afternoon light, feeling feline and spoiled in the warmth until it was time to go.

Ignacio had suggested we take his daughter's dog, Luna, for a walk into the hills. At the appointed time, I exited the hotel into the warm afternoon and made my way toward the Campanile (named for the Campanile in Florence)—the big bell tower in the center of the university—where he had instructed me to wait. I got there a few minutes early and sat on the steps, admiring the impressive campus, which seemed to radiate importance, intelligence, financial security, and answers to our complicated world.

After a few moments, Ignacio sauntered up, white hair blowing around his head in the evening wind. He was sporting a rose-colored button-down shirt, jeans, and brown, comfortable-looking shoes. He was pushing a bike with a helmet clipped onto the handlebars. His skin was supple and smooth and looked like coffee with lots of cream. His button-down was open at the neck to expose a smattering of dark freckles. He was friendly, if a little scattered, and I noticed, once we were standing close to each other, that he had almond-colored eyes. On the face of it, he wasn't a person who was extemporaneously articulate; like his chosen field of environmental microbiology, he focuses on minutiae rather than the big picture of what he's saying.

As the two of us walked through the lush campus, Ignacio admired the flowers that were in the midst of blooming—he pointed out a camellia and then a rhododendron, "Oh, look at the rhododendron! I hadn't even noticed it!" It was almost as if with someone alongside him, he was suddenly looking through fresh, clean glasses at the world around him.

We stopped at an archway dedicated to Phoebe Apperson Hearst (the American philanthropist, suffragist, and mother to William Randolph Hearst), which opens through the trees to a little bridge that crosses a trickle of stream descending from Strawberry Creek in the mountains behind and crosses to the arts and humanities buildings of the university. The bridge is meant to connect the sciences, Ignacio said, where we were standing, and the arts. Just across from the arch, he told me, is the building—on the sciences side—where the initial plans for the Manhattan Project and the nuclear bomb commenced.

After crossing the little footbridge, we came to a lush green courtyard in front of the Faculty Club. There we began an ascent up winding streets to Ignacio's home. We launched into a discussion of the state of the planet—climate change, the changes to our soil and environment from chemical overload, species extinction, etc. Ignacio surprised me with the snappy way with which he dispensed his opinion: "We've been telling students a lie: that the planet is dying. That is not true. The planet is fine, thank you very much. What we need to tell them is that the planet we *love* is dying. What kind of planet do we want? One with big animals and plants and beauty? Or the one we're creating? Which will not have the things that we love, the places that we love, and it won't have anything bigger and more soul satisfying than corporations." He told me that he predicts a planet in the not-so-distant future where none of us big creatures—bears, humans, even birds—exist, but where the fungi of the world rule. When he said this, I imagined a gray, furry planet, devoid of green, and covered with nothing more than a caustic soup of toxic oceans and landmasses crawling with mold. I felt an allergy attack coming on just thinking about it.

We continued our climb up until we reached Ignacio's small, low cottage, which he shares with his partner, Lisa (his daughter, Inés, is in college in New York State). The house sits perched above the Berkeley campus, where it can take in the immensity of the school in one glance. Luna, their small, black shepherd mix, came bounding out in that slightly neurotic and nervous sideways wiggly manner sheepdogs often have. Only a few rooms—a tiny kitchen, a living room, a bathroom, and a bedroom—come together to make up this slightly dark little house. Books were piled on most surfaces, including the top of a small dining room table, which was pushed to the side of the living room. On it sat a computer propped atop more books. An open bottle of wine sat next to a small stainless-steel kitchen sink. It was clear, just from the humility of his living space, that Ignacio's life had never quite rebounded from the difficulty of those years in the early 2000s; and that perhaps, compared to some of his colleagues, he'd therefore never quite arrived.

Leaving for our walk with Luna bounding ahead of us, Ignacio pointed out the houses that surrounded his—also low, hill-clinging structures, one of which was designed by Frank Lloyd Wright. He gestured up the hill and told me that the Sierra Club was "born there"—he pointed to one of the homes—and that John Muir finished his memoirs in one of the houses, too. "Right here in these buildings," he said with a sweep of his broad hand, "the environmental movement started."

I continued to follow Ignacio across a dusty gully and then up and into the mountains above the Berkeley campus. When we got to the top of The Big C, a promontory that sits high above the Berkeley campus and is demarcated by a big, yellow cement "C," the sun began to go down, a huge ball of orange over the San Francisco Bay. As it got dark and we were meandering back down the hill, Ignacio started to open up about his life.

IGNACIO CHAPELA was born in Mexico City in 1959, the last child of eleven. When Ignacio was three, his father, a newspaperman, was hit by a car and broke his femur, disabling him for the rest of his life. He died when Ignacio was eleven. His mother was a stay-at-home mom who was worn out when he was born, he said. And although "education was prized above eating, by the time I came along, the coffers were empty," so he didn't get the same private schooling his siblings had.

The family house was behind a great stone wall and behind it "was a derelict dairy farm with no cows." Inside those walls, though, he said, was a "paradise—trees and stumps and dirt to dig holes in," where he was left "largely unsupervised."

With a lack of structure at home—his father dead and his mother trying to keep it together with eleven children—the young Ignacio turned to the outdoor world to educate himself. As soon as he was old enough, he would take his bicycle and ride up and out of the city and into the mountains as far as he could bike, then he'd dismount and walk, observing the natural world at the slow, meditative pace of a child with few restrictions. On these walks he became fascinated with molds and fungi, he said, which had no roots and seemingly had no ends, either, because their ends continue ad infinitum. He realized, he said, that "there was a whole universe that was invisible" out there, and that thrilled him. When he was eleven, he told me, he first looked down a microscope and was hooked.

As Ignacio's life progressed and he began to show a strong preference and aptitude for science, he also began to hone his innate sense of injustice. When he was in college, by then an expert in fungi, he became intrigued and, by turns, saddened and outraged by a fungus that was killing the lush ash trees[1] around the city. He said that he "was interested in how the trees were sick" and wanted to find a solution, but that "nobody noticed the trees were dying" until it was too late. This

---

[1] Ash trees have recently been the subject of much discussion across America because they are being devastated by an invasive Asian beetle called the emerald ash borer, which is thriving because of climate change—it's not getting cold enough to kill the beetles. Ninety-nine percent of ash trees, it's predicted, will be gone relatively soon because of this beetle. The disappearance of the ash will affect entire forest ecosystems. This is just one of many ominous reports about the vanishing world we live in. Interestingly, as an aside, ash wood is used for baseball bats because it is so hard and straight-grained. What will we use for bats—for our great American pastime—if all the ash is gone?

perspective on life—from a position of moral outrage—he says, is what eventually got him out of Mexico and to Berkeley. "At some point in my life, I was supposed to be a well-positioned academic in the Mexican academic system. I was a good student and there were a couple of professors, especially one, that became very powerful, who said, *you*." He explained that in Mexico, if a professor marked you as a descendant, you would start working in their lab, knowing that you would be offered a position with them eventually and that you would begin to climb the ladder. "I said no. Oh, that was terrible, gosh. . . . How dare you? He was so mad. My reason for it was that I wanted to learn about fungi. And that was the most obscure, ridiculous, marginal thing."

Ignacio left Mexico and went to get his PhD in Wales from 1981 until '84. From there he went on to Cornell, where his wife, Laura, was studying for her PhD in English. At Cornell, Ignacio began studying rare kinds of fungi. And then he got a call from a biotech company in Switzerland called Sandoz Pharmaceuticals (Sandoz later became Novartis and, eventually, Syngenta, when it merged with the agricultural arm of the pharmaceutical giant Astra Zeneca).[2] They were interested in him because he had discovered a collection of fungi that nobody had ever seen. They felt that the possibility that he would find something new for them, too, was high, and finding new life-forms was becoming a growing interest for them. So they offered him a job.

He went to work for Sandoz in Basel in 1987. He said that it was there, in Switzerland, that he felt he was really "looking at the birth of biotechnology." This was when, he said, the drug companies were starting to diversify to include the patenting of new kinds of life-forms—which eventually became GMOs—and the creation of the chemicals that could be used along with the GMOs.

Ignacio had first heard about the possibility of GMOs in the early seventies when he learned about the research some scientists at Stan-

---

[2] When you learn of the connections between Big Ag and Big Pharma, you might wonder what Big Pharma stands to gain from an allergy and autoimmune epidemic caused by pesticides and/or GMOs.

ford were conducting to combine and transplant genes. In 1973, these scientists, Stanley Norman Cohen and Herbert Boyer, had discovered that they could transfer the gene for frog ribosomal RNA into bacterial cells, which would then express, or take on, the characteristics of the frog RNA. Ignacio said he was enthralled by these early chimerical forays into Biotech.[3] But not as a scientist. "It's as a kid," he says, "it's as a boy that you find it cool. That you say . . . oh my gosh, I can Tinkertoy with living things. To do whatever I want." Now, grown up and stationed on the cutting edge with Sandoz, it was exhilarating. Consequently, for a time, Ignacio enjoyed his job. He was making more money than he'd ever made and Laura, now pregnant with Inés, had flown over from Cornell to join him.

In late 1991, however, Ignacio began to tire of his work in Basel, and more importantly, he started to have ethical questions about what Sandoz was going to do with his discoveries. He wanted to go back to the safety and freedom of academia. So he started making plans to return with his family to the United States, where he was able to secure a position back at Cornell. In January 1992, he and his family uprooted from Switzerland and moved back to Ithaca in the middle of a snowstorm. But before he'd left Basel, some people in a remote area of the Oaxacan highlands had gotten in touch with him via fax. This connection would come to define the rest of his professional life.

"[My] first contact with them [the Oaxacans] happened because there were these Japanese people showing up—they called them Chinese. They said, 'These Chinese people are coming . . . who are offering huge amounts of money for [matsutake[4]] mushrooms in our forests. We're nervous because it's too much money and we feel there

---

[3] Ignacio says that GMOs really should be called "transgenics" because you take "DNA out of an organism and put it into another one." Furthermore, he says "it's not just engineering" in response to those who call the work of moving DNA between species "Genetic Engineering," or GE. "Pruning is engineering," he says. "Selecting your crop from year to year is genetic engineering. Whereas this [GMO] means taking genetic material from one organism and putting it in another without sex, right?" (Going forward in this section with Ignacio, we will sometimes refer to GMOs as "transgenics.")

[4] Like morels.

must be something wrong with this. Can you please help us figure out what's happening?'" When I asked Ignacio how they found him, in particular, he said, "You know, not many people knew anything about fungi, so they were saying, who can we contact who knows something about fungi who will speak Spanish?"

Ignacio said he took a cursory look into it and "it turns out it's a completely legitimate thing—that Japanese people are just crazy about these mushrooms and are willing to pay a lot of money. . . . At some point [the matsutake] were selling for fifty dollars a pound fresh. . . . So for people in Oaxaca, that's a huge amount of money for a mushroom they don't even eat." Assuming this was a small task that would be over and done with quickly, Ignacio said he got back to the Oaxacans and told them that he couldn't find anything wrong. But then they said, "'Will you come and help us negotiate with these people?'"

Why the Oaxacans needed a scientist, as opposed to a good lawyer, at this juncture is anyone's guess. However, Ignacio began to develop a relationship with them. He told me that once the Oaxacans realized that there was no way to cultivate the matsutake—they were only available through foraging in the forests (often done with leaf blowers, he said, which disrupted the forest floor)—it dawned on them that they'd need to care for their forests, and indeed police them because of poachers, in order to continue to supply the Japanese with matsutake. They were now, also, hip to the possibility that perhaps any—not just matsutake—mushrooms could bring in some serious amounts of cash. So they began getting interested in supplementing their matsutake business with oyster and shiitake mushrooms, which they could cultivate in a lab. The Oaxacans told Ignacio that they would invest their money, time, and people if he would help them set up a little lab to grow their own microfauna. He agreed. Consequently, their mushroom business—with Ignacio's help—became hugely successful, and the Oaxacans started to make good money from mushroom farming.

As the relationship grew, Ignacio says the Oaxacans then turned to him with questions about transgenics, or GMOs. "This is 1992 or '93,

I think. So it's really early." Ignacio admits it was still just hypothetical back then—most GMOs (primarily corn and soy at that point) were still in field trials in the United States. "The Oaxacans were saying, 'Okay, that sounds kind of cool that they will be doing that, but what happens if they put some pig DNA[5] into corn and then their corn mates with our corn?' And I said, 'I don't know.' And they said, 'That doesn't sound like a very nice thing. How can we find out?' And I said, 'You can't because you won't see anything different.' And then [they said], 'Well, but somebody must be protecting against it.'"

Ignacio guffawed audibly to show his incredulity at this idea. He said he knew, even back then, that there wouldn't ever be any such protection from the companies that were producing the GMOs or from the Mexican government. In any event, the Oaxacans decided to do something unprecedented: they wanted their own lab to have the capacity to detect GMOs in their own prize cornfields. Ignacio helped them make a list of the necessary equipment and began, himself, to get more involved because he thought they were asking an interesting question.

It took the Oaxacans and Ignacio a few years, and in the meantime, Ignacio and Laura had relocated to Berkeley, where Ignacio had landed a job. In 1997, the Oaxacans inaugurated their new lab (with mostly donated equipment from an international group of scientists). And then, a few years later, they were able to detect GMO DNA in their criollo corn. "And that was why that discovery was made in 2000 that completely turned my life upside down. I mean, it was a little bit like the Oaxacans did it, not me. I've stopped making this argument when people say, 'You made the discovery.' I say, 'No, I didn't do it—I helped people set up the lab, and of course I'm the one who could write in English and publish in *Nature*, but it really was their discovery. . . .' I've given up that one battle."

It wasn't until I heard the bigger story about how his piece in *Nature* was finally published—and the firestorm that surrounded it—that I

---

[5] They had heard about insulin at that point, which was the first true GMO, using pig-recombinant DNA to create insulin.

started to wonder if this last comment of Ignacio's was somewhat disingenuous. Maybe it wasn't for me to judge; complicated negotiations happen between people. It's clear the Oaxacans wanted answers because their indigenous corn—the criollo—was such an important part of their identity. But I couldn't get it out of my head that the renegade and morally outraged scientist in Ignacio was also drawn to this subject with his own agenda. That this was something he, too, wanted to understand and ultimately expose to the world. Would he have invested as much time and energy as well as his reputation into something this big and this politically charged if not? Would anyone?

BY THE TIME Ignacio and I were making our way down the hill, toward the lighted Berkeley campus, the sky had grown completely dark. As we traipsed, my feet sliding forward and jamming into the toes of my shoes, Luna carried a large stick that knocked me every so often behind my shins. She reminded me of Hopper, who did the same thing when we took him into the woods to walk.

We stopped for a moment at Tightwad Hill, a spot high above the football field where you used to be able to watch the game for free, though now the Berkeley administration has put a cannon up there, Ignacio said, which is fired during games. From there we continued on downward, walking, finally, through the campus and past students on their various ways to evening classes, dorm rooms, or meal halls.

There's something immediately nostalgic for me when I'm on a college campus; I loved being in college. Sometimes I can't believe it's been so long since I was walking around, my backpack slung over my shoulders, learning in such an open, unfettered way. I'm always wishing I could go back; but of course, "boats against the current."

Ignacio and I paused for a moment as we stood next to the lighted student center. He turned to me and wanted to discuss my piece in *Elle* and my illness, which appeared to prove to him that my body was especially sensitive to something in the transgenics. I could tell that Ignacio was curious—if not downright skeptical—about me. This was not new. I'd been through years of skepticism—of my own, of doctors, of friends and family, which was perhaps the hardest to take. When someone is sick with something no one can pinpoint, there's an odd "blame the victim" thing that takes hold; you almost can't help yourself from thinking their illness is psychosomatic. I understand this; I've done it myself, judged and juried.

In my case, after going back again and again to my GP, telling him something was wrong, that we needed to figure it out, I saw in his face, in the way he started talking to me, and in the way he turned to his notes rather than listening to me when I was talking, that he had become sick of me. Finally, he said, "You're just tired. Rest and come back next week." When I came back still tired, the pain radiating all over my body, making it hard for me to walk, he had a new theory: "You need to go on an antidepressant."

"Okay," I said. I tried one. It didn't work for the pain and it made me more tired.

"You need to go off the antidepressant," he advised. Then, "We need to test your thyroid again." Soon he said, "You need cortisone shots in your legs." Later, "You know what I think your problem is? Most people just live with this level of pain every day, you know. You've got an overly—*highly*—sensitive body. You need to stop focusing on it."

This diagnosis made me feel shame. *Toughen up*, I told myself.

Yet mental fortitude wasn't enough. I couldn't just *will* this away. My GP then, begrudgingly, farmed me out to various specialists in the Portland metro area. Looking over my medical records from that time, I see lists of test after test. And as my mind spins backward, flipping through time like an old Rolodex, it stops long enough for me to remember an elderly rheumatologist, Dr. George Morton, who has since retired. I remember his energetic and robust face. And I remember how assiduously he took notes, how concerned he seemed, how gentle. I remember being reserved with my story because I didn't want to make a big deal—I didn't want to bother this pleasant old man with my silly, childish, and probably female problems. *Let's talk about books or theater or anything else*, I thought. I was ashamed to have something wrong (I mean, what did this say about me, after all?) and I thought that if I downplayed it enough, even with a doctor, it wouldn't turn out to be anything.

Now, scanning my sheaf of medical papers—the file that preceded me from appointment to appointment—it feels almost voyeuristic and strangely discomfiting to read how that young woman, me—newly married, busy, career focused, ready to start this new stage in life— was perceived. In some of the notes there's a gossipy tone, as if it's an email written from one friend to another about this woman who lives down the road and has fallen into a yellow wallpaper vortex of illness. In Morton's notes there's a saddened, almost defeatist, tone that a "bright," "ambitious," "good-looking young woman," who was "casually but neatly dressed," is sick. Almost every record states that I was "worried" or "scared" by the severity of the symptoms and that "she wants to get well."

I did want to get well. I wanted answers, even if they were scary. Standing there with Ignacio, I remembered the horribly complicated feelings I had of wanting and needing help but also feeling such shame and anger. I remembered how, each time I met new doctors and had to tell them my story, just how exhausting it all got to try to fashion my narrative in a way that might not only interest them but also make a lightbulb go on in their heads, so they'd find a cure, or a drug, or . . . anything, really.

I understood, in the evening light, that although Ignacio was patient, belaboring too much of what I'd been through would shift something intrinsic between us; I didn't want his pity. Also, his skepticism about me made me respect him. Although he has become one of the most active voices in the anti-GMO movement, I could already tell that his scientific mind searches for data and patterns, and that he is naturally critical, even of someone like me who was there to write about him. That must portend a level of honesty, I thought.

I did tell him that I'm always looking for a way to prove or disprove this GMO corn theory for myself—something better than just feeling well—which in and of itself is a pretty convincing report. Then, almost as a caveat—but more as a way to put a period on what I was saying that left me wondering what he really thought about me that night—he told me about himself, shrugging my illness off like water sliding off a duck's well-oiled feather. "I'm like the cockroach. I can survive anything."

Two days later, when I was in his lab, he told me a curious story, however, which seemed to say the opposite. He said that he and his research assistant, Ali, had gone to a GMO cornfield to collect some specimens one day. The field had just been harvested but the farmer had left a good deal of corn on the ground. "As we walked through it," he told me, "Ali was covered, like with his hoodie over and just walking like this"—he pantomimed someone stiffly walking through a chemical war zone, not wanting anything to touch them—"and I was like, my usual stupid self—grabbing these corn-cobs. And as I walked, they were nice and fresh, you know, young corncobs. I was just chewing on them. I would just chew a few rows of one and then throw it and then get another one and keep going. And my God, did I get sick. This really horrible feverish thing. It wasn't really stomach problems; it was like this horrible reaction—like real pain, my body was in real, horrible physical pain in the joints and the muscles and bones. I got so spooked. . . ."

Here I interjected, "But I thought you were the cockroach?"

"Yeah, I thought so, too," he said.

chapter 20

The following morning I found a quiet table at the Berkeley City Club to have breakfast. I filled up on fresh fruit and green tea and ate some of the buckwheat hemp cereal I had brought from home. While I sat looking out the window, I translated my notes from the night before—as is my custom—writing down everything I could remember from my walk with Ignacio in the Berkeley Hills in a light yellow spiral-bound notebook I'd bought at a dollar store back home for 99¢. Then I put on my running shoes and went for a run around the campus, figuring I'd get my mind cleared before meeting Ignacio for lunch.

The sun was already hot by the time I hit the pavement. As I ran up the hill to the campus, I began to perceive a smell I remembered from living in Southern California when I was pregnant with Marsden: the slightly rotten stench of jasmine flowers mixed with the antibacterial smell of eucalyptus and the odd, tangy, fetid smell of the soil in California. The combination made my stomach turn. When Marsy was in my belly, I was so homesick for the clean smells of Maine—I wanted ocean breezes and pine trees, lilacs, lily of the valley, and dark, loamy earth.

But that day, on my run, the California stench was so pungent that it made me wonder if I might be pregnant with a second child. Dan and I had just started "trying" a little over a week earlier, a choice that we had vacillated back and forth about for the full five years of Marsy's life: Did we really want two children? Was it a good idea to add another child, considering the state of the planet? What kind of an environmentalist (or narcissist) adds another white, middle-class child to the already teetering consumerist overload of our world? Weren't we just too tired and old and our money too thin?

After Christmas, however, Dan had decided he wanted a second; our family is small, after all. Dan has little relationship with his family and Marsden is the only grandchild on my side. Perhaps this is what drives all living things in the end, this desire to make more of our kind, despite all the warnings against it. Nonetheless, it had taken me another month to come around to the idea. Then by the time I was ready, in February, Dan balked. Finally, in March, we just decided, "Hey, it's going to take a while, so might as well just start exploring this possibility now."

Around what we thought might be the right time of month (these things have always been a little murky to me), and just before I got on an airplane to go to Virginia to teach for a week, we did some "exploring." Ten days later I was in California, running. When the smell of that stinky California soil and cloying jasmine and sour eucalyptus hit me that morning, making me hunch over on the side of the road, I guessed that I was knocked up. I called Dan and told him what I thought. He laughed about it and asked me if I was sure that it could have been that easy (poor Dan never got the full benefit of "trying" with either child; it was turning out to be a one-shot deal with both). I told him I felt rather sure; there's just no feeling quite like being pregnant, and when it's not your first rodeo . . . you know. I walked back to the hotel and put on my swimsuit to go for a swim, preferring the smell of chlorine to the natural California ecosystem. As I swam in that pool in California, I thought about the salty ocean in Maine and had this flashback to the summer of 2010, when I was in one of the worst periods of my illness.

Somehow that summer, despite the illness—or maybe it was actually because of the illness—Dan and I had planned enough space around our work so that every morning we could take Mars and Hopper to Mackworth Island, a small state park off the coast of Portland, for a walk and a swim. It was an endlessly sunny summer (so sunny, my vitamin D level went up, according to a blood test, to 50 nanograms per milliliter that year, which is the best I've ever had, despite how sick I was). This was the kind of blissful plan I'd always dreamed of and it should have been nothing short of heaven. The island is only a mile and a quarter around, and the small beach where Dan and I like to swim from one end to the other is a half-moon-shaped inlet, carved by waves pummeling the rocky coast year after year.

We pushed Mars in the stroller—he was only one and a half then—until the beach, where he'd get down and squat on his sumptuous haunches and smash mussel shells with rocks, watching the blue and pearlescent colors powder together on a fat piece of Maine shale while we took turns swimming. Hopper would play the go-between nurse, swimming out to me, making a circle around me with a stick in his mouth, and then paddling back to Marsy to check on the mussel shell demolition.

And every morning, by the end of that swim and walk, I'd be walking like a ninety-year-old, my body stiff all over. It was such a peculiar pattern; I'd wake up feeling semi-okay, just tired, mostly. Dan would let me stay in bed as long as I needed. And then as the morning wore on, my body would start to feel like it was battening down all its hatches and closing off, a screw tightening it minute by minute until, by afternoon, I was on the couch leveled by the pain and exhaustion.

Even so, we went to Mackworth like Catholics to the Liturgy—the sun and the water felt like a ritual, something we needed; it was a kind of subliminal pause when we could try to suspend our fear for an hour, maybe two, in the transcendent sunshine.

One morning in mid-July, I was standing in the cold, clear water, the rockweed fanning out golden and brown around me, and I just knew that I didn't have the strength that day to swim the whole cove. I remember I looked up at the sky and prayed to whatever might be out there. I said, "Someone—ocean, summer, sun, world, God—take this away." Then I dove in; hoping that when I surfaced like a seal, I would somehow be magically washed clean.

When I came up for air, I was the same. In pain, exhausted.

Then a young woman, a stranger, arrived on the beach with her two small, blond sons. Standing in the water, she looked longingly at me and said, "I wish I'd brought my bathing suit." She looked healthy and happy and strong.

"Go in your underwear," I encouraged. "It's just us. I'll watch your boys. It feels terrific." She looked uncertain, like I was being radical. "Really," I said. "It's lovely. We come every morning and my day is just not the same unless I jump in. You only live once, right?"

And then she did it. She pulled off her shirt and shorts and went in her underwear and bra while her boys stood shyly near me on the shore.

When she came up, she shook herself and asked, "You really do this every day?"

"We do," I said.

In my head I was thinking, *If you only knew. I stand out here in this water and look back at that shore where my husband and son are smashing mussel shells and the gulf between me and them sometimes feels like I'm so far away. Like I'm already gone.*

THAT MORNING in California I felt blessed that this had turned around. That I wasn't gone. And now here I was, likely pregnant again—something that when I was sick I wasn't sure I'd ever be able to do again—and I felt strong and supple in the long, blue pool. Like the woman I'd encouraged to swim, it was possible, I imagined, that one day I'd be taking my own two children to swim on Mackworth Island. The possibility of this was almost too good to be true.

Giddily thankful, I pulled myself out of the pool and dried off. I went back to my room to shower and change and then made my way out of my room to reconvene with Ignacio for lunch.

Ignacio and I met downstairs, in the busy hotel restaurant called Julia's. Despite the fact that on the day I arrived a big Sysco food truck was pulled up to the door to unload, some of the items on the menu were labeled as organic and local. It was noisy in the restaurant, so we found a quieter corner and ordered simply: He got a Caesar salad that arrived on a square plate, the lettuce pieces arranged into a pyramid like a Mayan temple, and I ordered an organic burger with a side salad—no bun, because not only is corn often on the bottom of breads, rolls, pizzas, and such (usually so the dough doesn't stick to the pan), it can also be inside baked goods as dough conditioners and additives. Also, in 2013, I had stopped eating gluten after a terrible bout of acid reflux. My newest GP had told me that she takes all her reflux patients off gluten. It did seem to work, for the most part, though sometimes I can get reflux just from coffee, tea, or stress.

During our lunch, I wanted to hear from Ignacio how he got from setting up a lab with the Oaxacans to his piece in *Nature*. What were the actual steps in between and then how had he become as embroiled as he had in the GMO discussion for the last twenty years?

In 2000, Ignacio told me, in that rustic lab in the mountains of Oaxaca, he had discovered (with the help of a graduate student with whom he was working named David Quist) that the Oaxacans had "transgenic DNA in their local varieties of corn." By "local varieties of corn," Ignacio underscores, what we're really talking about are indigenous varieties of corn that have been cultivated by the people of Mexico for thousands of years. Not sure that this meant as much to the

Oaxacans as it came to mean for Ignacio, I asked, "And what did that mean to *them?*"

"That's a really important question," he said. "You know, corn is who they are . . . they are corn and corn is them. . . . So telling them that there is transgenic contamination [in their corn] is equivalent to coming to your house in the morning with a lab coat and some kind of distinguishing stuff that makes me a scientist, right, some kind of authority? And I knock at your door and I say, 'I just wanted to let you know that while you were asleep, somebody from this place that you also hate, you know, the U.S., just moved into your body and is living inside you.' And you say, 'I don't see anything, I don't feel anything, what do you mean?' And I say, 'That's all. I'm just telling you that, and good-bye.' . . . So they would say, 'So what's going to happen?' I would say, 'I don't know. I have no idea.' 'And how can I get rid of it?' 'I don't know.' 'And how much is there?' 'I don't know. I have no idea. Good-bye.' Which is basically what I did to them, which is horrible."

As a writer—a storyteller—this moment of discovery is compelling, because it has the painful human quality of innocent ignorance to it, ignorance of something that is, perhaps, right under one's nose but is invisible to the naked eye. That's really the crucial crux of this issue, I was coming to believe that afternoon as I sat talking to Ignacio: that GMOs are invisible. After all, we are creating, growing, and eating things to which we've given characteristics that are undetectable to our naked eyes and discerning noses—and for that matter, to the eyes and noses of birds, deer, butterflies,[1] and raccoons, too. And yet they look the same, smell the same, and seem the same as the regular non-GMO varietals, and, to boot, we're told by reliable-seeming officials that there is no difference. Maine's congresswoman Chellie Pingree had said to me, "Corn looks like corn." And yet, the question still lingers: Is all corn really the same? Might there be real, visible, and,

---

[1] Yes, butterflies can smell. Even better than humans!

perhaps, unintended consequences from GMOs? To our own bodies when we eat them? To the land on which they are grown? To the creatures with whom we share this planet?

To understand what this must have felt like for the Oaxacans, for whom Chapela was the messenger, I felt like I needed some CliffsNotes on corn and what it means to the Mexican identity. After some Internet surfing in my hotel room, I discovered that corn was first eaten as popcorn by the Mesoamericans, who began cultivating it in what is now Mexico as early as 5000 BC. It's said that in 1492 Christopher Columbus "discovered" corn and brought a corn plant back to show Queen Isabella, the queen of Spain, telling her court about how the white kernels, shaped like peas, could be ground like a grain. The court was intrigued.

In the following years, corn spread from Spain throughout Europe and to Africa. In North America, corn eventually made its way north of Mexico to America and Canada, where it was cultivated by the Native Americans, who showed the Pilgrims how to, in turn, cultivate it in 1621 (and then, of course, it became a part of our first Thanksgiving). As corn had its diaspora, it was recognized around the globe as a plant that would yield a lot of food—a big caloric bang for the buck. However, even as corn became a common staple in many countries, the Mexicans still held on to their deep association with corn as an intrinsic part of themselves. Today many Mexicans still refer to themselves as the "corn people." Michael Pollan writes in *The Omnivore's Dilemma*, "The phrase is not intended as a metaphor. Rather, it's meant to acknowledge their abiding dependence on this miraculous grass, the staple of their diet for almost nine thousand years. Forty percent of the calories a Mexican eats in a day come directly from corn, most of it in the form of tortillas. So when a Mexican says, 'I am maize' or 'corn walking,' it is simply a statement of fact: the very substance of the Mexican body is to a considerable extent the manifestation of this plant." (And, as we learned from Aaron Woolf's documentary, *King Corn*, a Bill and Ted–type adventure into the world of industrial corn, the fiber of the Mexican being probably *is* actually made of corn, as corn protein can show up even in our hair in America, according to the film, because of how much we ingest!)

Mexican farmers, I learned, often work small (20-or-fewer-acre) plots and yet their corn, in aggregate, accounts for more than two-thirds of the country's corn production. Most of their corn are heirloom varieties—in fact, today there are at least fifty-nine varieties that are still thriving and have been preserved for thousands of years due to seed saving and local farmers' simple breeding techniques between different corn plants in order to cultivate varietals specific to their little patch of earth. These corn plants have been developed "over millenniums," writes Peter Canby in an article in the *Nation*, "by indigenous farmers for different attributes; growth at high altitudes, early or late maturation, that ability to withstand drought or heavy rain" or "for particular dishes or shamanic rituals."

Because of this long and traditional history with corn, which Canby writes is "essential for the future of corn crops" worldwide, Mexico's official position—as of 1998—was that no GMO corn cultivation was allowed in the country of Mexico, since the Mexican farmers themselves could produce at least 80 percent of the corn needed to feed the nation. (Corn has long been referred to by Mexicans as "Vitamin T"—consumed in tortas, tostadas, tacos, tamales, and tortillas.) In 2003, Mexico signed the Cartagena Protocol on Biosafety to the Convention on Biological Diversity, an international protocol that was signed by various countries (many of which were in Europe) with the goal of protecting biodiversity from GMO contamination. The Cartagena Protocol also allowed some countries to ban not only the importation of some GMO products but also the cultivation of them.

However, back in the late '90s, because of both NAFTA, which Mexico signed in late 1993, and the globalization of food in general, the United States' GMO corn—which markets in Europe and Japan were summarily rejecting for human consumption—was coming into Mexico as animal feed for Mexican feedlots and, also, to be made into tortillas that were then shipped back to the United States for American consumption. According to Mexican scientist Dr. Exequiel Ezcurra (who was eventually appointed president of the Instituto Nacional de Ecología—the Mexican equivalent of the EPA—in January 2001), many scientists, himself included, became concerned at the advent of NAFTA about the future of Mexican corn.

Exequiel told me one afternoon on the phone, his voice as deep and sonorous as the character Esteben on the TV show *Weeds*, that in essence, they were worried about two things: that the United States' subsidized corn would unfairly compete with the Mexican farmers' corn, which is not subsidized, making the Mexican farmers vulnerable in the market; and that the native varietals of corn might, somehow, despite the ban on GMO cultivation, become contaminated by the new GMO corn that the United States was engineering. He said that he and others had urged the government to grind up all American corn at the border so that contamination would not be possible.

Their fears, as it turns out, were not so far-fetched: contamination did happen, as Ignacio's study showed. How it must have happened, Ignacio, Exequiel, and others theorize, is that sacks of U.S. corn intended as animal feed were being distributed by the Mexican government as a subsidized food into areas where peasants live. Ignacio stated that for the Mexicans—and perhaps in this case for the Mexican government—there was little differentiation made between the animal-grade food and the food fit for human consumption or, for that matter, for planting. "For people up there," said Ignacio, "the difference between seed and grain doesn't exist. A seed and a grain is the same thing."

This story becomes important because in 2000, during the exact same time period Ignacio was discovering contamination, a huge controversy erupted in the United States when StarLink corn made by Aventis CropScience (now a Bayer company)—approved by the EPA only for animal feed (and rejected for human consumption)—was found to have contaminated more than three hundred food products made for human beings (products such as taco shells and tortillas). The StarLink corn was genetically engineered with a Cryprotein, Cry9C, made from insecticidal Bt, which was thought to be impervious to stomach acid, and therefore would make it out of the gut intact. It, like all the Cryproteins, had been tested with the infamous test-tube stomach acid test, which many people have said does not simulate actual stomach acids, especially because of the overuse of proton pump inhibitors (PPIs), like Prilosec. However, Cry9C had even failed the test-tube stomach acid tests—failed so miserably that it was deemed by the FDA only appropriate for animal feed. Even so, somehow, a handful of people around the United States reportedly got sick from Cry9C protein, or Bt. Taco Bell–brand taco shells and other food products were then recalled and the FDA was criticized for not doing its job.[2]

A Cincinnati allergist whom I interviewed when I was first working on my *Elle* piece named Dr. Amal Assa'ad (whose practice is a short five-minute walk through long, gray hospital corridors from Simon Hogan's office) said that she never believed that StarLink corn should have been implicated. Dr. Assa'ad is a lovely smooth-skinned woman, with thick dark hair, who moved to America from Egypt, where she received her medical degrees. She has been interested in GMOs for quite some time, she told me, because of the hunger she has witnessed in her homeland (she said she's been disappointed by the African rejection of GMOs in general and sees no good reason for it). Assa'ad was part of a team, she told me, that, when the FDA said they were not going to do food challenges on the people who said StarLink had made them sick, stepped forward and offered to conduct the challenges in Cincinnati. She said that one patient came to stay in her hospital about two years after the incident when he said he'd gotten sick. In Cinci, she said, "We did what's called a food

---

[2] Aventis hired the consulting company Exponent to handle this crisis. Exponent, reportedly, also handled such disasters as the *Exxon Valdez*, the collapse of the World Trade Towers, and the space shuttle *Challenger*.

challenge. We put the [StarLink] corn in applesauce or something. One day he got an adequate amount, the amount that would be the equivalent to what you would have in a tortilla, because that's what he had said [that] he [had] reacted to—the tortillas, a couple of times. He had no symptoms either that first day, the second or third day; he had no symptoms whatsoever. This is really the only challenge that was ever done to corroborate the evidence that this person had an allergy. We did skin tests—they were negative."[3] In Assa'ad's view, corn has been unnecessarily "vilified." She did allow that "corn has been thought to be a major problem" in causing eosinophilic disorders—allergic disorders that cause an abundance of white blood cells, called eosinophils, to flood the body and attack tissues (which is what Mansmann had said ailed me).[4] But she also said she didn't believe that this was likely. In her practice, she is dealing with major allergies to things like peanuts, eggs, and milk. "I see a whole lot of patients with symptoms that one would get from a peanut allergy, for example: hives, lip swelling, eye swelling, throwing up, having really low blood pressure, anaphylaxis—[these] very rarely occur with corn. Having a corn-allergic patient is very uncommon." When I pushed Assa'ad a little harder on whether she thought that the GMO part—the Bt, which is the internal pesticide, or the proteins that DNA insertions create—in GMO corn could be indeed perturbing something in the body, she said, "What is wrong with chemicals? We are so afraid of chemicals because they are man-made, right? There are all kinds of chemicals, but a lot of chemicals have helped us." Furthermore, she said, "It's not the fault of the corn that because it's now resistant that people are

---

[3] I did point out to Assa'ad that I thought I'd learned from my research on allergies that two years between the initial episode and the challenge may have been long enough to desensitize the patient. She did not think that was possible if he'd gotten as sick as he said he had from the contaminated Taco Bell shells.

[4] Another allergist told me that many people with eosinophilic esophagitis (an allergic condition that causes eosinophils in the esophagus) test positive for a corn allergy. If corn is removed from their diets, he told me, all EE symptoms seem to improve.

using more pesticides than needed or that is safe. I think that is a totally different story. This needs to be controlled by the producers. The pesticides need to be studied in and of themselves. It's like, okay, you have food all over the place, the food is good, but if you feed your child more than they need to, they are going to get obese. Is it the fault of the food or is it the fault of the amount you are giving the child or the child having a big appetite? That's a different story."

Whether or not StarLink was truly the problem for the individuals who said they were allergic to it, for seven years after Aventis had taken its product off the market, Belinda Martineau, the GMO tomato scientist, told me that the EPA and the USDA monitored the U.S. corn crop annually until they found that levels of StarLink were low enough that they didn't have to worry about it anymore. "That's how long" it took to rid the commercial corn crops of StarLink residue, Belinda said. And, she continued, "That isn't saying that after seven years they couldn't detect it any longer. That's saying that the levels were low enough that they weren't going to worry about it anymore. So once it's out there, it's out there." She went on, "What is different about StarLink? There should have been research done to say, you know, 'Wait. What happened with this one? What did they change in the lab and why does this one behave like an allergen in these tests when these other ones didn't?' But no. They just throw it away, it's like 'Oh, that's a problem, we're just not going to look at that anymore.' And they don't even put it in [Rick Goodman's] database."

Ignacio's theory is that the StarLink event and what happened in Mexico are not necessarily discrete: "The U.S. was dumping bad-quality corn with an excess of transgenics [into Mexico for animal feed] . . . and then getting the Mexican government to distribute it to the most remote little corner. . . . By law there shouldn't have been any transgenics in the whole country of Mexico . . . obviously they [the government] were playing double-faced. Because they were saying, 'Well, we're distributing this only to be consumed [by animals] not to be planted.' But . . . who's going to enforce that?"

By now Ignacio had eaten his small though impressively constructed salad, and I had eaten up my burger. He seemed so calm as he ate, he was almost dainty. Though I didn't know that I was pregnant yet for sure, I did feel ravenously hungry. Throwing my pride to the wind, I told Ignacio I was going to order coffee—Peet's—and dessert. He followed suit. A vanilla and cara cara orange crème caramel for me and a warm orange marmalade cake for him.

As we dove into our desserts—mine so silken and creamy it was otherworldly—Ignacio told me that when the Oaxacans were informed of the contamination, they went berserk. "People were saying, 'Oh, that's why dogs are dying in our town. That's why people are losing their teeth now because of this,'" and, despite the absurdity of these claims, he felt an enormous responsibility to offer some kind of solution. Yet he had none. "Giving a message without a solution is something that's ethically questionable and difficult," he told me.

Inspired by the reaction—which seemed to portend the enormous consequences of their discovery—Ignacio and David Quist went back to Berkeley and began drafting the report that eventually ended up in *Nature*. "We all—any biologist—was worried about cross-contamination. But nobody had any numbers or any data," Ignacio said. Until now.

As they were penning the paper, Ignacio said he was already thinking through the political implications of what his data would mean on a global scale. Here he was about to submit a paper to the most influential science magazine in the world and he was saying two inflammatory and crucial things about GMOs: The first was that the DNA from GMOs will eventually contaminate other crops—organic, prized landraces that have been in existence for eons—whether by wind, birds, bees, human error, or some combination of all of the above. And second, his study indicated that the DNA from the transgenic corn was unstable, and had "become re-assorted" in the genome of the criollo—the local, indigenous corn—and might, in the words of Peter Pringle in his book *Food, Inc.*, "wander" and "produce all manner of unexpected and destructive results." What either one would mean for the local Oaxacan people—and the world—the study did not posit, but we can assume the news was not necessarily welcome from the point of view of sustaining biodiversity, at the very least.

Later, when I was home from California, I was still intrigued by Ignacio's theory that DNA from the transgenic corn would "wander." And as it turns out, this more novel idea had definitely become his detractors' focal point. Many of his critics chose to focus on that part of this study in their attacks rather than the more electrifying concept of contamination. Ignacio admitted to me, via email, that at the time he published his paper, this wandering idea was a relatively new one, one he had to fight to hold on to. He said that these days he thinks it's "generally accepted" by most scientists.[5] What his study proved, he told me, was that the GMO DNA could really go just about anywhere in the plant, despite what the "gene jockeys" (people who make transgenics in the labs) say.

To be sure I understood, I called Belinda Martineau to ask her some questions about the Flavr Savr tomato and the genetic insertions she had made when creating that GMO. I asked, "Could you, ostensibly, make a mistake and put the wrong DNA in a GMO? Or put the DNA in the wrong place?"

"Yes," she told me, "we actually know very little about what happens once you make a transgenic insert." She went on, "One thing we discovered when we were working on the tomato was [this]: The FDA came to us and said, 'You know, you say that only this little piece of DNA in this big vector [the vehicle that helps transfer the foreign genetic material] of DNA goes into the plant. How do you know the whole rest of the vector doesn't go into the plant? And, you know, I looked at them and I said, 'That's a silly question.' Ten years of plant molecular biology research indicates that only that piece of DNA will go in. . . . So my first response to the FDA was a literature review,

---

[5] Word to the wise: Saying that anything is "generally accepted" in terms of GMOs is fightin' words! Very little is "accepted" by everyone on both sides.

basically. I picked the expert at Berkeley and her latest review and said, 'Only that piece of DNA will go in.' And the FDA to their credit came back to us and they said, 'We didn't ask you whether you thought it would or not. We want you to look in the tomato plants and look for the rest of that vector DNA and make sure that it didn't go in.' So I did the experiment and lo and behold, thirty to forty percent of the time the whole darn vector did go into the plant."

"So," I asked, "what does that tell you?"

"That made me step back and say, 'Whoa, are we really ready for this?'"

But would most scientists know (or test to see) that something had changed? I asked.

Belinda said, "So if you're looking at your data and you say, 'Hey, I meant to put in this piece of DNA and it's changed in the plant. But this plant is the one that performs the best in the field and I've worked with it for four generations and I like the way it produces lots of seeds, it's really convenient for me to work with this particular plant. So I'm just going to tell the FDA this is the one I'm going to go to market with, even though something happened in the process of genetic engineering that altered the gene that I meant to put in there. . . .' I mean, it's their baby. This is their project, this is their livelihood, they've been working with this corn product for six years. Their paycheck depends on it, their promotion depends on it, they truly believe in their heart it's going to help farmers or somebody. And they don't want to admit it has any problems. It's just human nature, it's not a conscious decision, I don't think."

BACK IN BERKELEY and now on our second cup of coffee, Ignacio said that even when he and David Quist were finishing up the details of their paper, he knew that the wandering theory would be ground-breaking and the contamination piece would become a lightning rod: "I know it's going to be a big scandal . . . because I know the field. I know the forces, and I know that everybody's scared and worried about contamination. So I submit the paper. When I got the first peer reviews[6] that were very positive, I said, 'Now I'm going to start calling people on the phone.' So I made a list of people I thought would be involved in the response to this news, and I started calling them personally and [I] say, 'I want you to know that we're very likely going to be publishing this paper in *Nature* that you're going to be affected by.'" He said that on that list of people were heads of NGOs and government officials, though he couldn't remember off the top of his head who they all were.

I asked Ignacio point-blank: Why in the world would you send up smoke signals like that? After all, we were starting to get to know each other a bit better by now, and my courage to challenge him was growing (perhaps it was the caffeine), along with my desire to make sure I got the record straight. He told me that at the time what was going through his head was that if his study hit the airwaves quickly and without any advance warning given to the people who might be able to speak to it, or to contextualize it, it was "all going to be in the hands of reporters who have no idea what to do with it and no idea what it means and it's going to be a really bad scuttling of the subject." When I pressed Ignacio a bit further, he admitted that he was playing defense. "So my thinking was, everybody will run to them [the biotech companies] and—between reporters badly reporting the situation and Monsanto—they're [Biotech] going to manage the whole thing to their advantage and nobody will have any chance of exercising their intelligent analysis. . . . That's why I was making calls."

In an even bolder move, Ignacio accepted an offer to go down to Mexico to give a "closed doors, only with experts" seminar on his data before it was printed. This is now April 2001. He told me, "So

---

[6] Scientific papers in reputable journals are subject to a "peer review" process, which is meant to catch flaws or holes in the science prior to publication. Sometimes when flaws are found, the paper will not move on to publication. Other times the editors will suggest that certain clarifications be made, based on the recommendations of the reviewers, and at other times the study will be published despite questions and the scientific debate will ensue. I was told by many scientists while working on this book that this process is entirely normal to them and this is how the best science emerges—there are checks and balances along the way and the debate is necessary for new, reliable science to emerge.

they fly me in, and it's a meeting where the ministers and scientists for the ministers and everybody's there . . . but I speak to them on the condition of confidentiality because by policy, *Nature* will not publish something that has been touched by media."

Since I'm not the one going through it, I can see, hearing this story, how this might be poised to explode all over Ignacio. But remember Ignacio has a reputation for being something of a pain in the ass. I said to him, "It seems obvious to me at this point that this is going to hell in a handbasket. Why wasn't it to you?" In his defense, he said that scientists are always giving seminars on work that they're researching or that is on its way to being published. (I was able to confirm this from various sources. Dr. Exequiel Ezcurra also told me, "Scientists are always excited and want to let people know they've had important findings.") However, with the political din surrounding Ignacio's work, Ezcurra said, "Chapela tried to do it under the radar, but it got botched."

Over the next few months, things started to devolve with *Nature*. Despite the fact that *Nature* can accept a paper and publish it within a week, which Ignacio had originally hoped they were on track to accomplish, some of the later peer reviewers of the paper had begun to cast some serious doubts on his study. So, *Nature* asked Ignacio and Quist to recheck some of their results. They started working frantically—during the nights Pacific standard time to keep up with the London-based publication. Over the next few months, Ignacio and Quist endured "five rounds of back and forth," with *Nature*, which is unheard of.

Still no publication.

And then the story gets weird.

It goes like this: Ignacio goes back to Mexico for more meetings in September. And he gives another "closed doors" seminar on what his research has found. After the seminar, as he's leaving, "there's this big guy waiting there . . . and he says, 'Well, I'm here in representation of Mr. So-and-So, who is the chair of the committee on biosafety for Mexico, and my boss would like to talk to you. I said, 'That's why I'm here.' You know, I'm going to go talk to him. So what follows next is like a gangster story."

According to Ignacio, he and the big guy got into a green-and-yellow Mexico City taxi, a VW beetle. The big guy mutters an address to the driver, which Ignacio couldn't quite hear. As they started to drive, Ignacio says that he asked where they were going and the answer was, "We're going to the office." To which he asked, "Where's that?" And the response was, "Oh, it's not far." Then he said, "I'm taken into this really shady part of Mexico City where bodies are dumped and that kind of thing." He says he started to get really nervous when they arrived at what appeared to be a virtually empty building. "Maybe one or two floors were occupied with some kind of governmental offices, and it had a guard at the entrance. But it was completely empty by that time because it was after five. And we walk in and go up to the thirteenth floor. . . ." At that point, he said, he was starting to internally—and silently—panic. Then, he told me, "The elevator opens and it's this dark floor of an empty building . . . and there is a little light at the end of this dark hallway coming out of a room, and it's the boss with a big mustachio—it's kind of funny—in an office that is made of cardboard boxes, a door taken off the hinges on top of the cardboard boxes—that's his table. He has a cell phone, he has a laptop, there's a coffeemaker and a maid making coffee."

The man, it turns out, whom Ignacio describes as being like a *charro*—"the guy with the big hat, the big silken bowtie, and a horse who sings and plays the guitar and shoots in the air"—was a high-ranking government official, the executive secretary of the Commission for Biosafety and Genetically Modified Organisms of Mexico, by the name of Fernando Ortiz Monasterio. Ezcurra told me that Monasterio was "very flamboyant . . . very good-looking in his youth and . . . from a family of intellectual aristocracy in Mexico. He had bushy eyebrows and wore bowties that mariachi or *charros* wear."

According to Ignacio, Monasterio ordered that the maid leave, and he's "left with the bodyguard and this guy," Monasterio, whom Ignacio describes as "just the nastiest, nastiest person you can imagine." Next, Monasterio spent, he said, "about one hour berating me. Just telling me, you know, with really bad language what a big hole I've dug for myself. And what a big problem I've created and how I'm about to ruin the reputation of Mexico and . . . stop a whole technology that is going to save the world, blah blah blah. . . ." Then, says Ignacio, Monasterio offers him a solution to the problem: He tells Ignacio he's a great scientist, that "nobody denies the fantastic qualities of your research . . . and I've arranged for five of the best scientists in your field to get together and to try to deal with your fucking mess." So Ignacio asks who the other four scientists are going to be. And Monasterio reportedly tells Ignacio that they would come from Monsanto and DuPont. "So you and four scientists from the industry, we'll take you to this fantastic place in Baja California, you will not be disturbed by anybody and you will write the paper. You will get a publication in *Nature*. But what you're going to say is what you found is a piece of DNA that exists naturally."

Ignacio said that this was all just too unbelievable to comprehend. Suddenly he's being guaranteed a *Nature* publication (which is pretty darn elusive right about now), but not of the study he originally submitted. Instead, he's being asked to rewrite his own study with help from some industry hacks. He says that he told Monasterio that "I'm very happy to work with anybody, including industry, but I'm not about to let them tell me what I'm going to print. And also I have a job, you know. I have to go back to Berkeley and I have a class on Monday, and I'm not doing this. So he got really mad and he told the bodyguard, 'Show him the offices.'"

At which point, Ignacio says, he started to feel faint. He said, "The bodyguard started walking me through these completely desolate, messed-up spaces. The carpets were all curled up like there had been floods inside the building. . . . You could see this big dumpster in back [of the building]. I was just thinking, 'Gosh, am I going to be thrown out the window here? Is that what's going to happen next?' It was just so unbelievable, you know."

Ignacio paused and took a sip of coffee.

"And then what happened?" I asked. I was glued to my seat at this point, wondering what horrible thing was going to happen next. Tony Soprano around the corner? A Mexican drug lord? Guns? What?

Ignacio smiled for effect.

"Nothing happened," he said. "He just walked me through these empty spaces and then forced me to go down to the basement. I said, 'No, thank you, I'll just take a cab.' And he said, 'No no no, the boss insists that he has to give you a ride.' And so we went down to the basement where he [had waiting for them] . . . his black Suburban. And then he started talking about my daughter and insisting that he wanted to drop me off where my sister lives—basically just talking about my family and what he knew about, you know, my vulnerable points in my life or something. And that was it."

That was it? Really? Could Ignacio just have a majorly fictive imagination that made it seem scarier than it really was? I decided to call up Exequiel Ezcurra to ask him if this story seemed far-fetched. Could Ignacio Chapela truly have been threatened by Monasterio, I asked? "Yes," said Ezcurra. "It makes sense that he was bullied or threatened by him." As a caveat, Ezcurra said, "Between you and me, sometimes Chapela sees conspiracy where I might not see it. He sometimes seems to be overly concerned about the evilness of people. But that does not mean he was not bullied."

Even so, when I got home from California I tried to find Monasterio. First I found a famous plastic surgeon by the same name, from the same family, who happened to be dead. Then I found an architect who was Monasterio's son—also with the same name. Undaunted, I started writing and calling the son, trying to find El Papa. No one responded to me, though the son's secretary and I became friendly and I was getting to practice more Spanish than I had since I lived in Salamanca for a summer when I was fourteen. Finally, over two years later, just as this book was going to press, I was able to smoke the real Monasterio out.

On a brilliantly sunny and snowy Saturday morning at home in

Maine, the man himself agreed to talk to me via cell phone from a small village in the mountains outside of Mexico City. Not sure if he knew who I was, I started in. He cut me off and told me he knew exactly who I was, that he'd read all my emails. (FYI, he spoke perfect English, so thankfully we didn't need to wander around in the weeds of my old Spanish!) He told me that he had my most recent and long list of questions right in front of him. He said he was happy to go through them, point by point. However, he said, before we began, he wanted to make sure I understood what, to him, were two important considerations. I said, "Sure. I'm happy to do this however works best for you." He said thank you and then took charge. First, he told me, he wanted me to separate, in my writing, him "as a government representative fifteen years ago, and me as a name you publish in your book—as Fernando. I was a public servant," he told me, "who had a mandate." I agreed. "Okay," he said. Then, he said, he wanted me to understand the Mexican climate into which Ignacio unleashed his conclusions about GMO proliferation.

"Tell me," I said. "I will," he said. And honestly, he sounded quite reasonable and not at all scary, so I sat back with my pen scratching my notebook as he spoke, confident that with him in charge of the narrative I was about to hear, very little would be left unaddressed.

"Chapela's work is remarkable and it's commendable," he told me. "It is unequivocal that he found something widely known and widely expected. I have respected what he did and also what he went through. My position has always been in his favor. You must understand that at that time Mexico was importing several million tons of genetically modified corn from the U.S. every year. There was a vast distribution of the corn into the marketplace and everywhere in the country [of Mexico]. Can you imagine that that corn, sold for cattle, wasn't going to be planted? There is a contradiction [in the government] between saying we shouldn't [plant this stuff] and the harsh reality that we are invaded. I have said for fifteen years that Mexico should not plant

GMO corn. Mexico is the center of diversity for corn. The big companies of course want this market. But no country of origin should plant GMOs—just like the U.S. and Canada should not plant GMO canola and Peru should not plant GMO potatoes. Countries of origin of any plant should not allow GMOs of that species."

Points taken, I told him. "Now that I've said those two things, we can move on to your questions," he said.

He told me he had had Ignacio brought to him for a meeting. And yes, he said the offices were "under construction." "We had no furniture and no salary, no rooms—it was tough luck, bad conditions of work for such an important job."

"Did you really have your desk on top of cardboard boxes?" I asked, suddenly feeling a surprising combination of protective toward him and also just embarrassed that I was asking what seemed to me to be such a first-world question.

"Yes," he said. "It was hard." But, he said, what our offices looked like "is irrelevant."

What was the tone of your meeting? I asked.

"Direct," he said. "I had to explain the position of the Mexican government. And this is not the same tone with which I am talking to you, Caitlin. We were not meeting as friends. The information he had was a cherry bomb for biosafety."

Did you threaten him? I asked. "I have heard this before," he said, "the fact that Ignacio felt threatened." But, he said, he could assure me that "I was professional but not friendly. It's completely wrong to say I threatened him." However, he went on, he feels that these details of how the meeting did or didn't go are "irrelevant" to the bigger point. "Don't lose yourself in the details," he instructed, "when what is important was the meeting between a public servant and a scientist who brought to life an important reality."

Did you swear at him? I asked. "No." He said he did not swear.

Did you feel that Ignacio's discovery would hurt biotechnology and

NAFTA? I asked. "Yes," he said. "His information would change public policy in the country and probably the world—it was very important."

Did you ever intimate that he should redo the study with industry scientists in Baja? I asked. "I don't remember Baja California," he said. "But I did say that he should do this again with university scientists, government scientists, and yes, since Monsanto has better labs and techniques, their conclusion would be important so [they would give] us more evidence of what we were sure was happening [to corn] in Mexico," he said. Did you ever suggest that he change his evidence? "No. Absolutely no. This is out of this world. It was in the interest of biosafety to say, 'Look, we're in danger.' We all knew he was right. Is the implication that I didn't want him to tell the truth?" "Yes, that's the implication," I said. Not true, he told me. To retread a bit, I asked, "Did you or a bodyguard ever imply physical threat to Ignacio?"

"A bodyguard?" He snorted. "We were without offices. A body-guard is completely out of context."

"But I understand you come from an aristocratic family. Did you have a chauffeur or some family staff who might have been helping you that day?"

"I had some friends who helped me. That's maybe who brought him here [and back]. But no family staff was involved."

"Then what happened?" I asked.

"Well, then Ignacio left."

"Does it bother you that Ignacio tells a story that's different from yours?"

"No, it doesn't bother me," he said. "It's irrelevant and it minimizes the point that there are higher levels of debate which are urgently needed on [GMOs]." Again, he said, "what is relevant is that he changed public policy on GMOs—that is more important than the driver or no driver and what part of town we met in."

"Not to be a pain in the ass, but can we address once more that he felt unsafe?"

He said, "Look, the fear is real . . . revolutionary scientists are going to change the world. And if you go to war to change the world, you better not be afraid. Chapela's work threatened international perception of science, and he was not supported by his government or his university, and he fought for his study like Quixote and the windmills. Chapela's contribution to understanding the problem of GMOs in the world is a turning point. If he likes me or not, that's another thing. What he did was courageous and stood against the wind. He was *right*. It's in everything. It's everywhere. I honor and value and respect his position. His work made a difference. Period. In the world."

ACCORDING TO IGNACIO, the day after his meeting with Monasterio was a Friday. He says he was scheduled to fly back to California. While he had been in Mexico the situation with *Nature* was reaching a fever pitch of dysfunction. The stress, Ignacio said, that he and Quist were feeling was unimaginable, as their careers—if not their lives—appeared to be dangling over an abyss. Apparently, in the morning, as he was getting ready to fly home, he was called by an official from Greenpeace who alerted him that Ortiz Monasterio had leaked the news of his study. Monasterio had, apparently, told the Greenpeace official that the criollo corn contamination was a discovery made by the Mexican government (not Ignacio). The official told Ignacio that at that point a variety of NGOs were planning on going public with Ignacio's information about Oaxacan contamination, and that the press would follow suit. No one could abide by Ignacio's request to keep the study quiet anymore.

Dr. Ezcurra says he remembers when this happened. He said that when Monasterio leaked the information, it was a move of terrible faith between scientists: "That's a basic moré of good behavior between colleagues and scientists—that you don't disclose." Nonetheless, Ezcurra said, suddenly, "This guy who doesn't know the difference between DNA and RNA is calling the NGOs and disclosing the whole thing. And at the time his argument was 'we're telling The People.' . . ."

"In all likelihood," Ezcurra told me, "he [Monasterio] was

concerned [about NAFTA] and of not doing something [with information] that would damage the companies." In other words, if he didn't precede Ignacio with this news, the powerful multinational companies that had everything to benefit from NAFTA would have no recourse to explain themselves; Monasterio did it this way so that damage could be controlled. However, Ezcurra said, "Monasterio damaged Chapela's chances of getting published." When I asked Monasterio if this was true, he said that Chapela's information was not news to him, and that the Mexican government already had this information and that it was public information at that point. "We all knew [this]," he said. "Chapela just confirmed what everyone knew. This was not a tight secret [that needed to be protected]."

That may be, but Ignacio said that as soon as the information was out there, like pollen on the wind, it spread. And he knew immediately that this was the end of his publication in *Nature*—which, remember, has a strict policy that they will not publish anything that has appeared already in the press. So, in a move of incredible hubris, Ignacio called Rex Dalton, the West Coast correspondent for *Nature*, and told him the story of what was going on—the weird meetings in Mexico, the fact that his study wasn't being published but that the news of it was about to be released, and the back-and-forth with *Nature*. Dalton then published a piece in *Nature* about the study—or, actually, explaining the results of Ignacio's study—despite the fact that *Nature* had not yet published the real study itself (nor had anyone else at that point). Dalton also called out Monasterio in his piece for leaking the information in a "meeting of an international food-safety organization." Dalton went on, "Ortiz denies breaching confidentiality, but acknowledges that he did reveal Chapela's research results in a public forum."

According to Ignacio, it became an absurdly bizarre situation at that point, where the editors of *Nature* were saying, "We're rejecting the paper, we're not going to print it," while at the same time "*Nature* was breaking news about the discovery. . . . And so it's this completely contradictory situation where the same magazine is printing news about the scientific discovery without printing the scientific discovery. . . . Completely crazy." Ignacio said that, in the end, the reason *Nature* gave for not publishing the paper, was that "it just wasn't interesting."

Even so, like a domino effect, the perhaps "uninteresting" news of Chapela and Quist's study suddenly started appearing in many major news outlets, including the *New York Times*, arguably the world's most powerful and thorough newspaper. The *New York Times* led their report, dated October 2, 2001, this way: "In a finding that has taken researchers by surprise and alarmed environmentalists, the Mexican government has discovered that some of the country's native corn varieties have been contaminated with genetically engineered DNA. The contaminated seeds were collected from a region considered to be the world's center of diversity for corn—exactly the kind of repository of genetic variation that environmentalists and many scientists had hoped to protect from contamination. The result was unexpected because genetically modified corn, the presumed source of the foreign genes, has not been approved for commercial planting in Mexico." The *Times* went on to explain, "Mexico's Ministry of the Environment and Natural Resources made the announcement on Sept. 18 that contaminated corn had been found in fifteen different localities. The announcement credited Dr. Chapela with the initial discovery but described only the results from government-led research. Neither Dr. Chapela's team nor the Mexican teams' work has yet been published."

That same day, according to Ignacio, a friend traveling in Paris was sitting in a café, reading the October 2, 2001, edition of *Le Monde*. He saw Ignacio's name in an article by Hervé Kempf on the front page of the paper, just below an article about the widening 9/11 investigation into Europe. Ignacio said, "All I had to do was to take that PDF that this guy had sent me of the front page of *Le Monde* to Phil Campbell [the editor in chief of *Nature*] and say, 'Phil, tell me again that this paper is not interesting. It's been covered on the front page of *Le Monde*.' Next thing I knew, they [the editors of *Nature*] were saying, 'Okay, we're printing it.'"

chapter 21

Despite all the hullabaloo, Ignacio's final printed study in *Nature* comes across as very sober and straightforward, not at all hyperbolic. It's only two succinct pages long, but it delineates and breaks down the central thesis that "Here we report the presence of introgressed[1] transgenic DNA constructs in native maize landraces grown in remote mountains of Oaxaca, Mexico, part of the Mesoamerican centre of origin and diversification of this crop." Furthermore, "Concerns have been raised about the potential effects of transgenic introductions on the genetic diversity of crop landraces and wild relatives in areas of crop origin and diversification, as this diversity is considered essential for global food security."

Then, in scientific terms, Quist and Ignacio simply lay out their analysis of grain samples from the criollo corn grown in the Oaxacan mountains, some grain from Diconsa, the organization that distributes subsidized food throughout Mexico, some blue corn (that was clean of transgenics) from Peru, some seed from a historical

---

[1] The movement of a gene from one species into the gene pool of another.

collection obtained in the Sierra Norte de Oaxaca in 1971, and two samples of Monsanto's Bt corn—YieldGard and Roundup Ready. The blue corn and the historical collection seeds were the "negative" controls (i.e., had no contamination) and the Monsanto seeds were, obviously, the "positive" controls. They claimed that they used the PCR—polymerase chain reaction—testing method, to date the most effective and sensitive way of testing for GMOs (still the current standard necessary for anyone to determine whether GMOs are in a product).

Interestingly, in a later email volley between myself and Ignacio, he told me that when he and Quist went to a seed bank to get some corn for their "negative" controls, they "*also* found that the seed banks are contaminated with GMOs, but that is another matter (and it has not been published)." This issue of the seed banks is actually a very important one. One hopes that these vaults that are said to house any number of seeds for our futures will preserve the diversity our planet may need if we get in a tight spot. Walter Haefeker, my German beekeeping companion across Belgium and Germany during the preceding fall, laughed when he described the absurdity of the "doomsday seed bank" in Svalbard, Norway, which is supposedly the planet's best safe box for the world's seeds. Walter likes to point out that if bees can't be saved, the banks themselves may become useless, because there will be nothing to pollinate the plants. Furthermore, there are legitimate questions about who actually is going to benefit from the banks in the end, because it turns out that DuPont/Pioneer, Syngenta, CropLife International, and Monsanto have all donated millions of dollars to Svalbard. Another seed bank, in Colorado, is said to be maintained and controlled exclusively by Monsanto.[2]

---

[2] This story, according to Reuters, has an interesting twist: The government-controlled National Center for Genetic Resources Preservation in Fort Collins, Colorado, which was created as an inclusive seed bank, was found to have been storing Monsanto's not-yet-approved GMO wheat among the other natural seeds. It was discovered when crops in Oregon were found to contain the restricted grain. After an investigation, all the known GMO seeds at the storage facility were destroyed.

. . .

NOT UNEXPECTEDLY, once Ignacio's study was finally printed, despite accolades from many, there was also a quick and ferocious backlash from some members of the scientific community. This isn't necessarily unusual with any study—it's part of the process. But what was unusual were the harsh critiques from some faculty at Berkeley, who were also Ignacio's peers. Ignacio's methodology was peremptorily called into question and the work itself was dismissed as ideological and poorly executed science. Letters were written to *Nature*—and two were published right away—by naysayers. In response, Ignacio and Quist themselves wrote a letter to *Nature* in which they admitted that they had made a mistake in their breakdown of the "wandering" DNA, but only in two DNA sequences; the rest was right and Ignacio stood firmly by his larger claim about the DNA. He wrote, in a letter to the *Guardian* newspaper in London, that, in the words of Galileo, "*E pur si muove*" (And yet it moves), which Galileo supposedly said under his breath after being forced by the Inquisition to recant his theory that the earth moves around the sun. In the meantime, some reviewers clamored for *Nature* to retract the paper.

Instead *Nature* asked Ignacio and Quist to once again recheck their science. Trying to stay cool, they were thinking about one reviewer's point, which they thought was a good one. The reviewer had written that the blue corn from Peru might not have been a good control because there would be many other inherent differences between the Peruvian sample and the Mexican samples. So, taking that note, Ignacio and Quist got an older Mexican variety from a seed bank to test as their negative control. "This was how we solved the last legitimate technical question about the paper," Ignacio wrote me in an email.

As background, he wanted to tell me about both the personal and professional climates into which he unveiled this study by way of explanation for his Berkeley peers' attack. In 1997, he told me, a year after he was hired by Berkeley, when he was still an assistant professor, he was appointed to the chair of the executive committee of his college. He said, "It was an incredible responsibility. At the time, I was so proud of myself and so full of myself that, 'Oh my God, my colleagues just elected me to do this, they must think I'm so great.'"

But, according to Ignacio, within a week of taking over the chairmanship, the dean, Gordon Rausser, called him and said, "I'm hereby advising the faculty, since you're the representative, that we are going to sign a fifty-million-dollar agreement with Novartis"—the same company (Sandoz) that Ignacio had been working for in Switzerland that later merged with AstraZeneca to become Syngenta, Tyrone Hayes's nemesis. Ignacio was told to "show up in half an hour" to convey faculty opinion on whether the university should sign the agreement.

According to Ignacio, when he worked for Novartis in their previous incarnation as Sandoz Pharmaceuticals, they had been trying to get a foothold on the West Coast of the United States with a college or university for years. He said, "We tried to go and buy Scripps [Research Institute] in San Diego. And that attempt was so outrageous . . . that Senator Al Gore and Bernadine Healy, who was actually head of the NIH, held hearings in Washington, D.C., in Congress, where they told Sandoz, 'You cannot possibly do this.'" The *Los Angeles Times*, reporting on the Sandoz/Scripps deal, writes, "In unusually strong language, Dr. Bernadine Healy denounced the deal between Scripps, a prestigious research organization in La Jolla, and Sandoz Pharmaceuticals, a major drug manufacturer, as an 'aberration,' a possible violation of federal law, and a 'dangerous exception' to the normal dealings between industry and research institutions that use federal funds."

Ignacio continues, "This is now years later, my dean is now telling me that we're about to sign a fifty-million-dollar agreement with this company and all I had the presence of mind to say was, 'Gordon, that's great, but I just hope it's not another La Jolla [Scripps].'" In exchange for the money, Novartis wanted first look at all research coming out of the plant biology department at Berkeley.

As soon as Ignacio hung up with Rausser, he started making calls to ask other faculty groups and individual members if they supported him, as chair, in condoning this agreement. According to Ignacio, the other faculty members he talked to were not in favor of the Novartis deal (Rausser says most of the faculty he talked to were). So Ignacio showed up at Rausser's meeting and said he wouldn't sign "off on behalf of the faculty." Ignacio reports that Rausser got furious and started pounding the table. Ignacio told him that he believed his job was to represent the desires of the faculty and also to do what was best for the faculty. He felt he was doing just that.

Morally outraged, Ignacio left the meeting and began organizing a movement. Over the next two years, there were fights and demonstrations and a push-pull between the university and Ignacio (during one demonstration someone tossed a pie at Rausser). Almost overnight, Ignacio was leading a loudly dissonant group of faculty and students against the Novartis deal. The discussion eventually escalated to the state level, where hearings were convened. Finally, after two years of fighting, the university was given $25 million by Novartis, which gave twenty-three Berkeley researchers access to the company's research and trade secrets, principally in genetics, in exchange for "first dibs on potentially lucrative discoveries" made in the university lab, reported the *Sacramento Bee*. The *Atlantic*, reporting on the fiasco, called Berkeley "The Kept University," stating that the biggest concern in a situation like this was "the possibility that behind closed doors some corporate sponsors are manipulating manuscripts before publication to serve their commercial interests."

When I spoke with Gordon Rausser about the Novartis events, we were connecting on his cell phone on a Saturday morning while he drove north of Berkeley to his cow-and-horse ranch outside of Grass Valley, an incredibly hip and nostalgic Gold Rush town near Nevada City on the South Yuba River. Nestled in the foothills of the Sierra Nevada mountain range, Grass Valley is known for its vineyards, white-water rafting, and gourmet restaurants. Rausser, no longer a dean (he was dean from 1994 to 2000), is now the Robert Gordon Sproul Distinguished Professor in the Department of Agricultural and

Resource Economics at Berkeley. If his CV is any indication, he has been enormously successful in his career. Rausser told me, incidentally, that he's a GMO advocate.

Rausser's version of events, in my opinion, didn't actually deviate much from Ignacio's—except that he did say that, to his mind, there was nothing negative about the Novartis deal at all (and he quibbled about the $50 million number, saying that the university of course wanted more money if they could get it but that the number Ignacio had given me was never seriously on the table; the fact that they got less, he says, had nothing to do with the brouhaha). Rausser did say that when the Department of Microbial Biology, under his jurisdiction, decided to put out a proposal to fifteen biotech companies—Monsanto, Dow, and DuPont among them—to receive funding, the goal was just to secure money that some faculty at Berkeley needed to proceed with some of their studies in plant and microbial biology. He says that the timing was critical. The biotech companies, he realized, "were all in a race to make major innovations on drought resistance, for example." To his mind, he was offering his scientists a collaboration that could only propel Berkeley to the forefront of scientific discovery. (In fact, in the years since the Novartis deal, the biology department at UC Berkeley has become the top in the nation.)

The only big roadblock, Rausser said, when the deal was coming together, was the one of publication; Novartis and the university eventually agreed to a ninety-day delay for any scientific discovery, which some faculty felt was too long, Rausser admitted. But Novartis also thought it was too short. In the end, he said, Novartis had no say about whether faculty published things that might be seen in a negative light. Academic freedom, he argued, was always protected.

Despite all the initial furor, Novartis didn't end up using any of Berkeley's research. And a final assessment made by an independent council advised that such a model should not be repeated because of the incredibly high-profile—and negative—attention the situation received.

However, many people I spoke with for this book say it's gotten worse, not better, in academia. Congresswoman Pingree told me, "Commercial investment [in] research, particularly at land grant and agricultural colleges, has gone way up. So, you know, you don't have pure research that isn't 'possibly tainted'—you get all this commercial research. And I think at all levels you could find a lot of people who would say that's really changed the field for scientists." Tyrone Hayes, in his dry, succinct way, said simply, "The best place to get funding is the industry . . . but they won't publish it. . . . And if you're industry and you know there's a scientist out there who's trying to study your product, you should buy them off to silence them."

Ignacio said that looking back he now believes he was used by the university to rubber-stamp this agreement because of his Novartis ties: "All of a sudden comes this young guy who will not have the guts to jeopardize his career and stand up and say, 'Well, let me ask this question.' So to me it's obvious why they elected me. Stupid me thinking they [liked] me . . . that I was good at something." For what it's worth, Gordon Rausser told me this was ridiculous; he said that Ignacio was elected because no one more senior wanted to take on the time and work of the chairmanship.

However, no sooner had the Novartis rumpus died down, Ignacio was denied tenure. He then launched into another huge battle, even staging himself in protest with his desk, books, and a teapot outside of University Hall. Rausser told me that Ignacio waged this battle based on the fact that one of the naysayers of his *Nature* study happened to be on the panel that reviewed his tenure application. This was deemed to be a conflict of interest by the university, Rausser said. Eventually Ignacio filed a lawsuit against the university and hired a high-powered attorney to aid him, while further irritating the university by making every step of his legal process transparent to the press: "So every letter I got, as soon as it said 'confidential' on top, I would pass it on to reporters, and [it] would appear in the newspapers and, you know, it was, like, a completely public process."

By now Ignacio was widely viewed as a nuisance—not only at Berkeley but further afield—and as an ideologue, which is, perhaps, the worst word that can be slung at a scientist; he or she might never be found credible once that word has been used. Though, when I asked him if he felt that Ignacio was just a huge pain in the ass, Rausser generously said, "No. I don't think so. If he's a pain in the ass, then there are lots of faculty members who are pains in the ass. If he's contributing real science to Berkeley, he's not a pain in the ass." On this last point, however, Rausser had a few sharper words: "I don't know whether he's been promoted to full professor. Is he still an associate professor?" he asked me.

"Yes," I said.

"Then, if he's still not a full professor," he said, "that's a bad signal about his science."

IN JUNE 2002, almost a year later, *Nature* was still abuzz with Ignacio's study. By then, the editor of *Nature,* Phil Campbell, had asked Ignacio and Quist to retract their paper and they had refused. Campbell then disavowed the paper. In the meantime, *Nature* continued to publish letters still addressing the study. The most interesting of them accuses some of the original critics of the study of having received industry funding from Novartis: "The eight authors of the two published criticisms of Quist and Chapela's paper have had all or part of their research funded by the Torrey Mesa Research Institute (TMRI), an offspring of the agricultural biotechnology company Novartis (now Syngenta)," say the authors, two of whom were also scientists from Berkeley. This letter goes on to say that this connection would have been less "noteworthy" if Ignacio and Quist had not been "leading critics" of the Novartis/ Berkeley deal four years earlier. Peter Pringle (the author of *Food, Inc.*) reports that Campbell "denied that a campaign against the two researchers influenced his decision to disavow the paper."

From the distance of time, it's hard to believe that the undeniably intense pressure from Biotech and the voices of a few heavy-hitting scientists attacking the study did not have any influence over *Nature.*

It's not like the press is impervious to outside pressures. Meanwhile, to add to the din, an Internet campaign was mounting from strident defenders of Biotech to defame Ignacio and Quist's work. A damning email smear campaign was later traced to a D.C.-based PR firm, The Bivings Group, with Monsanto listed as one of its biggest clients.

To come back to Dr. Ezcurra for a brief moment: his role in all this became more critical after all the hoopla had exploded. In April 2001, when Ignacio came to Mexico City to elucidate his findings in Oaxaca for the people in the Ministry of the Environment, Dr. Ezcurra, then president of the Instituto Nacional de Ecología,[3] first learned of the contamination. He said, "I was really alarmed by his findings," though since NAFTA had been signed, he had expected as much. He then sent a colleague named Sol Ortiz to the same hinterlands where Chapela had gathered his Oaxacan samples. She came back with samples, which they sent to a lab in Mexico that confirmed Chapela's work. "There was a lot of [GMO] DNA in the corn," he said. So, later that year, in November 2001, after Chapela's piece had been published, he went to an international meeting in Raleigh, North Carolina, full of scientists and press people. There he told the audience, "We've duplicated Chapela's work and it's true." He told me that they sent their own study to *Nature* but that "*Nature* didn't want to touch it with a ten-foot pole." His study was rejected because, he said, *Nature* had told him that the PCR might have been contaminated. When I asked why *Nature* might have said that, Ezcurra said, "There's an unwillingness of leading journals to publish something like that because of the economic consequences—and also because of the level of political activism that surrounds this."

But what's interesting is that Ezcurra did not stop there. Over the next year and a half, he sent colleagues back to gather more seeds. By then, he said, the Oaxacan people were well abreast of the situation. Since receiving Ignacio's news, they had jumped into action. "[They]

---

[3] He's now the director for the University of California Institute for Mexico and the United States and holds the position of professor of plant ecology with UC Riverside's Department of Botany and Plant Sciences.

are very self-organized and they started generating ideas and recommendations to the members of their communities on how to plant corn and what to avoid. Since 2001, [there was] an avoidance of U.S. animal feed—they don't do it anymore. And then another thing is that if you plant transgenic corn from Iowa in Mexico . . . it doesn't grow well outside of the Corn Belt. They need huge amounts of fertilizers and water and long summer days of Iowa—Oaxaca has shallow soil and no water. . . . Why would you need Roundup Ready corn in an area where no one uses Roundup? The same with Bt plants. The corn borer is not a problem in Oaxaca. . . ." His second sampling, which was then sent to Genetic ID, a highly specialized lab in the United States, showed absolutely no presence of GMO DNA. How does Ezcurra explain this? "The Zapotec people[4] were able to turn this around," he said. In a short amount of time, they put a stop to the contamination. Ezcurra's story is elucidating, because it means that with the right kind of isolation and avoidance, GMO contamination does not, necessarily, have to spread rampant across the world.

Ezcurra, however, is not overly optimistic for the future. The future that he's concerned about is not just about GMOs, it's about food in general: "I believe we are in the middle of a huge food crisis in the world—not food quantity but food quality induced by modern agriculture. This problem exploded in Mexico after NAFTA. [We went] from a healthy population to [ranking] third in the world [after the United States and Saudi Arabia] in obesity and diabetes. The diet of the Mexican people, as a result of going from small farmers' to . . . industrially grown food, GMO corn, and chicken and beef in feedlots[5] with lots of antibiotics and growth hormones, has taken a huge toll on the Mexican population. We have a huge problem on our hands—GMOs are part of the whole package. . . . [But] . . . the enemy is larger than the GMO problem. It is more related to the multinational companies."

---

[4] The Zapotecs are indigenous people in Mexico who reside primarily in southern Oaxaca. In pre-Columbian times, the Zapotecs were one of the most developed cultures in Mesoamerica.

[5] Ezcurra later referred to feedlots as "concentration camps."

chapter 22

I t was now the end of our lunch and Ignacio looked visibly exhausted, despite the numerous cups of coffee we had just imbibed. Like "The Rime of the Ancient Mariner," he had told me his tale, long and winding as it was, and I had listened—I was the first person, he said, he'd told the entire thing to. It had been more than ten years, he said, since everything had fallen down around him in an avalanche of discord: his fight against the Novartis/Berkeley deal, his marriage ending, his fight for tenure, the fight for his scientific integrity with the Mexican corn study. In those long years, he had lost not only standing at Berkeley but also the financial success some scientists like him who make discoveries, publish, and get tenure at one of the best universities in the world might have gained.[1] Tyrone Hayes says that he knew Ignacio during these extremely hard years. He said, "Because I knew him personally, I knew he wasn't crazy. You know when you

---

[1] This is an aside, but Ignacio was so scrupulous in our lunch meeting that he insisted on paying for his own lunch, as he never wanted to be seen as being someone paid off by me for a story. He was the only interviewee during the course of this book who mentioned this concern.

hear these kinds of things when you're on the outside, that, for example, the big companies and the tactics they'll take and their entanglement with the university and their entanglement with government agencies, you know, this kind of conspiracy stuff sounds kind of crazy. But it's very real and I experienced it myself."

With that in mind, on the third day I was in California, I woke up early, swam in the pool, ate a bowl of fruit, and walked up the hill from the Berkeley City Club. I made my way across the Berkeley campus, which was overwhelmingly aflower, the air scented like a thick and languorous perfume, to find the Life Sciences Building—a huge, stately bastion of intellectual rigor—to meet Tyrone Hayes in person. By then I had spoken to him many times (and he'd led me to Ignacio) and I'd also read both a *Mother Jones* article by Dashka Slater that beautifully encapsulated the bizarre and caustic dynamic that had developed between him and Syngenta and a 2014 profile in the *New Yorker* about the bullying tactics of Syngenta.

Inside the Life Sciences Building, a cast of an enormous fossilized T. rex skeleton engulfs the stairwell, its capacious mouth roaring (or grinning, depending on how you look at it) at the students who make their way up and down the stairs to their classes and labs. I passed through a gleaming hallway studded with doors that open into sprawling labs. Eventually, I came to Tyrone's lab.

Tyrone is about five foot three, African American, portly around the middle, and has long hair in a ponytail. He was wearing a sweatshirt and shorts, showing his muscular legs from walking every day from his home in Oakland to UC Berkeley—a trek that takes him at least three hours, but which he enjoys because he likes walking through downtown Oakland (even at 3:30 a.m., when he needs to leave home to get to work on time). He radiates calm and goodwill in person and is soft-spoken. After introducing me to some of his graduate students, who came and went as we talked, Tyrone offered me a chair and told me more about the struggle he had with Syngenta and how it might relate to Ignacio's story.

Tyrone said that in 1997 he was first approached by a consulting company called Ecorisk, based in Washington State, which was working on behalf of Novartis (which later gave birth to Syngenta). He was already a professor at Berkeley. This was in the middle of Ignacio's vociferous struggle to halt the university's proposed financial entanglement with Novartis, which didn't take effect until 1998. Syngenta said they wanted Hayes to look into atrazine, the chemical herbicide, which was undergoing a product reapproval process mandated by the EPA. (Atrazine has been used since 1959 on corn, sugarcane, Christmas tree farms, golf courses, and lawns. Other than Roundup, it is recorded as the most prevalently used pesticide in America. Atrazine sales are estimated to bring in about $300 million a year.) Tyrone said he figured there wouldn't be much there; this stuff must have been vetted. Anyway, why would the company ask him to study it if it was dangerous? "When I first started working with the company, I was sort of naïve," he said.

But when his studies with frogs began to prove that male frogs exposed to atrazine had shrunken voice boxes, which put them at a disadvantage for courting females, or, even more disturbingly, that some frogs' gonads were malformed or castrated and that many were "gay" or hermaphrodites—as we discussed earlier in the book—he began to think something else was going on. He said that it occurred to him then that Syngenta just wanted someone to test atrazine so they could say, essentially, that tests had been done and they "just wouldn't be liable."

In Dashka Slater's *Mother Jones* piece, she wrote, "Gender deformities were present among frogs exposed to as little as 0.1 part per billion (picture a thousandth of a grain of salt in a half gallon of water). That's thirty times less than the 3 ppb the EPA allows in our drinking water." Indeed, some of Tyrone's studies were showing that atrazine, even at extremely low levels, was causing some male frogs to "become" females—complete with female parts. This was an electrifying and terrifying discovery.

Eventually, Tyrone was able to show that atrazine was activating an enzyme, which was converting androgens—male sex hormones—to estrogens. He said, "You can expose genetically male frogs to atrazine, which causes an increase in estrogen, and some of those frogs will identify themselves as females. And by that I mean they will always copulate with other males, as a female. . . . It sets up in early development and it's irreversible."

In Elizabeth Kolbert's book *The Sixth Extinction: An Unnatural History*, she writes about the "mass extinction"—"fast," "global," and "vast"—of frogs, and amphibians in general, which scientists and biologists have been concerned about since the 1980s. Kolbert quotes a biologist in Panama who has been working to save the frogs—and harbor them in an ark of sorts—as saying, "Unfortunately, we are losing all these amphibians before we even know that they exist." Because of this trend, based on his research, Tyrone was starting to think that part of the problem might not just be that something was in fact *killing* frogs but that, instead, in some cases, the endocrine systems of males were getting so disrupted by chemicals like atrazine that they were no longer able to function as the gender they were born with. Therefore they were unable to procreate.

Eventually Tyrone speculated that if frogs, as Slater writes in her *Mother Jones* piece, are "steeped in an aqueous environment" that is similar to "amniotic fluid," and can become gender confused due to the atrazine contamination, that means there could be an effect on us, too. And he said he began to wonder if some gender confusions, resignations, and abnormalities, which are becoming more common in humans—especially those that are on the rise in small children—could also be the result of atrazine exposure.

Syngenta was not exactly thrilled with Tyrone's work or his questions. They canceled funding for him to continue and asked him to, essentially, hand over his research. "The reason they paid me to do it is because they didn't want me to publish it," he said. In other words, the money was intended to silence him. He said no, breaking his contractual agreement, and then published his research.

To be clear, Tyrone's wasn't the first research that showed some negative effects of atrazine. But it certainly became the most famous. In the loud and peculiar showdown that followed—which, Tyrone said, became a "certain sort of macho thing"—his work went everywhere and he became known as the "hip-hop scientist" for his raps, some of which he would extol (in a refreshing ownership of his ethnicity and the cultural importance of hip-hop in the black community) at dry scientific meetings. The most caustic—and foul—raps he wrote were sent in emails to Syngenta, as the temperature went up in the intellectual battle between himself and the biotech giant, like the two below:

> *everywhere i go*
> *i cause a ruckus*
> *act like you know*
> *that's how i do it m*th* f*ck*s*

Or:

> *my abstract for e.hormone below. . . .*
> *strike like lightning*
> *voice like thunder*
> *i hear the fear when you call my name*
> *oh so frightening*
> *makes you wonder*
> *if the second coming done already came*
> *tyrone*

One gets the sense that Tyrone is not overly willing these days to discuss the email volleys. It was a crazy time—one, he says, that is past him. And it seems fair to say that most people wouldn't have been brave (or energetic) enough to take on Syngenta. (Tyrone's battle sucked away years of time and money from his life.) Tyrone brought me back to, what he considers, the salient points: "Syngenta claims, for example, that there have been thousands of studies on atrazine [by them]. None of those are public, none of those are published. You and I haven't seen them. So that's their claim. So their documents and tests and studies do get turned in to the EPA but I don't know that anybody necessarily reads them. Even when I worked with the company I never saw these documents."

In terms of GMOs or the pesticides that go along with them, Tyrone says that we should never be fooled by the reams of tests any company is saying they are submitting to the government agencies: "All the government requires is that they do testing—that they move papers. You need to be able to say, 'I spent x million dollars a year on this testing.' But that doesn't mean you published it and it certainly doesn't mean it's safe." Remember those two tractor-trailer trucks full of data that Bruce Chassy told me about? Dr. Eric Chivian said to me, "What would the American people think if the government relied on secondhand smoking studies done by Philip Morris? If they knew that the testing on the pesticides used to grow GM crops to determine their safety for human exposures was done by the companies making them? Would they trust the results?"

Tyrone went on to tell me that when he was going through his enormous struggle with Syngenta, he at least had tenure "prior to shit hitting the fan." In hindsight, regarding studies that take on Biotech, he said, "If I were early in my career and still trying to get tenure [as Ignacio was], I'm not sure I'd do it . . . there's a lot of risk to a career."

In the end, Tyrone said, the incredible and systematic backlash against him, and for that matter Ignacio, was about money and really boiled down to the industry protecting its product. Biotech did not want the public to think atrazine might be turning little boys gay or deforming their genitals in utero and they didn't want anyone to think about the GMO contamination Ignacio's study proved would spread across the globe. Considerations like those would get in the way of the enormous profits they stood to gain. "I think the bottom line with GMOs or with pesticides is that the biotech companies will protect their product by any means necessary. And in my experience I think that means that if there are harmful effects, if there are concerns, they will go to every effort to hide those and make sure they don't come out," said Tyrone. Along those same lines, Pringle quotes Don West-fall, a biotech industry consultant, in his book *Food, Inc.*, as saying that in terms of GMO contamination, "The hope of the industry is that over time the market is so flooded [with genetically modified organisms] that there's nothing you can do about it. You just sort of surrender."

Tyrone told me that he, like Ignacio, had no interest in surrender-ing or backing down—even when Syngenta sent "goons" to stand at the back of the room when he was giving public talks or lectures, and even when, as Dashka Slater writes in *Mother Jones*, they alluded to threatening his wife and children. Slater writes that a Syngenta rep accosted Hayes at a meeting where he was set to testify on the dangers of atrazine: "'Who's taking care of your family and your lab when you're traveling so much, Tea Bag?'" the rep allegedly said. "'Don't you worry about that?'" The episode ended, Slater writes, with the rep saying: "'Next time you give a talk, I'm going to bring some of my good old boys and let you tell them how atrazine is making them gay. That should be fun. How about that, Tea Bag?'"[2]

When I asked Tyrone how he was able to sleep at night knowing his own life or his family's might be at risk, he told me that the author Theo Colburn, who wrote the book *Our Stolen Future*, about chemicals that are endocrine disruptors and can harm developing fetuses, had

---

[2] Interestingly, Tyrone was also attacked by Jon Entine, the journalist with ties to Big Ag who attacked my *Elle* piece. According to the illuminating 2014 *New Yorker* piece by Rachel Aviv that explores Tyrone's ordeal with Syngenta, Entine is listed as a "supportive third party" by Syngenta.

been worried about him because she, too, was harassed by the chemical companies. "She would tell me," he said, "don't go home the same way twice, you know, and things like that." Even though Tyrone said he grew up "in a pretty tough place, in South Carolina," there were times—like when he was alone in Nebraska—that he did wonder if someone might do violence against him.

Did he ever want to quit, cry uncle, just get out of Syngenta's way? I wanted to know. "Well, that may have been one of the things that drove Syngenta crazy is that I don't give up on things. I knew that there was a problem, I knew something was wrong, [and] I knew they were behaving improperly," Tyrone said.

These days, Tyrone has not let up. He's just changed tack, shifting his focus to chemical mixtures and synergistic combinations. Someone has to do this job, he figures, since there is no governmental task force assigned to this problem. He said he has to be creative for funding, because "most studies like that come from industry—they're not going to pay anybody to publicize negative data . . . if you look at federal agencies, the National Science Foundation only funds basic science, the EPA also won't fund anybody to look at individual products or compounds . . . there's [just] no federal funding. . . . And then [if you choose to study it and somehow can fund it], there are risks to one's career, like I experienced." Another scientist I interviewed while working on this book said, point-blank, "There's a research recession out there and no one will give you the kind of funding you need to answer the questions you're asking."

Tyrone told me that he's keeping his head down while he works, aware of the shit storm that will, undoubtedly, come his way when he starts publishing. But, he told me, in many ways the *Mother Jones* and *New Yorker* pieces managed to certify his experience; he feels, finally, like someone was able to get down in black and white what really happened to him. Aside from those two articles, his Facebook feed is filled with comments from "fans" who want him to comment on everything from pesticides to GMOs. He spends little time commenting on others' posts but does post funny photos and dry remarks on everything from his dinner to an odd hotel mirror that had a TV inside of it when he recently visited Harvard to give a lecture.

Although GMOs themselves are not his field, I asked him if it could be true what the biotech companies tell us, that GMOs are entirely safe. He told me first off that "they have fields and fields in Nebraska of experimental crops—long before they hit the market, long before they're registered for human consumption or to be sold." Fields, he told me, which are out in the open air and potentially contaminating nearby nonexperimental crops with inevitable drift. So, "honestly?" he said. "No, they can't say that. Of course they can't. Even today, for example, I mean here at the university—I should probably shut up but I heard somebody. . . . Actually, nope—that was sort of a confidential meeting. . . . No, I'll get into trouble. . . ." He gave me a funny look, and then he was quiet and thoughtful for a moment. Then he started again. "I guess the bottom line is whether it's a GMO or a new chemical, there's no way you can put anything into the environment and say, 'Oh, it'll be completely harmless.' Right? You know, that was the same thinking that went into, 'Hey let's release mongoose on Hawaii, they'll kill the rats.' I mean, you can't predict what it will do. You can't say with certainty, 'This is absolutely harmless.' Especially when you're talking about chemicals. Especially when you're talking about chemicals that are designed to kill things. There's no way you can say, 'Those will have no unwanted circumstances.' I wouldn't believe it for a second."

chapter 23

fter meeting with Tyrone, I made my way across campus to
meet Ignacio in his office on the top floor of Hilgard Hall.
Hilgard Hall is a gray stone building situated on a small rise
a few minutes' walk from a stand of eucalyptus trees and across a
skinny footbridge that spans Strawberry Creek. On the outside of Hilgard Hall, etched in the stone above the front door, are the words TO
RESCUE FOR HUMAN SOCIETY THE NATIVE VALUES OF RURAL LIFE.

With the windows open to his little balcony, and the college green
below, Ignacio sat across from me at his cluttered desk. Behind him a
deep sink was piled with dishes, beakers, and wineglasses from a class
celebration. He told me that, for a time, when the loudest fighting
was over, after he was finally granted tenure and the mayhem over his
corn study was beginning to dissipate, he was somewhat lost as to
what to do next. The years that preceded him hovered like thunderclouds, threatening to erupt no matter what move he made.

But in his small lab, just below his office full of beakers and white-
boards, he kept coming back to the Oaxacan people. He was still pained
by his role as a messenger to the Oaxacans who, he felt, had no real

solution. He said that he wanted to do something "proactive and creative" that would give people like the Oaxacans—indigenous, farming peoples—"the capacity to see" what had initially been invisible.

What he came up with, finally, was simply to make a "gadget" that poor people all over the world could use to answer a definitive "yes or no" as to whether they had GMOs in their honey, in their cornfields, in their rice paddies, what have you. This was a departure from the kind of sciencey science he was normally steeped in, he said, and was more of a "technological intervention."

His gadget, which is named the Turtle, needed to meet a variety of criteria: it needed to be disposable or recyclable and it needed to be nontoxic. He didn't want any radiation, electronics, heavy metals, or even electricity to make it work (he pointed out that some places in the world still don't have electricity). The object of this effort "was to produce something that is incredibly simple, incredibly cheap, and disposable . . . [that] doesn't have a footprint of waste afterwards," and would not have any planned obsolescence, which creates a dependence (the heroin model of selling the technology of anything, from GMOs—you need to rebuy your patented seed each year—to iPhones, a business model Ignacio finds despicable).

More than anything, said Ignacio, his device needed to do away with the expensive PCR testing that requires specific lab gear and also the expertise in how to run the equipment. (The equipment alone costs around $10,000, and, as Ignacio said, that's "a lot of money for your everyday housewife or farmer to be doing this.") Having PCR testing done at a lab is also expensive—usually anywhere from $300 to $500 a pop—for one small sample of honey, one leaf, one sample of corn seeds. Ignacio said, "So you can imagine nobody can do that on a regular basis. If you have a field, even if it's a tiny field, like this"—he motioned with his hands to the green outside his window—"you would like to know, you know, what percentage of these plants here is transgenic. . . . How many of them have picked up contamination? If you really wanted to have ten samples from this field, you would need to pay five thousand dollars. . . . And if you wanted to do it again next week to see if something happened, you'd need to pay again five thousand dollars." The end result, says Ignacio, is that "people are living in darkness, in this blind world where they're not allowed to see . . . because you need to go through these experts to get to know. So if I ask you even here in the U.S., where is the nearest GMO to where you are standing right now? You cannot tell me." It occurred to me, listening to him, that he was taking the Right to Know campaign to a whole other level; if his gadget worked, consumers might no longer be dependent on labeling from food manufacturers, the government, the Non-GMO Project, or Whole Foods. They could find out on their own. That might prove to be rather revolutionary.

Ignacio went on to tell me that at this point there are only two highly respected companies globally that do GMO analysis (though this is a growing field and a quick Google search pulls up a handful of labs putting their shingles out). One is here in the United States, and is called Genetic ID. It is run by an outspoken critic of GMOs named John Fagan (who has been criticized as a little too "out there" by many GMO opponents because of his ties to Maharishi University of Management in Fairfield, Iowa, where transcendental meditation is a tenet). The second is in Luxembourg, and is called Eurofins Scientific. Both have made highly precise GMO testing their business. The dependence on these two companies—especially Genetic ID—rubs Ignacio the wrong way: "If you are the only person who can see, then you're in business. And it's in your interest that there is contamination so that people will call you from both sides." He goes on, "His [Fagan's] business depends on GMOs existing in the world and contaminating, because then they become a problem and he becomes necessary."

As Ignacio was talking, I remembered a conversation with Jim Gerritsen, the organic potato and corn farmer I visited in northern

Maine at the start of this book. Jim had told me that he sends a small sample from his corn every year to Fagan's company, Genetic ID, to see if it's been contaminated. Gerritsen said that despite his relative isolation up in Aroostook County, there is a farmer growing GMO corn a few miles away, just over the border in Canada, and with birds, bees, and wind, he's never certain he hasn't been contaminated. "We always test our seed at our expense even though ethically it's not our responsibility . . . even though we have go to the expense of a couple hundred dollars a sample." I asked him if his sample—which includes ten thousand kernels of corn—answered his question. He said slowly, "No." And then elaborated: "We can't offer one hundred percent guarantee. We'd have to empty a silo or bin and then use it all up— the corn would have been destroyed in the testing so it would have been an exercise in futility."

This problem—of guaranteeing that any grain or legume is clean of contamination at this point—was elucidated by the 2011 uproar over Monsanto's GMO alfalfa, a common crop grown for livestock. It was deregulated by the USDA amid incredible controversy; opponents said it would spread like wildfire, contaminating non-GMO alfalfa, taking off across fields and prairie and making it almost impossible for the organic and grass-fed dairy and meat farms to boast that their animals received only "organic" grass. Maine congresswoman Pingree had this to say about the GMO alfalfa: "My first term on the agriculture committee was when we had, I think, the one and only hearing about alfalfa, and, you know, it just didn't get very far because—I can't speak for the administration or the USDA—but I just think the climate in that room on the agriculture committee from Republicans and Democrats was just like, 'We're not taking up any rule, legislation, conversation that has anything to do with restricting the use of GMOs.' And I don't think there's been any meaningful public hearing in Washington around this topic for the last four years."

Because of Pingree's story and others, I was interested in the

USDA's position on contamination, especially because I had been told by one source that the USDA is, essentially, "toothless" in terms of what it can do to the big biotech companies, which have captured the regulatory process.

So I called up the USDA. Eventually I was given to Michael Gregoire, the associate administrator of the unit that regulates the introduction of genetically modified crops at the USDA. Gregoire took umbrage immediately when I asked him if the USDA really was toothless, or captured. "We, in fact, have a lot of teeth under the plant protection act," he snapped. "We have the authority [to] and do conduct field [inspections] of GE crops. We can seize, hold, or treat any crop and there are criminal penalties. Last year we performed seven hundred inspections of field trials." When I asked him to tell me more about the criminal penalties, he sent me a list of incidents where the USDA had discovered that the biotech companies were not doing what was agreed upon in the USDA paperwork. But the fines the USDA imposed and recorded were so paltry and so few and far between, they almost made me laugh. In one instance, Syngenta Seeds released twenty-nine pounds of corn that had not been approved for deregulation by the USDA and was still in development, and it somehow got mixed in with approved corn. (In other words, a test crop went into the normal food supply.) Their penalty was $13,125. In another, Monsanto had a mix-up when they harvested "non-regulated cotton" with regulated cotton and let it go to market, never having told the USDA this had happened. They were fined $18,690. There were more examples like some field trials that were supposed to be in Puerto Rico but were found by the USDA to actually be in Texas, and more of grains being mixed up and entering the food supply. In every single instance the fines were relatively tiny, when you consider that these companies are huge multinationals and that their seeds are contaminating the outside environment, perhaps irreversibly. It made me wonder what "regulation" really means, anyway, when we're talking about living things in the environment. I remember the poet and environmentalist

Wendell Berry's famous words: "You cannot regulate an abomination. You have got to stop it."

Farmers, breeders, and food makers are starting to come to the unfortunate conclusion that it will be difficult—if not impossible—as the seed companies continue to develop transgenics, to guarantee absolute purity for many grains and legumes now grown in the United States. Too many factors work against purity: pollinators, human error, sloppy practices, and wind.[1]

Belinda Martineau told me that in her experience working on the Flavr Savr tomato, it was absurd to think you could control these products. "I mean, the squirrels get in, the birds come in, the insects . . . you can't keep all those guys out of there! And they're going to go and spread your seed when they eat your tomato. When we first did our taste tests before the USDA approved the tomato, we wouldn't let people swallow because they could take the seeds and, you know, deposit them elsewhere," she said.

In light of contamination and what Pingree described as a standstill in Washington, there are many farmers, Ignacio believes, like Gerritsen, who would like to know more about their operations and are willing to take this question into their own hands. For them, he says, the Turtle will be a personal and inexpensive GMO detection device.

That afternoon, Ignacio pulled a model of the Turtle out of a cupboard and showed it to me. To my eyes, the Turtle looks like a cardboard cylindrical toilet paper roll, held horizontally, with little pegs that come off it and look like insect legs. Inside, it's a more complicated doohickey. Ignacio told me there are actually two cardboard cylinders,

---

[1] Also, the biotech companies are coming up with products with such an incredible rapidity that keeping track of what's contaminating what is almost impossible. As I was writing this book, Syngenta came out with a new corn called Enogen, which has high levels of a heat-resistant enzyme that would help in ethanol production. Corn chip and cereal makers were concerned because if it contaminates regular corn that's made for food, it would ruin those crops since it would change the consistency of the food-grade corn, making it crumbly and soggy, impossible to shape into Doritos.

one inside the other, and both cylinders are aligned by the pegs. Then, there are three little tubes, which go through both cylinders and hold them together, each containing an optic filter. On one side of the gadget it is labeled "Sun." It looked (sort of) like this:

The way the Turtle works is complicated. I felt like I needed a PhD in genetics, biology, and probably physics, too, to understand the larger part of what Ignacio was talking about, but I tried to hang in there. Ignacio patiently outlined how the various factors worked on a whiteboard with red, green, and blue markers while I smiled gamely. What I gleaned was that the Turtle uses fluorescence (the property of absorbing the light of short wavelengths and emitting the light of longer wavelengths; think of glow paint) to give light signals that will tell you whether a chemical compound you are searching for—GMO DNA, for instance—is indeed in your sample. "So you get a yellow light signal when you expose that substance to blue light. If you see yellow, you say 'Aha, that substance is there.' So it's a way of reporting the presence or absence of a substance. . . . The whole trick is to get this light signal to light up whenever there is whatever we are looking for, and not to be on when it's not," Ignacio said.

To illustrate this point, Ignacio took me out on his balcony (I thought, *How nice to have an office with a balcony*) to show me his invention in action. And, indeed, when I held the Turtle in the sun, I did see through the viewfinder a blue/purple light and then a yellow/orange light, indicating one contaminated substance and one "clean" substance—in this case we were using honey (as part of the project, he has been testing honey samples from all over the world, including honey for the embattled beekeepers in Germany).

Ignacio hopes that each device will ultimately cost only a few cents—"or fractions of a cent, with the goal of having these things just dropped in the world so that people can start asking [about GMO contamination] on their own." He says that this is not a moneymaking venture. And he hopes that he'll be able, as results are recorded, to start making maps of where GMOs have contaminated other crops around the world, thereby giving him, his team, and the general public information about the scope of GMO proliferation worldwide. This is, obviously, an ambitious goal—and, again, like his study in Oaxaca, one that has steep political implications. What will happen when people get a sense of the expanse of GMO cultivation and contamination? Will they care?

It's possible, he said, that his gadget will go out there into the world and mean nothing. Perhaps, he said, people who use it will "find that, my gosh, we're all surrounded by it and nothing happens. So then they stop worrying maybe. I don't know. I personally don't think so, but it's not up to me to make that decision. Science is about asking whether you can be wrong, not whether you're right. People believe it's about being right but it's not. It's about always doubting yourself."

I asked Ignacio if he was concerned that a new backlash, almost fifteen years later, could bring him back to those proverbial ditches that he was digging late at night in the early 2000s, when everything was falling down around him. He said, "I know whenever I show my head over the parapet, people will start shooting, right? They don't forget who I am." That being said, he hopes that this time his science is the focus, and that it doesn't spin out of control. In the end, he said, he's uncomfortable with the role he's been given: "I'm against GMOs for a whole set of reasons, but I do not want to be cast as an anti-GMO ideologue. . . . I refuse to join that crowd."

I wasn't sure, sitting in Ignacio's office that afternoon, if he meant this in earnest. As far as I could tell, he's already been cast as an ideologue. Whether he can undo this label with yet another foray into the GMO discussion, I'm not sure.

What did occur to me, however, was that what he meant might be that he somehow wants to undo time, to go back to some neutral place where he can shed his reputation as an embattled and disenfranchised scientist and again be appreciated as an academic who is making a contribution to a greater good, whatever that may mean. In the end, it occurred to me, that's what all the scientists I'd interviewed for this book wanted.

Gordon Rausser, the dean with whom Ignacio had fought in the late 1990s over the Novartis deal, told me that he doesn't begrudge Ignacio for their battle. In fact, he said, "I like him as a person. I like his engagement." To me, this said something about an intrinsic quality of the American Dream: we are always remaking ourselves, and there is endless room to regroup and try again.

On my way home from Ignacio's lab that night, I was hungry. The wind had picked up and my hair was blowing around and I was tired and ready to go home, where it was easier to feed myself. I missed Dan and Marsden and Hopper. I had seen a "Grass-Fed Burger" sign on my way to Tyrone's lab that morning, and I decided I could use something substantial to eat. Inside, I ordered a burger with guacamole on top of lettuce. When it came, despite how promising it seemed, it was disappointingly greasy and rubbery. *Ack*, I thought, *it's late and I'm pregnant—for all I know, this tastes great and I just don't have the normal taste buds to recognize it!* Leaving it half eaten, I went back to my hotel and packed to leave the next morning.

In the morning, when I boarded my plane in San Francisco, I found myself going back over my sick years and the winding and confusing journey I'd made from my private and consuming illness to this bigger concern that was growing in me about the cost of GMOs and pesticides to not only ourselves but also to every creature we share this planet with. To me, as a mother, this was becoming an issue not of who's a good guy and who's a bad guy, really, because that can be vague. Or whose science is the most valid, because all the science, to date, seems to have complicating factors, and one of those complicating factors is the ideology of the people involved—on both sides. Instead, as our plane crossed over the Sierras below, the shadows of the clouds looking like massive bear-paw prints on the face of the earth, I was thinking about who's benefiting and who will undoubtedly lose. And, newly pregnant with a second child, it was becoming clear to me that the losers will be our children. Sitting there and feeling small and mortal on that plane, the truth of this suddenly felt like it was going to just break my heart.

Epilogue:
Invisible Monsters and Tender Mercies

"Unless someone like you cares a whole awful lot,
nothing is going to get better. It's not."

—Dr. Seuss, *The Lorax*

"And if there are fears, know also that Nature has its
unexpected and unappreciated mercies."

—Henry Beston, *The Outermost House*

When I was in the throes of writing this book, five-year-old Marsden was having trouble sleeping. It was the middle of a hot summer and I was seven months pregnant with my second child.

Just when I'd dragged my tired, swollen feet downstairs and was starting to relax into the idea of ten minutes to myself, I'd hear a tentative and forlorn "Mommmmmmy?" Up the stairs I'd tromp.

When I got there, I'd do my best to be more Mary Poppins than Miss Hannigan.

"Yes?" I'd ask.

"I'm scared," Marsy would say, his voice tremulous.

"Of what?"

"Monsters."

It's not like I didn't remember the monsters from my own childhood. They were probably the same ones: big-toothed and shaggy-haired with long, curled fingernails. They surfaced, for me, during the summers and resided in the ice machine located in the hall outside the room I shared with my brother in my grandparents' cottage on Nantucket. Somewhere deep inside the machine's fake wooden door—which we'd open about a hundred times a day to grab ice for our Coca-Colas, Tabs, or just to suck on—they crunched bones. At night, I'd lie awake listening and get more and more terrified until I heard my grandfather, Pop, make his late-night shuffle—when he assumed everyone was sound asleep—from the TV room to the bar to make himself one last little nightcap of Popov vodka on the rocks. After his brave journey, hearing him shuffle back to the TV room unscathed, I'd fall asleep. I eventually grew out of my monster heebie-jeebies when I began sharing a bedroom with my cousin Jane. I found I could parlay my own distress into scaring the shit out of her with stories about werewolves hiding in the laundry room.

I told Marsy, "Look, any monsters come your way, I'll wrestle them with my huge belly and pin them down, like this. . . ." And I pretended to throw a monster on the floor, growling like a hyena, my hair flipping around like I was Hulk Hogan.

This made him laugh. And lie back down. Success.

I started down the stairs, thinking, *Okay, this is really going to be fine now.*

But a few moments later, just when I'd start doing something as scintillating as laundry folding, I would hear, "Mama . . . ?" Back up the stairs. Now I was asked to peer inside the closet, under the bureau, and behind the curtains. I was to do it once, then twice. Then Daddy needed to do it.

This routine would go on—nightly—sometimes for two hours or more. The conversations, the monster checking and wrestling, and more and more lights illumed—the hall light, the bathroom light, and the small lamp at the end of his narrow room next to the window that looked out into the Norway maples in the backyard. Inevitably, I'd start to get grumpy. I began to protest, "For the love of God, Marsy, you are safe. I am here. Daddy is here. Hopper is here." Not only was I tired and desperate for some time to myself, but I would also start to feel a sort of irrational fear for him, for his exhaustion the next day at camp, for his growing body, for his psyche.

When he finally did fall asleep, his lips pursed, his tawny hair tousled on his pillow, I felt guilty for my grumpiness and sighs. I felt guilty for my protestations.

One morning, propelled by guilt (as many a moment of good parenting is), I had the presence of mind, as I was driving him to camp, to finally ask, "What do you think is making you so afraid, buddy?"

"Well, Mommy," he said, "when I lie on my side, I'm afraid there's something behind me. When I lie on the other, I'm afraid it's behind me there."

"What might be there? Behind you?"

There was a pause and he looked thoughtful in the rearview mirror. I waited. "The monsters I'm worried about are the invisible monsters, the ones I can't see."

I took in his face, at once thoughtful, intelligent, vulnerable, and open. My heart filled with love. And then I said, "I understand that, buddy. We're all afraid of invisible monsters. Even Mommy. Things we can't see that might hurt us are the worst things to consider, aren't they?"

"Uh-huh," he said quietly.

After I said good-bye and left him at camp, I felt wistful. I wanted all that time back when I'd been annoyed. His problem was so understandable to me now. I myself had endured almost four years of an illness that no one could find the answer to; it was invisible to everyone but myself. This was also the exact same fear the Oaxacans had had when Ignacio Chapela told them that GMOs were contaminating their criollo corn. It's the same issue that beekeepers in Germany (and all of us consuming honey, for that matter) have: How can you see a GMO or, for that matter, a pesticide, inside your honey? It's the same problem a mother in the supermarket has when she wants to buy food for her family that she knows is safe, without a shadow of a doubt, no matter what the circus of scientists or policymakers tell her. And, if you think about it, it's what a farmer like Zach wants to know, too—that he's growing something that won't hurt anyone, least of all his own children.

To take this a step further, I'd argue that this invisible monsters situation is our modern-day crucible: As parents, we cannot discern the chemical flame retardants that come to us packaged in innocent baby PJs and sleep sacks and Johnny Jump Ups—or for that matter those that are steeped into the foam cushions of our couches and chairs. We can't see the endocrine-disrupting chemicals used to make those vinyl bins in which we store our kids' clothes in the attic, their microscopic dust getting all over everything as they sit and degrade; and we can't see them in the vinyl that's used in replacement windows that rub up and down and make a fine dust on the sill that's perfect for little hands that travel, disconcertingly, straight to little mouths. We cannot see the BPA on everything from receipts to food-storage containers and water bottles—not to mention BPS, a chemical that has been used to replace BPA but is almost the exact same chemical and is no more safe, though companies can use it and affix a "BPA-Free" sticker to the label. We cannot see the lead in the chocolates we purchase for our kids' Easter baskets, and we cannot see the toxic chemical PFOA coating our nonstick Teflon pans. We cannot see the pesticides and fertilizers our neighbors spray or sprinkle on their lawns and flower beds, or the drift from Raid they might be using to kill wasps. We cannot see the trace amounts of neonicotinoids that have been found in the baby foods we are feeding to the most innocent members of our families.

I could go on with 85,000 examples of the things we cannot see but with which we are deluging our water, air, food, and earth daily. But I don't need to. Because you understand and I understand that the situation is impossible. For mothers, in particular, the fact that we cannot protect our children even when they are still inside us, is just mind-boggling. Our placentas, which are intended to filter out toxins, cannot keep 85,000 chemicals at bay. They are not designed for this kind of dire situation.

No parent *chooses* this.

And do the plants and animals around us choose this? If we humans can't see or smell or taste those chemicals, can they?

In my family, once we had knowledge of the invisible, our lives changed drastically. But it was not an easy transition. Before we consciously went off the food grid and stopped eating GMOs and the pesticides that come alongside them, we just trusted that the food that was out there must be safe for our family. In fact, that trust might be the biggest internal and external revolution we experienced. Because once we started to make the shift to an entirely local, organic, and non-GMO diet, we began to ask a fundamental question: Why, Dan and I wondered, had we ever thought that a company would feed our family carefully and healthfully? And what about the modern world had allowed us, and everyone we knew, to become disenfranchised enough from the food we ate that we no longer knew very much about where it came from? An allergist I interviewed while I was on this book's journey said to me, "You're eating what somebody in some office has decided is good for you rather than what your grandma would have told you is good for you. There's something scary there."

Now, it's not like this is an easy way to live. It requires work— from all of us, even little Marsy who helps peel and core apples to make sauce and removes the stones from peaches to can them (the most sublime treat in January is a canned peach, just by itself, a little orb of yellow sunlight, in a bowl). We need to pay ahead for that grass-fed cow. We have to make the extra trek to our egg farmer's wide, fragrant, *Charlotte's Web* barn, where we buy three dozen eggs rather than one, so that we have enough to get through. When we go on trips, we pack a cooler of food from home, even though it's certainly more inconvenient than stopping at Mickey D's. During October, I spend my nights sitting at our dining room table and tying up herbs and hot peppers I've grown to dry in front of the windows. Then, when they are dry, I crumble them into jars to use all winter in soups and stews and teas. Dan loves that I dry our own herbs. Each year he laughs and says, "I never could have imagined I'd marry someone who is drying our own herbs!" And without Dan, frankly, none of this would be possible: he's become an inveterate—even proud—canner and stays up countless late nights, long after I've thrown in the towel, to can apple and tomato sauces; to make plum, strawberry, peach, and blueberry jams; and to pack jars full of pickles and sauerkraut.

If this all seems like too much, I will tell you that there are hidden and true joys in all this labor: our jams, pickles, and sauces become gifts for family and friends during the holidays. And we are connected in a real and tangible way to almost everything we eat; we know where it comes from, what loving hands touched our food and helped it grow. And there is nothing, to my mind, as comforting as going down into the basement on a cold winter night and coming up with a few jars and a hunk of frozen meat to make a warm and cozy dinner. Knowing that I have it all right there, at my fingertips, to feed my family, is a blessing, even a mercy, in a world full of pressures.[1]

To get down to brass tacks, this isn't actually more expensive than buying premade food at the supermarket. The costs are just more

---

[1] One of our favorite cookbooks is Martha Stewart's *One Pot*, which helps us turn our food stores into easy yet satisfying meals.

condensed. That one big order of beef can be around $700 to $800. But it's for the better part of a whole year—and there are all kinds of cuts in that one order, like pot roast and steaks and hamburger.[2] If you were to buy grass-fed beef at your local supermarket, you might spend, on average, $9 to $13—or more—per pound. Let's say you eat some of that beef one or two times a week. You could spend close to $1,400 in one year—that is almost double the amount we're spending. With CSAs, farm shares, and bulk buying groups, it's possible to buy chicken and eggs and vegetables for less, too. But all of this requires planning and budgeting. And lugging of large quantities. That's the part no one tells you, which is that you have to carry that big box of peaches home, with or without Dan there to help you. The upside is you don't have to live in Portland, Maine, to make this shift in your food. Farmers markets full of organic comestibles have sprung up everywhere across this country—in cities and suburbs. And, believe me, those organic farmers want to meet you, they want to feed you, and they want you to support their choice to grow food on a smaller, more conscientious scale.

All that being said, I will be the first to say that this can be a really daunting shift. And also that this is not a pure science; purity in our modern world is probably out of the question. For instance, the chickens and turkeys (and the eggs, too) we get from our friend Daniel, who owns Frith Farm down in Scarborough, eat some corn in addition to their mostly foraged diet of bugs and plants. (Our initial corn-free

---

[2] A quick and easy recipe for the busy mom or dad (Dan, who grew up eating Chef Boyardee, likes to call this "Chef Cait-R-Dee"): Wilt half an onion in a skillet with olive oil and a sprinkle of good-quality sea salt and some coarsely ground black pepper. When the onion's soft, throw in a pound and a half of ground beef. Begin browning. When the beef is almost completely browned, add 2 or 3 collard leaves that have been shredded into ribbons and cook them along with the beef until they are dark green and shiny, about two minutes. Now add in a big jar of tomatoes—one full canning jar (4 cups, or 32 ounces). Add a finely chopped garlic clove and a sprinkle of hot pepper flakes to taste. Add a tablespoon of sugar. Simmer until the flavors meld and the sauce is thick and fragrant, about ten minutes. Meanwhile, cook up a pot of penne or your favorite pasta—two packages should be the right amount. When it's cooked, drain it and coat with a little olive oil, then toss in the sauce. Serve with salad and crusty bread (your choice on that—homemade baguette is always best, but not always possible! I've started making a tapioca starch, milk, and cheese "baguette" that I quite like for its chewy lightness). We eat this meal at least once a week because it is fast, easy, and healthy.

chicken farmer eventually got tired of raising a small amount of chickens on the more expensive oats, which did, he felt, a poor job of fattening up the chickens the way he wanted. He's hoping to switch eventually to sprouted barley.) And although the corn Daniel's chickens eat is organic, I know too much at this point to believe that there isn't some tiny bit of contamination along the way there, so I've had to reconcile myself with the realization that it may be impossible to ever feel totally secure about my food. There's just too much coming at me in the form of rain, pollen, water, farming practices; the list goes on. And also sometimes I just need to buy the conventional dairy because it's Sunday and I need butter or cream or yogurt for a cake I'm baking and my grass-fed dairy guy only shows up on Wednesday at the market. And sometimes I just need something cheaper this week or month or year. Also, to be honest, there are foods in our family that we miss and crave, such as corn tortillas or creamed corn or corn on the cob. Sometimes, when we've really needed a fix, we've gotten some organic popcorn, which likely comes from flyover country, and made that, figuring it's the corn with the least possible contamination. I've had mixed results (sometimes I wake up the next day with stiff hands and my IBS flares), but Dan and Marsden seem to handle it fine as an occasional thing.

Once, while working on this book, we spent a night on Cynthia and Bill Thayer's Darthia Farm, way up the coast in Downeast Maine. Cindy served us fried chicken and corn on the cob that night. Both the chicken and corn came from their farm. I was concerned about the corn, but Bill told me he'd been growing his own seed since the sixties and that they were darn isolated—for miles and miles of ocean and trees—from any other farms that could conceivably contaminate them. That night, we slathered our cobs with butter and salt and muckled onto the sweet corn kernels. I have to say it was the most sublime-tasting corn I've ever tried, like sunlight and summer in a bite. And nothing happened. I was just fine.

Socializing can often be a whole other problem. Friends seem afraid to cook for us. This is a bummer for a variety of reasons, of course. But in order to have some semblance of a social life, we often offer to pot-luck dinner or just tell them the major foods we'd like to avoid—corn and gluten, knowing they are in many things—but that we'll love whatever they make. To stave off total isolation, we enjoy hosting feasts that showcase the lessons we've learned from gathering fresh, local ingredients and preparing them.

What I came to understand these last few years was that it was all about making as much of my diet as GMO- and pesticide-free as I could. Perfection with food, over the long haul, would not be possible; I had to strive for the best I could do for myself, for my family, for my budget. And with this effort, I had to acknowledge a gray area, one that you might have wondered about as you read this book: Is it possible that it wasn't the GMOs that made me sick? Is it possible that in my road rage to take out GMOs, I somehow actually became a study on pesticides? (Dr. Eric Chivian at Harvard told me he thought this was plausible. He said, "It is very unlikely that one can eat a GM food product without being exposed to pesticides. Neonicotinoids, glyphosate, and other systemic pesticides are inside our GM food, in the cells and fluids of treated fruits and vegetables. So one can't wash or peel them off. And there is almost no data about chronic human exposures and long-term health impacts. What data there is, however, is deeply disturbing. So, in a sense, we are all test cases.")[3]

Still, could there have been something else that was making me sick and just because of the weird synchronicity of the world, when I took out GMOs, I got rid of it, too? Like a vitamin or an over-the-counter medication? Or did I force some other condition into remission with a radical change to my diet? I don't know for sure. It's a chicken-and-egg kind of situation. I mean, I have Dr. Mansmann, who said what he believed (and the hard proof that not only did my eosinophilia disappear

---

[3] Rachel Carson: "What makes one person allergic to dust or pollen, sensitive to a poison, or susceptible to an infection whereas another is not is a medical mystery for which there is at present no explanation."

but I hardly ever even get a virus anymore), and I have the theories of the scientists that I talked to, and I have the evidence right in front of me of both Dan and Marsden being healthier than I've ever known them. But do I intrinsically know all this to be true for myself? Do I know enough to quiet down that natural, pain-in-the-ass skeptic inside my head? Not really. Not yet.

But then it's in my DNA to always ask questions. I'm always going deeper.

When I was a sophomore in high school, I took a class in Western civilization taught by a guy named John Greene, who was widely understood to be one of the toughest teachers in the school. I remember the day he looked at me and realized I was going to be an absolute nuisance. We had been studying the nomadic peoples who had migrated across Asia. As he was explaining the Diaspora, I raised my hand and asked, "Why?" Everyone sniggered. He asked me what I meant by "Why?" "Well, why did they do that? What *made* them do that? What were they responding to? What were they *feeling*?" I asked.

This was deeper than he had anticipated going on that bright fall morning. "What were they feeling?" he asked, visibly annoyed.

What he wanted was to get on to the "Western" part of the whole civilization deal. He sighed and looked helpless for a second. And then tried to answer me. (Unfortunately, I don't remember what he said, so I'm still not sure what those people walking across Asia into Europe were thinking.)

If I'm honest, this behavior of mine, as it pertains to the subject at hand, is not just about a lack of trust. It's a matter of fear. I'm always waiting for my illness to come back, to threaten to take me away from my family again. Every year when I get my physical, I persuade my doctor to check my rheumatoid levels again, wondering if rheumatoid arthritis might turn up and put my wandering mind to rest. It is always negative. So I wait, in the quiet, lonely moments before sleep, or the early hours of the morning when my family is deeply breathing, for the day it doesn't work anymore. For the day something happens and I have to admit Dr. Mansmann was wrong or I am wrong. Until then, I hold on, like a lifeline, to the diet to the best of my ability, despite the inconveniences and cravings and difficulty of it. Because it's the best I've got.

And, after five years of learning everything I did about what goes into making a GMO, I know I am on the right track. Because when I consider the pesticides, the unpredictable and numerous proteins, the mineral chelation, the lack of independent university studies that any of us can actually see (not to mention the absence of the modifying proteins on Rick Goodman's allergen database), the lack of testing on animal models that is equivalent, at a bare minimum, to that of testing drugs, I feel confident that most GMOs are probably dangerous.[4] And probably to differing degrees to not only us but also to the creatures   both plant and animal—we share this planet with (to say nothing of the climate, which is getting changed drastically and permanently by our excessive burning of fossil fuels, a huge portion of which are used by industrial agriculture either in the form of pesticides or in the energy used to create them).[5] Ultimately, from the

---

[4] It's possible that some GMOs like the wheat that's being developed in China to be mold-resistant—the goal being to eliminate the use of dangerous, petroleum-based fungicides—may end up being a good thing. Or that disease-resistant GMO papaya is actually okay, or even some rice varieties, like those golden rice grains being developed with funding from the Gates Foundation to give poor people in developing nations more vitamin A. But these products are a tiny fraction of the moneymaking GMOs that blanket our world—corn, soy, and cotton, which are made to work in concert with pesticides—like neonics, glyphosate, and 2,4-D. Not to mention the scary new frontier—like something out of *The Lorax*—of GMO trees, which are now being planted on enormous plantations all over the world. Actual forests, teeming with life, once stood where these fake forests now reach to the sky. And when those original forests were demolished, the CO_2 that was released was enormous. These GMO plantations are sterile un-forests and are highly sprayed to keep the bugs at bay. Their wood is used for pellets and paper worldwide. (Jonathan Franzen wrote in a 2015 *New Yorker* piece that a GMO eucalyptus plantation, for instance, is "secretly appealing to human beings, because, having so much less life in it, it would certainly have so much less death.")

[5] Monsanto recently acquired a company called The Climate Corporation. On its website they claim that this acquisition represents their investment "in supporting farmers by offering them novel options in the way they manage risk on the farm—including weather, which is the single biggest risk farmers face on an annual basis." The Climate Corporation, they say, will advise them on how to create seeds that "maximize yield" for a changing planet. To me, this is another indication that Monsanto is trying to own and control every angle of the conversation.

research, on the health front, I have come to believe that it is likely GMOs do disrupt our immune systems just like those of Hogan's mice—or, to put it in Mansmann's words, our immune systems are sensitive enough that they recognize the genetic shifts in the substances we are eating and can go haywire, as mine did. These immune perturbances, I think it's reasonable to believe, activate allergies and help create autoimmune disorders; the overstimulated immune system can no longer keep the overabundance of chemicals, toxins, food proteins, and environmental stimuli that are coming at it in any kind of order that makes sense, so it's all fair game for attack. And my guess is that GMOs and their accompanying pesticides likely damage our gut microflora, which could lead, among other things, to obesity, autoimmune disorders, and any number of inflammatory issues. GMOs may create antibiotic resistance. And they may do more. After all, data in situations like this—especially about health—is often trivial, anecdotal, and circumstantial at first. Warning signs are missed. And then, suddenly, someone figures it out. The bottom line is that we just don't know enough yet.[6] And one of the things we don't know is which is more dangerous, the genetic insertions inside the plants or the pesticides they are bred to withstand.

My friend the environmentalist and writer Steven Hopp once said to me, "GM only makes sense if you freeze evolution." He is right, I've come to believe: once you invent these things, you lose control. They are living things, after all, unleashed into the environment where they will undoubtedly have consequences.

Now, the advocates of GMOs would have us cleverly parse and separate the pesticides from the inserted DNA and the human toll from the plant and animal and vice versa. They'll never want us to connect GMOs to the climate or our water or fossil fuel consumption. But we cannot continue to be confused by this line of thinking.

---

[6] Talk to any allergist or immunologist out there and they'll tell you that we don't even understand how the immune system really works yet. Let alone how the immune system responds to proteins in regular foods, not to mention those in GMOs.

Arguing the virtues of one aspect of GMOs while ignoring the dangers of the whole dangerous system does no one any favors. What I feel sure about now is that there is, essentially, one undeniable truth: as we modify the environment, we modify ourselves.

And if the natural world is our bellwether of things to come, consider the following: just while I was finishing this book, in the summer of 2014, "A Worldwide Integrated Assessment of the Impacts of Systemic Pesticides on Biodiversity and Ecosystems" was published after review by fifty-three scientists from fifteen countries on four continents of more than eleven hundred scientific studies. The study said that neonics are as dangerous as DDT and are affecting birds, fish, worms, pollinators, bugs—you name it. Their study also found that traces of neonics have been found in fruits, vegetables, cow's milk, and honey. This is the first comprehensive compendium that seems to point the finger, without a doubt, to the trouble neonics, used primarily on GMO crops, could be wreaking. A 2014 Harvard study, published in the *Bulletin of Insectology*, found that neonics are likely to blame for the bees' CCD. And a 2015 study, published in *Environmental Chemistry*, found that more than 70 percent of 219 pollen and 53 honey samples were contaminated with neonics. A Swedish study found that when people—in whose urine countless pesticides were found—were put on an organic diet, after two weeks 70 percent of the pesticides were gone. By the time you're reading this book, I'm sure there will be more evidence. It is coming fast.

In light of the studies that we already know about, many researchers and scientists are stridently calling for a closer look at the chemicals we are saturating our planet with. Effective in 2016, the U.S. Fish and Wildlife Service has banned the use of neonics in the National Wildlife Refuge System, and in 2016 the EPA made some unprecedented moves to try to restrict or cancel their approvals of some pesticides. Even so, Tyrone Hayes told me that he's feeling pessimistic that we can turn this around. He said, "I just published a paper with twenty-one other scientists from around the world—twelve different countries—that all show atrazine has these sexual effects. Still, in the market, we're still fighting. I mean: tobacco. We're still arguing about it. Why are we still arguing about tobacco? We know what it does. Why is it even still available? I guess the difference is if you're a smoker, it's your choice. You're choosing to take that into your body." But those 85,000 chemicals? The GMOs in our baby food (even the organic kind)? We are not choosing those. We and our children are enduring them because we need food to live.

The French philosopher and biologist Jean Rostand once wrote, "The obligation to endure gives us the right to know." This may be. But the fight for the right to know, I've learned, is an enormous, uphill battle. For instance, by the time I was finishing this book, the Parliament had overturned the European Court of Justice decision Walter had fought so hard for. Honey was exempt again from labeling, just like meat and dairy, and there would be no protection for beekeepers whose honey could be contaminated by GMO crops and no way for a consumer to have any idea how pure their honey was or wasn't. Tireless, Walter told me, "Now we're getting EU member states to go to court." He told me he will continue to fight for honey worldwide. In that vein, in one of this last emails to me, he said he had begun an initiative to reach out to beekeepers in the Syrian refugee population, using a common love of bees to build bridges between Europeans and Syrians.

And, back here on the relative home front, Lisa and Dave of Food Democracy Now! moved to Boulder—where Lisa has dreamed of living for years. But they have split up. Lisa is tired of the incredible stress level of working against the multinational companies with far deeper pockets than what she and Dave can ever raise. She's sick of the fact that their work consumes every corner of their lives. She wants something else, something more fun. Who can blame her? Dave, on the other hand, refuses to give up. "We're going to make this a national issue," he told me. "We have to fight these companies. I can't stop until we get some kind of victory."

Like Dave, Jim Gerritsen says he's unwilling to back down from the front lines of the fight. For him, this means that on top of his farming he's often staying up late into the night writing emails and making phone calls and on weekends he's traveling to demonstrations and meetings. Where some might throw up their hands in the face of massive corporate power, and some pretty convincing evidence that we have rendered much of our earth toxic, Jim still says, "This is not a lost battle. We haven't gone too far down the road. Because it's only six major industrial crops, it's not the end of agriculture." Here his voice caught a little in his throat with obvious emotion. Deliberately, he told me, "We have the ability to change course and right our ship." To his mind, there's one grain out there—barley—that still hasn't been tinkered with, that's still pure, and he's willing to go down punching for it. "A farmer can switch to barley," he told me. "We've raised barley in other places; it's roughly equivalent in feed value [to corn]."

Rick Goodman, on the other hand, keeps fighting from the other side. But I detected a hint of defeat when he said to me, his voice weary, that labeling, if it succeeds on the federal level, will "drive the biotech companies out of business." And then, almost as an aside, as if I weren't still on the phone, he said quietly, "Maybe that's the point."

He's not the first to suggest that labeling GM foods would be a mortal wound to the biotech companies; Dave Murphy also fervently believes it will be the beginning of the end for Monsanto, DuPont, Syngenta, and the others. But there were just as many I interviewed—including Rick Goodman's colleague Steve Taylor—who said that people, after seeing the label for a while, honestly won't care. "I think people will say, 'I've been eating that all my life,'" he said, "'and I seem to be fine.'" Because of that, he admitted, that labeling wouldn't be the worst thing to happen. "On the face of it," he said, "that's a good civil right to know." My own rank opinion is that I think it's unlikely that Biotech will suffer much from labeling. The industry still has its chemicals to peddle, which, until regulated better, will be major cash cows.

But when I spoke with Ignacio Chapela around Thanksgiving in 2015, he told me he thought I was wrong. He said, "I never thought I'd say this, but I am coming to believe that 2015 is the year GMOs and pesticides start to go. It feels like the old dinosaur is finally dying—they [the biotech companies] are on the ropes—they are desperate." I asked him why he thought that and he rattled off a variety of examples, among them the increasing tide of public opinion across the United States, into Mexico and Europe, the fact that in Germany and Switzerland Roundup has been taken off the shelves in response to the World Health Organization's announcement that Roundup likely causes cancer. He also told me a personal story: he said that executives from the Big Box chain Costco had recently approached his department, asking to be kept up-to-date and educated about GMOs because they want to think about phasing them out of their stores, he said. (Costco has already taken a stand on this issue and said no to the new GMO salmon.) He says this is a sign that a huge shift might be coming. I have to admit that Ignacio sounded more optimistic than I'd ever heard him; not only did he see the beginning of the end for Biotech, but he also was busy publishing his papers on the Turtle, and all publications were going easily and well. He and his assistant, Ali, were busily getting the Turtle into the hands of people in Mexico and they had more requests and samples to analyze than they ever thought possible. He was moving on to his work of synthesizing and making maps.

As I was wrapping this book up, I called Zach to check in. He told me that he continues to farm and raise his family out in flyover country but that his farming is changing. As of the fall of 2016, "a couple" of his fields will be planted with non-GMO corn for the first time. He told me, "Now the market needs non-GMO." He said that he has always assumed that GMOs are safe and that there are "no immediate medical problems" associated with them. But, he said, "At what point do we call it long-term? You can have long-term problems with food no matter how it's grown or how it's used. There are no studies right now to the contrary [that GMOs are anything but safe], but the thing that gives me pause is that in our industry we can be one hundred percent sure it's safe but at the end of the day, we're producing it for customers. I can scream till I'm blue in the face, but I'm going to grow what the public wants. . . ." The market, he said, is "giving us pause about whether we should grow GMO anymore." When I asked him if he might transition to organic, he said, "Never say never." Also, he told me, he's scaled back on some of his pesticides since I was out there. He told me the number one reason was that his fields need less of it at this point. He said his fall spray of 2,4-D is "pretty rare" now. And that he's spraying the "minimum that is necessary." Not because, he told me, carefully, he thinks the pesticides, when used correctly, are dangerous, but because he doesn't want to use them unless he has to. And then he told me a personal story: He said that when I was out there, his brother, Brandon, was in the middle of some dire health problems. And that eventually they discovered that his brother couldn't eat grains, including corn. He said, "This was ironic given he's on the Corn Growers Association." He said watching his brother go through this made him realize that there was credence to my piece in *Elle*. He said, "There are people out there that legitimately have sensitivities to these things, and to the person who's going through it, it's pretty important." These days, he says Brandon can eat some grain and still be okay. But in his own nuclear family, he told me, his eldest son became allergic to Red 40 and now reads food labels "better than most adults." He and his family now shop some at Whole Foods (an hour away) and they do buy some organic if it's available, though like many of us, his family pays attention to prices and only buys organic when they can. This phone call inspired me. I was impressed with how Zach was slowly and quietly shifting his farming practices, keeping his chin up and staying open to all options while he does it, all the while tweeting iconic missives and photos of farming the Great Plains out to the rest of the world.

And, finally, in one of my last conversations with Simon Hogan, he told me he had come up with a study that he felt would answer some questions about whether GMOs could be creating allergies. He said he'd figured out a way to use a mouse model that he thinks will work and will be credible, even to the pooh-poohers of animal models. Because of his work at the University of Cincinnati, he has a lab and everything he needs to make the study go. He just needs independent funding—to the tune of $500 thousand—to pay for the mice and get his research off the ground.

As I sit here today, snow is falling outside my window in big white flakes. My baby, Lev the Lion Cub, a second boy whom we named for Konstantin Levin, the agrarian idealist in *Anna Karenina*, is curled up and sleeping in the Moby wrap—a long, flexible piece of fabric that you wrap around yourself eight hundred times and then stick your baby in like a mummy attached to your chest. His breath comes in and out, hot and reassuring. It makes sense that he is here with me as I pen these final sentences. After all, he has been with me since I was finishing my research in California and then starting the first few sentences of this book.

As I feel the little thrum of his heart against my chest, my mind scans through all the voices I listened to and the stories I was told, the images that were conjured and the passion in the various arguments for and against GMOs. And I have to admit to feeling an enormous weight to what I'm writing here: This matters. To my kids, to your kids, to the planet. Overstating the danger would be irresponsible; and by the same token, understating the dangers would be equally as irresponsible.

So I find myself stopping on a conversation I had with an oft-quoted apple expert named John Bunker who lives in an old farmhouse in Palermo, Maine—inland, near our state capital of Augusta. John spends his time searching for and identifying and writing about heirloom apple varieties across Maine and New England. Sometimes John can be found, uninvited, in someone's old farmyard, having suddenly pulled his truck over to hop out and inspect an apple tree he's never seen before. He'll pick an apple, slice it open with his knife, peer at the inside, and then taste it.

I called John when I was first starting this book to ask him about the Arctic apple, a GMO apple that has been bred by some gene jockeys to never go brown after it is sliced. The idea is to put it into snack packs for kids at school or for fast-food restaurants to carry it in little plastic containers. The makers of the Arctic apple have given it the tag line "The perfect fruit just got even better," and the website features a lovely little blue-eyed boy eating a big, delicious-looking slice of our all-American fruit. In the news, pundits were wondering whether mothers would want to pack GMO apples for their kids, when they know full well that all they had to do to make regular apples stay fresh was to sprinkle a little lemon juice on the slices. Do we need a nonbrowning apple? reporters were asking. Do we really need any of these things, actually, when it comes right down to it? I wondered. When we consider the risks?

When I got John on the phone, I asked him this question. He laughed. First, he told me, in his craggy and frank voice, that it wasn't necessary: Even though America's apple consumption has been dumbed down to the Red and Golden Delicious, McIntosh, Granny Smith, and a few others, there are actually thousands upon thousands of varieties out there that have developed any number of traits anyone would want, not to mention the advantages to the planet (and the future of apples, themselves) if this biodiversity were embraced. "It's absolutely irrelevant," he said. "There is absolutely no reason for them to have done what they did."

John went on, "Secondly, what they are doing is they're producing an apple that doesn't turn brown as it *rots*. I'll just leave that one there." He paused for effect. "And thirdly," he went on, "there's two reasons they're doing this: One is they're too lazy to go back into history and find those varieties of apples that did so well and could still do so well. And second is it's about profit. They can make a lot of money doing this."

When the Arctic apple first hit the papers, I had gone on my yearly apple-picking trip with my family to Ricker Hill farm in the hills just north of Lewiston. After we had loaded up with enough apples to make sauces, apple butter, and pies to sustain us all winter long, and had enough to eat fresh in lunches until Christmastime, I asked the owner, whose farm has been in his family for hundreds of years, what he thought of the new GMO apple. "The only thing I can say about that," he said, "is that food is king. When this country goes down, the one with the food is gonna win. It's all about food sovereignty."

We turned and looked together across his lush orchards, which seemed to stretch all the way to the mountains in the distance and beyond. I said, "You must feel so lucky to have this farm."

"I do," he said.

When we drove home that afternoon, the sun going down and Marsden, Dan, and I all crunching on delicious crisp Macouns as we went, I was thinking about something John had said to me about this whole business of GMOs: "We either have a responsibility to now do something *about* what we've done. Or we could also say we have the opportunity now to do something *with* what we've done."

What that opportunity is today, I cannot say for sure. But I do feel that the responsibility is ours. We, like Jodi's bees gathering pollen and nectar, must remember our hive, and the long winter ahead we have to survive.

A Note About Resource Material

Dear Reader,

It took me—on and off—just over five years to bring this book to fruition. When I first starting writing it, I was doing so just to get down on paper how sick and scared I was. I was trying to write myself out of a box and find words for what was happening to me. On the weekends, I would find myself poring over the "Diagnosis" column in the *New York Times Magazine*, wishing I could be the test patient or that I'd find, some sunny Sunday over scones and tea, my answer. In some more depressing moments I carried around Rabbi Harold Kushner's *When Bad Things Happen to Good People*, though I couldn't ever bring myself to read it. It was my unlucky talisman.

When I was finally diagnosed by Dr. Mansmann, long before I was sure I had a book in me, I began to read. I needed to know more about GMOs, corn, pesticides, and Big Ag. I plunged myself, like Alice through the Looking Glass, into a full immersion—trying to learn from those who'd blazed the path ahead of me. What follows here is by no means a comprehensive list; it's just a few of the things that particularly spoke to me as I worked. If you are excited about this subject matter, you will undoubtedly find endless directions to go from here.

The first book I turned to was Rachel Carson's *Silent Spring*. Though I have the same old dog-eared copy from college and vaguely remember being taught it in a terrific American History course with a professor who was a crusty Mainer wearing tweed vests and who had an accent as thick as the fog off Cobscook Bay (which made me feel like I was at home, despite being away at school in Providence, Rhode Island), reading it a second time, as an adult, was revelatory. If you've never read it—and do not be ashamed, you are not alone!—you won't regret taking the time. Over half a century later, this book is still relevant—even prescient—moving, beautifully written, and important. It will make you weep for all the things that could have been but were not done.

From Carson, I moved on to Michael Pollan. First I read *The Omnivore's Dilemma*, which is The Book about our corn-driven food system. After reading *TOD*, I turned to Barbara Kingsolver, Steven Hopp, and Camille Kingsolver's *Animal, Vegetable, Miracle*, which is the real-world application of Pollan's paragon. In *AVM*, the family of four (there's a younger child, named Lily) went off the food grid for a year and grew everything they ate on their sprawling, rustic farm in the foothills of Appalachia. In *AVM* I found kindred spirits in the comforting voice of Kingsolver and a ton of information about our current food system, doled out by both Kingsolver and Hopp. Then I turned back to Pollan to read *The Botany of Desire*, an in-depth look at four crops: apples, potatoes, tulips, and marijuana. "The Apple" and "The Potato" were especially illuminating ("The Potato" is all about the GMO potato). I then read Pollan's book *Cooked*, about how the food we eat is transformed from raw ingredients into comestibles. In the midst of all this, I watched Jeremy Seifert's documentary *GMO OMG*, a fresh and honest look at GMOs and an attempt by one dad to understand them and explain them to his children.

The night before I left for my first trip out to the Great Plains, shortly after committing to writing the book you've just finished reading, my friend Matt Moon handed me Ian Frazier's brilliant, moving, beautiful and *funny* road story, *Great Plains*. This has become one of my all-time favorite books—you will learn everything about that part of the world, from the Native American history to the history of agriculture—there's nothing he doesn't touch on. When I was done with *Great Plains*, I diverged to read my friend

Mike Paterniti's book, *The Telling Room,* which is one writer's adventure to learn the history of the world's greatest piece of cheese—in a small, far-flung town in Spain. Like my book, Paterniti was following the trail of something elusive—a foodstuff with a complicated history—and it took him twelve long years to get the book down. I remember telling Dan not to talk to me as our plane landed in Boston after our long flight from Rome—"I'm almost done," I said, "and I'm not getting off this plane until I read the final sentences." Paterniti left me with tears in my eyes—I didn't want his book to end. When I went to California, I took Gretel Ehrlich's *The Solace of Open Spaces* with me and reread it on the plane, bringing back the first time I read it when I was in my early twenties and living in New York City but dreaming of being a cowgirl. On all three trips, I packed a bird book appropriate for that place in the world and, at night, in bed, I would look up the birds I saw and try to ID them.

My research over, as I began writing "Flyover Country" on April 1st of 2014, I first turned to Peter Pringle's amazingly detailed and intelligent book *Food, Inc.: Mendel to Monsanto—The Promises and Perils of the Biotech Harvest.* I think I read this book three, or maybe four, times throughout the writing of my book. He is the authority on the history of GMOs in this country, in my humble opinion. As I started my section about the Dust Bowl, I reread *The Grapes of Wrath* so that I could relearn some of the history from a human perspective. I looked at a ton of photographs, too: Walker Evans, Dorothea Lange, Frank Gohlke. Then, as I got into the parts of the book about pesticides, I turned to Sandra Steingraber's *Living Downstream,* which, despite its seemingly dry subject matter about chemicals in the environment, is easy to read and incredibly illuminating. After that, I turned to Aldo Leopold's posthumous classic, *A Sand County Almanac,* a collection of essays about living in the natural world and about conservation. I then reread my friend Terry Tempest Williams's book *Refuge: An Unnatural History of Family and Place* because it was dawning on me that I was working on a book not just about food but about the environment. While writing this section I also watched the following movies: Aaron Woolf's *King Corn;* Ken Burns's *The Dust Bowl;* PBS's *Rachel Carson's Silent Spring; Food, Inc.; The Farmer's Wife* (a touching—and at times harrowing—PBS documentary about a couple trying to make a go of farming in Nebraska); *Ingredients; To Make a*

Farm; *Scientists Under Attack* (which is sort of an alarmist movie, but very interesting nonetheless); and the brilliant film *The Corporation*.

As I moved on to write about bees for the second section of my book, I started with *Beekeeping for Dummies*. I truly had no idea how to even talk about bees. Then, when I was in the hospital with Levin, my friend Susan gave me one of the most beautiful books I've ever owned, called *The Bee: A Natural History*. Marsden and I have spent many a bedtime poring over that book together, taking in the photos of every kind of bee on the planet, reading about the history and challenges to bees. I also read Bill McKibben's memoir, *Oil and Honey*, about his activism against the fossil fuel companies and his tangential journey into supporting a beekeeper. I then read Martin Blaser's *Missing Microbes* and David Michaels's *Doubt Is Their Product*—all important books worth spending the time with. When I was writing this section I watched two terrific documentaries: *Vanishing of the Bees* and *More Than Honey*.

When I began the "West of Eden" section, I read Elizabeth Kolbert's *The Sixth Extinction* (and made Dan read it, too, so that we could talk about it), Belinda Martineau's *First Fruit*, Dan Charles's *Lords of the Harvest*, Emily Anthes's *Frankenstein's Cat*, Theo Colburn's *Our Stolen Future*, and John McPhee's *The Control of Nature*. As I wrote, I found myself circling back to Charles Darwin's *The Origin of Species*.

Along my journey, I also listened to everything I could by the aforementioned Dan Charles, who reports on agriculture for NPR; I read magazine pieces from all over the world about bees, the Great Plains, Mexico and corn, GMOs, agriculture and chemicals; I read and carried around with me from writing spot to writing spot (whether it was my dining room table or a friend's spare room) two banana boxes full of scientific studies; I read political speeches, transcripts of bills put before different committees in D.C., poems by Wendell Berry and Mary Oliver; I listened to music that inspired me—music tied to the landscapes I was writing about or just music that set my imagination free; and whenever I could, I pored over photography books and maps to learn more. I got into bed with cookbooks by Alice Waters, Melissa Clark, Martha Stewart, and the old standards *The Joy of Cooking* and *The Fannie Farmer Cookbook*, and came up with ways to make meals that would satisfy my family and were GMO (and indeed most grain) free. And I spent a lot of time on the following websites: beyondpesticides .org, gmo-compass.org, The Endocrine Disruption Exchange (endocrine disruption.org), The Environmental Working Group (ewg.org), Environmental Health News (environmentalhealthnews.org), National Pesticide Information Center (npic.orst.edu), epa.gov, fda.gov, and usda.gov.

I hope these sources will inspire you, too, and that from here you will go out and find things I did not find. Or even write the next book that picks up from where I've left off, as this is all about—in the end—handing off the baton.

Best,

Caitlin Shetterly

April 1, 2016

Acknowledgments

When a person like me—without staff or even a particularly clear road map, as the journey is a part of the story and what the story *is* is unclear until the journey gets made—embarks on a book like this, there is an unseen supporting cast of many, encouraging and giving time, money, energy, ideas, friendship, and just general kindness to make it all possible. What follows here is by no means everyone who touched my life as I worked on this book. For instance, I don't know the name of that L.L. Bean employee who, upon learning, the night before I left for Europe, that a bag I had purchased had a hole in it, so generously sent another employee to my house late at night to drop off a new bag. Or the kind staff at the Berkeley City Club who made my stay there just that much more comfortable. Or Graciela, the cook in Italy who made us beautiful food and took Marsy under her wing.

So, here goes. You may want to play that Oscar music . . . but what was it Julia Roberts said when she got the Oscar for *Erin Brockovich*? "Sir, you're so quick with that stick, but why don't you sit, because I may never be here again!"

This book could not have been written without two people. The first is my agent, Lisa Grubka, who is not only the most organized and practical person I know, but is endlessly encouraging while always being extremely frank. (My editor, Kerri, and I liked to say, "Tell us how you really feel, Lis.")

I don't know of many agents who read every draft of a proposal for a book and then go on to read every draft of the manuscript, too—helping; refining; spending long hours thinking deeply about not just big-picture questions, but also willing to go down rabbit holes into discussions of actual sentences. Without Lisa seeing something that was book-worthy in that very first proposal and then staying by my side at every step—with intelligent and kind advice along the way—I can't imagine we'd be reading this book today. Thank you, Lisa. You are my most trusted adviser and a good friend, too.

The second person to come on board, who was also tirelessly energetic, supportive, intelligent, funny, sharp, and just there for me, was my editor, Kerri Kolen. Together the three of us became a tightly run "Team Modified," and although there were hurdles, it certainly felt as if nothing could bring us or this book down when we were standing strong together. Kerri could not have been more patient as I went and got pregnant and then had a baby in the middle of all this (though I like to think I won a *few* brownie points when I was in labor with my second child—two and a half weeks early—and I told the hospital staff to give me two hours, that I needed to hand in the last section of my book in before I had this baby. I somehow managed to do this in the midst of contractions and Dan gently suggesting that, perhaps, now was the time to put the computer down . . .). Kerri, like Lisa, read many, many drafts of this book, and together we worked hard to make the science readable and the concepts understandable because, more than anything, we all felt that we, if no one else, needed a book that explained this GMO thing easily and carefully. Kerri had solutions to every problem and was always good humored and cheered me on when I flagged. Thank you, Kerri.

I had three readers for this book. They were Susan Conley, Steven Hopp, and Jessie Moon. These three people read a middle-of-the-process, extremely long draft (was that thing 500 pages?) and each one gave me feedback that made the book what it is today. They all took an incredible amount of time to write notes, to encourage, to think ideas through, to look at rewrites, to listen as I yammered about the intricacies of science interfacing with the written word, and to be there for me. Thank you all. I am forever indebted.

And then there were the people who just gave and gave and gave: my father, Robert Browne Shetterly Jr.; my uncles, Jay and Tom Shetterly; Jamie and Beth Kilbreth, who gave me a room of my own in which to write in their lovely townhouse in Portland (and Joan and Dan Amory who did the same when the Kilbreths needed my room for guests one summer)—thank you especially to Beth for playing such beautiful piano music as I worked; your music became my muse and soundtrack. Bruce Blumberg, the scientist at UC Irvine, who became an advisor, helping me parse studies and evaluate scientific language, and who introduced to me to Tyrone Hayes who, in turn, introduced me to Ignacio Chapela; Lily King, Kate Christensen, and Bill McKibben, who all agreed to give early blurbs when the book began its journey from draft to finished product and needed some certification; The Falmouth Memorial Library, where I finished a crucial piece of the writing; Stan Smith, of the MacSmith, who fixed my computer more than once, and twice actually saved the manuscript, which appeared to have been lost in the ether; The Maine Arts Commission for giving me a necessary and important piece of funding; endless support and love from the most optimistic person I know, Tim Rhys, and my dear friend, his wife, Jessica Rhys; Craig Pospisil—always there for me despite children and jobs and partners and busy lives; Jodi Moger—there are no words to thank you enough for your friendship, care, and time spent listening to me perseverate about everything from food to the book to family, and then for all you have taught me about organics and bees and honey and gardening and plants—thank you.

There were all the people in this book whom I interviewed, who gave me time on top of more time: especially Leslie and Paris Mansmann, Simon Hogan, Richard Goodman, Walter Haefeker, Jim Gerritsen, Zach Hunnicutt, Eric Chivian, Belinda Martineau, Dave Murphy, Lisa Stokke, Chellie Pingree, Severin Beliveau, Karl Heinz Bablok, Wolfgang Koehler, Tyrone Hayes, Ignacio Chapela, Exequiel Ezcurra, John Bunker, and everyone at Spannocchia.

To everyone at Putnam who helped me bring this to fruition, especially Ivan Held, who believed in this book and supported both me and it; Karen Mayer, who did endless legal vetting; Alexis Welby, Karen Fink, and Stephanie Hargadon for publicity; Ashley McClay and Anna Romig for marketing; Claire Sullivan for numerous copy edits; Tanya Maiboroda and Claire Vaccaro for a beautiful design; and Alise Hofacre and Sofie Brooks for support.

Thank you to my two incredible research assistants, Emma Deans and Caitlin Allen. And Bethany Flannery for all things web.

Fact checking was done by Hilary Elkins and Keith Bearden. Thank you, Keith, for your hard work, your positive personality, and for catching as much as you did. You came on at just the right time.

Many more people supported me behind the scenes, sending me words of encouragement, helping me in small and large ways, or just opening doors as I went: Laurie Abraham, who took my piece for *Elle*; Robbie Myers, who wrote and published a crucial support of my *Elle* piece after it was attacked; Kate Lee, who sent me to Christy Fletcher, who handed my proposal to my agent, Lisa, who ran with it; Daniel Wenger and Debra Spark, who both read an early draft of my proposal; Ed Seldin, who saved a relationship with a source; Steve Drucker, who graciously read a late draft; Seth Rigoletti, who helped me believe in the power of my message; Michelle Bolduc, who found me great outfits for all my trips and photo shoots; Sandy Johnson, our realtor and friend; and Susan Hand Shetterly, Maggie and Eric Miller, Sally Shetterly, and Aran and Margot Lee Shetterly. My babysitters, without whom, forget it, just not possible: Bella Bergeron and Melanie Ross.

Thank you to Ryan Adams and Greg Brown for writing music that continues to inspire me, no matter what continent I'm driving across.

Thank you to the incredible, intrepid farmers in Maine and to MOFGA, our state organic farmers and growers association; you all feed me and my family healthy, organic, beautiful food and continue to inspire me that there is hope for our seeds. You also help me believe that as Maine goes, so will go the nation. . . .

And to Dan, who did dishes and took care of our children when I was working numerous weekends, doing this on top of his own demanding career; who patiently listened to many drafts of this book, which I read out loud as our children slept; who cared for me, brought me tea, and made us beautiful fish-fry dinners on Saturday nights to give me a break from cooking; and who loved me through the lean times this book presented us with. It was a lot, I know, Dan, to believe in me and this book when I was toiling away with not a penny to show for it. But you kept us in food and clothes while I went out there to fight this fight. Thank you.

Marsden and Levin: You two, you happy two. You are my inspiration and my cause—I wrote this book for you. Not only did I want you both to see by my example that we can exert change, in small and big ways, just by going out there and asking important questions, but, also, that we should never be afraid to take on any behemoth. My hope is that, with what we now know about our food and the planet, together we can make the planet a slightly better place. As the poet Denise Levertov writes, "We have only begun to love the earth."

Finally, to Hopper: Our beautiful, smart, gentle, and intelligent dog, who died when I was near the end of this book. I can't thank Hoppy enough for his constant companionship with me on runs and walks in the woods, gentle babysitting of our children (it's true!), and just lying by my feet as I wrote (often warming them). Although I cannot prove this, I believe that Hopper got cancer and eventually kidney disease—which killed him painfully and quickly—from the pesticides that were being sprayed by our neighbors in Westbrook. These pesticides, which he undoubtedly took in on walks, gulping water from puddles, in conjunction with the neonicotinoid-based top-spot tick treatments we used on him, I think, did him in. I see no other explanation for what could have felled, with such alarming rapidity, such a strong and healthy dog—to whom we fed an all-organic homemade diet—other than toxic overload. In the weeks after Hopper's death, we found a new home and soon thereafter moved to a safer street, where no one uses pesticides. Of course, Hopper's situation has made me wonder what our kids were exposed to, too. This may never be traceable or provable, but it nags at my heart.